CLINICAL

AROMATHERAPY

CLINICAL AROMATHERAPY

ESSENTIAL OILS IN PRACTICE

SECOND EDITION

JANE BUCKLE, RN, PhD

COMPLEMENTARY HEALTH THERAPIES CONSULTANT
NEW YORK, NEW YORK
UNITED STATES

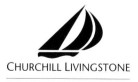

CHURCHILL LIVINGSTONE

An Imprint of Elsevier Limited

Edinburgh London New York Oxford Philadelphia St Louis Sydney Toronto

CHURCHILL LIVINGSTONE
An imprint of Elsevier Limited

Published 2003
  Reprinted 2003, 2004 (twice), 2006, 2007, 2008 (twice)

ISBN: 978 0 443 07236 9

NOTICE
Complementary and alternative medicine is an ever-changing field. Standard safety precautions must be followed, but as new research and clinical experience broaden our knowledge, changes in treatment and drug therapy may become necessary as appropriate. Readers are advised to check the most current product information provided by the manufacturer of each drug to be administered to verify the recommended dose, the method and duration of administration, and contraindications. It is the responsibility of the licensed prescriber, relying on experience and knowledge of the patient, to determine dosages and the best treatment for each individual patient. Neither the publisher nor the editors assumes any liability for any injury and/or damage to persons or property arising from this publication.

Library of Congress Cataloging in Publication Data

Buckle, Jane, RGN, MA, BPhil, Cert Ed, MISPA, MIScB.
  Clinical aromatherapy / Jane Buckle.—2nd ed.
    p. ; cm.
  Rev. ed. of: Clinical aromatherapy in nursing / Jane Buckle. c1997.
  Includes bibliographical references and index.
  ISBN 0 443 07236 1
  1. Aromatherapy. 2. Nursing.   I. Buckle, Jane, RGN, MA, BPhil, Cert Ed, MISPA, MIScB. Clinical aromatherapy.   II. Title.
  [DNLM: 1. Aromatherapy—methods. WB 925 B924ca 2003]
  615'.321—dc21   2003043823

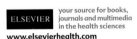

Working together to grow
libraries in developing countries
www.elsevier.com | www.bookaid.org | www.sabre.org

ELSEVIER   BOOK AID   Sabre Foundation
           International

Printed in China

Publishing Manager: Inta Izols
Development Editor: Karen Gilmour
Project Manager: Peggy Fagen
Design Manager: Mark Bernard
Design: Sheilah Barrett Design

This book is for all those who walk the path with me.
Thank you.

FOREWORD

Aromatherapy is possibly the most simple of all complementary therapies to integrate because when we inhale air, we inhale aroma, although we are usually unaware of it. However, aromatherapy is rarely presented in a cogent, scientific way; as a result, it has been difficult for physicians and nurses to take the field seriously, or to understand how we could use it in our practice. Here is a book from a health professional who writes about aromatherapy in a way that we can understand and apply.

As a small boy growing up in Turkey, I had my own special paradise—my grandfather's walled garden—where I became aware of the power of the senses; in particular, how the fragrance of plants made me feel good. Now, as a cardio-vascular surgeon, I work on repairing the heart. I know the heart is perceived by many to be more than a pump, the epicenter of emotion, and I continue to be aware of how important our senses are to our well being, and how *feeling* good can help recovery. The very smell of many hospitals is unpleasant, alien, or distressing to our patients. Patients feel at their most vulnerable in a hospital's high-tech surroundings, so a familiar and comforting smell can do much to put them at their ease. In common with several forward-thinking hospitals in the United States, we now use aromatherapy at Columbia Presbyterian, and we have been working with Jane Buckle on research since 1995.

Our sense of smell is located in the catacombs of the most primitive area of the brain and is extremely powerful. Smell can produce all sorts of physical reactions ranging from nausea to napping. The amygdala, the brain's emotional center, is located in the limbic system and is directly connected to the olfactory bulb. Rage and fear are processed in the amygdala and both contribute to heart disease. Our studies at Columbia have found that diluted essential oils rubbed on the feet affected some volunteer's autonomic nervous system within minutes.

Clinical Aromatherapy is presented logically, with considerable background information given at the outset. I expect many readers will go straight to the clinical section and look at their own specialty. In each specialty, a few symptoms or problems have been explored, and the way in which aromatherapy might help treat those symptoms or problems is clearly outlined. The information will be of particular interest to readers working in that clinical specialty. However, I think the book will also be of great interest to those who want to know what aromatherapy really is, and how it can be used in a scientific way.

Jane Buckle is well qualified to write this ground-breaking book. She brings a wealth of knowledge and clinical experience acquired over 25 years in the field.

With a PhD in health service management, a background in critical care nursing, a teaching degree and a fistful of degrees from the world of alternative medicine, she writes authoritatively, and she speaks from the heart. Jane was a co-presenter with me at The World Economic Forum in Davos, Switzerland, a few years ago. We were invited to talk about the economics of alternative medicine and its impact on globalization. I was impressed by Jane's passion, as she also hosted four different events that helped bridge the divide between big business, alternative medicine, pharmaceutical organizations, and political leaders. An underlying question permeated all her presentations: What can we do to get the caring back into healthcare? When Jane speaks, people listen.

Jane Buckle is a pioneer and she uses writing, researching, and teaching to get her message across. Her message is one of holism and she inspires those in healthcare to evaluate how they use simple things like smell and touch to help people heal. In the United States, many hospitals are beginning to integrate clinical aromatherapy and use Jane's program. She is involved in numerous hospital research programs (apart from our own) and has been a reviewer for NIH grants.

Under her guidance, hundreds of students have carried out small pilot studies in American hospitals. She has written templates for aromatherapy policies and protocols that are being used by hospitals. More than any other person, Jane Buckle has labored to integrate clinical aromatherapy into hospitals, not as a possible add-on but as a legitimate part of holistic care. That achievement alone is remarkable. But, she has another string to her bow. She has pioneered a registered method of touch, called the "m" technique. This technique was tested in our laboratory at Columbia Presbyterian on the legs of students and found to have a pronounced parasympathetic response in some. The technique is very relaxing (I have experienced it myself!) and eminently suitable for hospital patients (with or without the use of essential oils), so I am delighted to see a section on the "m" technique in this book.

Essential oils offer extraordinary potential from a purely medicinal standpoint, and the recent studies on MRSA and human subjects show just how powerful they can be. That an essential oil can be effective against resistant organisms is medicine indeed and I think the chapter on infection will be of great interest to pharmacists as well as those involved in infection control. When nausea is relieved through the inhalation of peppermint and insomnia is alleviated through the inhalation of lavender or rose, we are witnessing clinical results—not just the "feel-good" factor. The studies on alopecia and topically applied essential oils, or *Candida albicans* and teatree, show that aromatherapy can work at a clinically significant level. However the strength of clinical aromatherapy is that it offers care as well as, in some instances, cure. This is of particular relevance in the field of chronic pain where the perception of pain can be altered using smell and touch.

The subject of clinical aromatherapy is vast and will be of interest to nurses and physicians, chiropractors and massage therapists, pharmacists and naturopaths, pharmaceutical companies and herbalists. I share a goal with Jane Buckle—to enhance patient care and give the best of what we have to offer, whatever that may be. As a physician, I believe clinical aromatherapy has an important role to play in integrative medicine. Jane Buckle gives us a glimpse of the future, and it smells good!

MEHMET OZ

Mehmet Oz, MD, is a cardiac surgeon. He is the Director of the Cardiovascular Institute and Vice Chairman of the Department of Surgery at Columbia Presbyterian Medical Center, New York, NY.

PREFACE

This book is intended for health professionals in the United States wanting to use aromatherapy in a clinical way to enhance their practice. It draws from *Clinical Aromatherapy in Nursing* (London: Arnold, 1997) but is a different book as it is no longer written from a nursing perspective and has been substantially expanded to meet the needs of *all* health professionals. Things have changed since 1997. I have gained a PhD (which helped my thinking!) and much has improved in the aromatherapy world. Several clinical studies have appeared in peer-reviewed medical journals. Aromatherapy is finding its way into wellness clinics, hospices, and hospitals, and courses are being taught at leading universities. Aromatherapy has become part of everyday language. Despite this, popular misconceptions abound. This book was written to try to correct those misconceptions and to indicate the important role that essential oils could play in future healthcare.

The book is laid out in a similar way to the first book but with several important differences.

1. The book is no longer written from a nursing perspective, although there is a section on aromatherapy as part of nursing care.
2. The text has been reviewed and edited by experts in the field (see *Acknowledgments*).
3. The text includes many new tables to help the reader assimilate the information.
4. The chemistry section has been expanded and improved and includes molecular drawings.
5. There are new sections on psychology, psychiatry, and aromatic medicine (which covers internal use). There are specific sections for the physician, massage therapist, chiropractor, and naturopath.
6. The individual clinical sections have been updated and expanded, especially the part on immunology.
7. The book is intended for U.S. residents and so OSHA and JCAHO requirements are covered and education in the United States is addressed.
8. The number of references has almost doubled.
9. The reference system has been changed to make it easier to identify the references in the text.
10. There is an extensive index.

The book is divided into two broad sections. These are *Overview* and *Clinical Use*. The overview begins with a background section, which covers such topics as historical use, where essential oils come from, how they are obtained, what they consist of, how they work, and how they are absorbed into the body. Then there is a short introduction to the psychology of smell. This is immediately followed by contraindications, toxicology, and safety issues. After this broad introduction, the book begins to become more specific, with sections on how aromatherapy could be used by nurses, massage therapists, and physical therapists, or as part of prescriptive medicine used by physicians, chiropractors, and naturopaths. A general hospital section follows, addressing how the generic problems of infection, pain, insomnia, nausea, and stress could be relieved by essential oils. Finally the clinical section is divided into departments found in a medical setting, and there is a discussion of how aromatherapy could alleviate some of the common problems found in each clinical section with reference to published research, my own clinical experience, and that of my students.

I am greatly indebted to the many physicians, nurses, and other professionals who edited and reviewed these sections. At the end of the book there are appendixes covering OSHA and JCAHO requirements, training and education in the United States, and some recommended reading, websites, and essential oil companies.

This book has been a labor of love. I hope you enjoy reading it as much as I enjoyed the journey. If one piece of good research is carried out because of this book, all the hours will be have been well spent.

Jane Buckle

ACKNOWLEDGEMENTS

I would like to acknowledge the following people who edited specific parts of the book. Thank you for your generosity of spirit and your nurturing editorship.

Ann Adams, RN, CMN
Elizabeth Barrett, RN, PhD
James Duke, PhD
Charlotte Eliopoulos, RN, PhD
Ben Evans, MSN
Claire Everson, MSN
Debbie Freund, RN, LMT
Howard Freund, PhD
Ron Guba
Diana Guthrie, RN, PhD
Sue Hageness, MSN
Bob Harris
Rhi Harris, RN
Dorothy Larkin, RN, PhD
Michael McCrary, MA
Lee McGunnigle, DC
Lori Mitchell, RN, MSN
Gayle Newsham, RN, PhD
Tom Numark
Mary Poolos, RN, PhD
Ganson Purcell, MD
Scottie Purol-Hershey, RN, PhD
Linda Scaz RN, PhD
Kurt Schaubelt, PhD
Paul Schulick
Neal Schultz, MD
Keith Shawe, PhD
Kay Soltis, MSN
Brenda Talley, RN, PhD
Mark Warner, MD

CONTENTS

SECTION I

Overview

INTRODUCTION TO SECTION I

Section I is an overview covering the foundations of aromatherapy. This section opens with an examination not only of the history of aromatic medicine and the emergence of a new, complementary therapy in the 1940s but also of the "what, how, why, and when" aspects of essential oil production from plant to bottle. Next is a two-part chapter on toxicity and contraindications (the "when and why not" aspects of aromatherapy). Following this is a chapter on the psychology of smell. The next part of Section I covers the use of aromatherapy within the context of specific healthcare fields—nursing and manual therapies—including a discussion of the oral and internal uses of essential oils.

The author is grateful for the input of many reviewers in this section whose help and advice was most appreciated. The reviewers include: Tony Balazs PhD; Elizabeth Barrett, RN, PhD; James Duke, PhD; Howard Freund, PhD; Ron Guba; Bob Harris; Dorothy Larkin, RN, PhD; Lee McGunnigle, DCh; Gayle Newsham, RN, PhD; Tom Numark; Mary Poolos, RN, PhD; Scottie Purol-Hershey, RN, PhD; Brenda Talley, RN, PhD; Kurt Schaubelt, PhD; Keith Shawe, PhD; and Neal Schultz, MD.

I

INTRODUCTION

The scent organ was playing a delightfully refreshing Herbal Capriccio—rippling arpeggios of thyme and lavender, of rosemary, basil, myrtle, tarragon; a series of daring modulations through the spice keys into ambergris; and a slow return through sandalwood, camphor, cedar and new-mown hay.

Aldous Huxley
Brave New World

O F ALL the complementary therapies, aromatherapy is perhaps the most misunderstood. It is maligned, misrepresented, and can be very confusing. Even the name *aromatherapy* is a misnomer. Contrary to popular belief, aromatherapy is not just about smells! It is little wonder that orthodoxy ridicules what the perfume industry guards so well.

Despite the misunderstanding, aromatherapy has become very popular in the United States (Jacknin 2001) and was even part of the millennium celebrations in Times Square, New York. Two million celebrants were each given a $4^1/_2$-inch square scent strip that bore a global bouquet representing the aromatic choice of every nation—the culmination of 10 years work by Gayil Nalls, a New York artist who works in multimedia. Her work was endorsed by the United Nations Educational, Scientific and Cultural Organization (Kyle 2000). The United States chose pine, England chose sweet grass, and France chose lavender.

Aromatherapy is the fastest growing of all complementary therapies (Buckle 2001). Although not mentioned in David Eisenberg's groundbreaking 1993 study on alternative medicine, aromatherapy was clearly in the picture just 5 years later when it was being used by 5.6% of the study cohort (Eisenberg 1998). Aromatherapy is now an all-time favorite with UK nurses (Thompson 2001) and is becoming popular among nurses in the United States. In a recent survey of

3

certified nurse-midwives in North Carolina, 32.9% had recommended aromatherapy (Allaire et al 2000).

There are currently 761,000 web sites on aromatherapy. This is hardly surprising. As Larry Dossey, MD, states in his editorial on the impact of smell (2001), "Throughout history people have responded to aromas." Clinical aromatherapy has been described as the "most exciting of all complementary therapies" by Andrew Weil, MD (personal communication). At the Nurse Practitioner Associates for Continuing Education conference in 2001, Tieraona Low Dog, MD, stated, "If you think herbal medicine is exciting, wait for clinical aromatherapy!" Mehmet Oz, MD, cardiothoracic surgeon at Columbia Presbyterian Medical Center and pioneer of the first complementary medicine center in New York city wrote, "Aromatherapy appears to impact perceptions of pain" (Oz 1998); chronic pain is big business.

The effect of complementary therapies in general, and aromatherapy in particular, is economic. I was one of the speakers at the World Economic Forum in Davos, Switzerland, in January 1999. The economics of herbal medicine (in which clinical aromatherapy has its roots) is exciting and global. Americans spend an astonishing amount of money on health care, approximately $4000 per person in 1997. Americans and others in the Western world are growing tired of pharmaceuticals as the "cure all" and are yearning for a more holistic approach that would enable them to use more natural products. "People's perception of the chemical industry is belching chimneys, acrid smells and toxic waste products, not an enticing prospect" (Brooks 2001). The recent Fen-Phen debacle, involving hundreds of thousands of people whose heart valves were damaged by the drug, is more evidence of a pharmaceutical industry that is accused of seeing itself above federal regulation (Mundy 2001). The 44,000 to 98,000 deaths that occur each year because of medical error (Pear 1999) also are encouraging people to try complementary therapies, or at least to be wary of hospital visits.

Despite aromatherapy's popularity, some important questions remain. What is aromatherapy? Does it work? Is it safe? Where is the research? Many licensed health professionals (LHPs) have been using aromatherapy in clinical settings without really knowing exactly what they are using on their patients (Buckle 1992). There are few specialized training courses for LHPs who want to use clinical aromatherapy to enhance the care they provide. Most training programs are intended for the lay public. Some universities have begun to bridge the void, introducing a more academic voice. A discussion on the different types of training available appears in Appendix I.

Some critics of clinical aromatherapy have cited the paucity of research (Vickers 1996). This is a fair criticism. Until recently, research has been limited mainly to studies of animals or in-vitro systems. However, in the last 3 years many pilot studies have been carried out and published, as a search on the National Library of Medicine's journal search engine, PubMed, indicates. Many of the studies on human subjects have been carried out by nurses, many of whom were not trained in research and had little or no funding. Often, the patient population was small and the study modest. However, these studies demonstrate that aromatherapy is being used clinically in many hospitals throughout the world. The results of these studies also indicate that aromatherapy is safe, efficacious, and, most importantly to managed care, less expensive than orthodox drug therapy.

Perhaps orthodox medicine might be more open to the published research available if they were to look hard at their own research. A Canadian study evaluated 4000 medical papers, applying 28 basic criteria that should be met in scientific papers; the researchers concluded that only 40 of the 4000 papers met all of the criteria. This analysis went on to state that only 15% of medical interventions are supported by reliable scientific evidence, that most therapies applied daily in doctors' offices have never been tested by the scientific method, and that these therapies are not supported by any evidence at all (Smith 1992). Peter Gotzsche, a Danish statistician, chose for his thesis in 1990 the title "Bias in Double-Blind Trials." Gotzsche is director of the Cochrane Collaboration, which reviews clinical studies; he made headlines in 2001 with his suggestion that mammograms did not show evidence of reducing the number of deaths resulting from cancer (McNeil 2002).

Although aromatherapy has been ridiculed by some, a growing group of practitioners believe that aromatherapy has a valid place in integrative medicine. Integrative medicine includes complementary and alternative medicine (CAM). CAM has been around much longer than Western medicine (Buckle 1999a). However, the growth in CAM's popularity has precipitated a power struggle between the believers in Western medicine and the believers in CAM. Both appear to be entrenched in their philosophies, but share the idea that if one is correct, the other one is wrong.

Orthodox medicine may save lives, but it does have considerable drawbacks: expense, serious side effects, and a considerable loss of life. Orthodox medicine prides itself on being reductionist. It treats everyone more or less the same regardless of age, sex, ethnicity, diet, stress level, or weight. Orthodox medicine talks about the "average" patient and claims to be rigorously scientific. However, some well-promoted procedures such as appendectomies and tonsillectomies have, over time, proven to be of little value. Even bone-marrow transplants, the much-lauded treatment of the 1990s, received a major setback in 1998. Results presented at a world conference in Atlanta, Georgia, indicated that in four out of five major trials there was no difference between the survival rate of patients receiving chemotherapy and patients receiving chemotherapy plus bone-marrow transplantation (Kolata & Eichenwald 1999).

Some orthodox treatments are invasive and some can go badly wrong. In the United States in 1998 there were between 44,000 and 80,000 deaths caused by the misuse of pharmaceutical drugs. This exceeds the number of people killed in car accidents (44,500), who died from breast cancer (42,300), or who died from HIV/AIDS (16,500) (Pear 1999). Success in orthodox medicine is measured by how quickly patients return to work. Few follow-up audits of orthodox treatment have taken place, and if a patient "breaks down" again, it is classified as a new occurrence rather than as a reoccurrence.

The rationale behind CAM, including aromatherapy, is quite different. These therapies are multidimensional and are not aimed at one specific body system. They are not usually invasive. CAM therapists are interested in the individuality of the patients and what has led each patient to his or her particular disease process or set of symptoms (Hildebrand 1994). CAM therapists feel that when the patient is balanced, homeostasis can return and the disease will be unable to survive. They believe that the world is full of viruses and bacteria but that it is mainly individuals whose immunity is compromised because of emotional, spiritual, or physical trauma who tend to succumb to disease (Gasgoigne 1993). Thirty years of orthodox research into cancer, with relatively little progress toward an overall cure, support this viewpoint (Beardsley 1994). Currently, 3% of the US population (9 million people) is living with the diagnosis of cancer (Okie 2001).

Success in CAM therapies is based on a long-term view. Practitioners look at the "patterning" of the disease process: how often a patient has been ill during his or her lifetime, and whether the incidence and severity of the disease has increased. All diseases are taken into account, not just those of the same system. Patients are warned that treatment may take time. Emphasis is placed on teaching the patient preventative medicine to avoid a relapse and on providing support during the healing process. The patient is encouraged to rest, and not to work, while the repairing process is in progress. The old-fashioned idea of convalescing is stressed.

Is it possible for the two opposite positions to merge? Possibly. Certainly, the term *integrative medicine,* coined by Andrew Weil, MD, conveys that vision. Perhaps CAM is the yin of medicine and orthodoxy is the yang. Together yin and yang make a circle, each needing the other to complete a whole. Yin is often perceived as intuitive, feminine, spiritual, and artistic. Yang is often seen as masculine, dominant, invasive, and scientific. Together, there could be a strong symbiotic partnership between orthodox medicine and CAM, each bringing out the best in the other. Acute illnesses and trauma could be treated with Western drugs or surgery, and chronic illnesses (e.g., arthritis, insomnia, and irritable bowel syndrome) could be helped with CAM.

So what is the place of clinical aromatherapy? Clinical aromatherapy can be used to encourage healing and promote relaxation, but it can also help fight infection and chronic illness. Clearly it has a role to play in integrative medicine. Angela Avis (1999), chair of the Complementary Therapies Forum of the Royal College of Nurses (the largest union in the world with approximately 330,000 members), suggests that an aromatherapist (normally a lay person) is not "an aromatherapist" when essential oils are being used clinically within the parameters of a recognized license. In other words, aromatherapy is a tool used by LHPs, and, as such, requires more specialized training than most lay practitioners receive.

Approaches to aromatherapy can be herbal or chemical. Aromatherapy is rooted in herbal medicine. Many orthodox medicines also are derived from herbs, for example, aspirin, atropine, codeine, curare, digitalis, ephedrine, ergometrine, ipecacuanha, morphine, papaveretum, podophyllum, quinine, senna, theophylline, and vinblastine (Hollman 1991). Even the contraceptive pill was originally derived from a plant, the Mexican yam (Ryman 1991). Herbalists are vitalists; they believe in the synergy of plants (i.e., the whole is more than the sum of its parts), and they also understand that plants are adaptogens (i.e., that their therapeutic effects are affected by the "terrain" of the patient). Chemists believe that the chemistry of a plant indicates its therapeutic properties. A chemist is more likely to have a reductionist viewpoint similar to orthodox medicine: Eradicate the symptom and the patient will be cured. An herbalist might have a broader and more holistic approach to the patient, stressing the patient's background and intrinsic make-up. Both approaches have validity.

In the United Kingdom, aromatherapy has been closely associated with massage. Perhaps this confusion arose because aromatherapy emerged in England via the beauty therapy industry. However, aromatherapy has become sufficiently accepted as a therapy in its own right and the massage element has become less important. Certainly, applications of essential oils in massage have their place, particularly in stress reduction, but there are many other ways essential oils can be used in health care. It is troubling that the only systematic review of aromatherapy examined 12 studies targeting relaxation and combining essential oils with massage (Cooke & Ernst 2000). Double-blind, randomized studies of essential oils used topically, through inhalation, or orally, instead of in conjunction with massage, were ignored.

In France, aromatherapy is seen in a different light. Essential oils are often diluted in vegetable oil and given orally in a gelatin capsule by a medical or herbal doctor. The oral use of essential oils is often called aromatic medicine; it can be an effective treatment for gastrointestinal complaints or to combat an acute or chronic infection. Essential oils can also be given rectally or vaginally; the essential oils are absorbed through the "internal skin" of the body. Dermatologist Neal Schultz (2002) suggests that there is a clear difference between the modus operandi of essential oils that are ingested and those that are absorbed through external or internal skin. However they are used—topically, through inhalation, or orally—the use of essential oils goes back several thousand years.

Because often only one or two drops of essential oil are used, aromatherapy is known for its gentleness and is important in stress management (Buckle 1999). Aromatherapy can produce tremendous relaxation in a relatively short period (Mathers 1991). Many nurses use aromatherapy to help their patients relax. However, aromatherapy is not just about relaxing patients, improving their comfort level, or reducing pain. Essential oils can also help fight infection, also an acceptable nursing diagnosis (Carpenito 1993).

Essential oils are multitalented, and it is possible to use the same essential oil for relaxation and for infection. This can pose a problem: Is the essential oil cure or care? Florence Nightingale once said "the cure is in the caring" (Dossey 2000). (Nightingale was adamant that patients should be removed from malodorous odors.) During illness and following surgery relaxation can be a vital key to recovery (Nightingale 1859), and the ability to relax can be greatly enhanced by aromatherapy. By helping patients relax and feel better, they may actually get better. Shames (1993) suggests that "we need to put more caring back into curing so we can create a less costly, healthier system that will empower us all."

This book is not intended to be a substitute for training. I believe strongly in education, preferably in a hands-on class. There is a need for a clinical focus; the "recreational" issues can be left to the perfumers and soap makers. Safety concerns, as listed by the US Department of Labor Occupational Safety and Health Administration, need to be addressed. Health professionals need to be aware of the position on aromatherapy taken by the Joint Commission on Accreditation of Healthcare Organizations (JCAHO). JCAHO is in favor of complementary therapies that have a positive effect on pain and improve patient care. Protocols and policies need to be written. With these guidelines in place, aromatherapy can enhance patient care and reduce costs. This last point is important in a health care business desirous of a rapid, reliable turnover.

This book is about aromatherapy in clinical settings. It describes the use of essential oils in health care: as part of nursing care and as an aid in massage and physical therapy. It also covers the oral use of essential oils for physicians, nurse practitioners, pharmacists, and chiropractors. The chapter on the psychology of smell will be of interest to clinical psychologists, neurologists, behaviorists, and psychiatrists.

REFERENCES

Allaire A, Moos M, Wells S. 2000. Complementary and alternative medicine in pregnancy: a survey of North Carolina certified nurse-midwives. Obstetrics and Gynecology. 95(1) 19-23.

Avis A. 1999. When is an aromatherapist not an aromatherapist? Complementary Therapies in Medicine. 79(2) 53-124.

Beardsley T. 1994. Trends in cancer epidemiology: a war not won. Scientific American 270, 130-138.

Brooks M. 2001. Turning chemistry green. Worldlink. Accessed April, 2002, from http://www.worldlink.co.uk/stories/story.

Buckle J. 1992. Which lavender? Nursing Times. 88, 54-55.

Buckle J. 1999a. Aromatherapy in perianesthesia nursing. Journal of Perianesthesia Nursing. 14(6) 336-344.

Buckle J. 2001. The role of aromatherapy in nursing care. The Nursing Clinics of North America. 36(1) 57-73.

Carpenito, LJ. 1993. Nursing Diagnosis, 3rd ed. Philadelphia: J.B. Lippincott.

Cooke B, Ernst E. 2000. Aromatherapy: a systematic review. British Journal of General Practice. 50: 493-496.

Dossey B. 2000. Florence Nightingale: Mystic, Visionary, Healer. Springhouse, PA: Springhouse.

Dossey L. 2001. Surfing the odornet: exploring the role of smell in life and healing. Alternative Therapies in Health and Medicine. 7(2) 12-15, 100-107.

Eisenberg DM, Davis RG, Ettner SL et al. 1998. Trends in alternative medicine use in the United States; 1990-1997. Journal of the American Medical Association. 280, 1569-1575.

Gasgoigne S. 1993. Manual of Orthodox Medicine for Alternative Practitioners. Richmond: Jigme Press.

Hildebrand S. 1994. Aromatherapy. In Wells, R. (ed.), Supportive Therapies in Healthcare. London: Baillière Tindall, 124-125.

Hollman A. 1991. Plants in Medicine for the Chelsea Physic Garden. London: Chelsea Physic Garden.

Jacknin J. 2001. Aromatherapy. In Smart Medicine for Your Skin: A Comprehensive Guide to Understanding Conventional and Alternative Therapies to Heal Common Skin Problems. New York: Avery Penguin Putnam, 73-79.

King. J. 1994. The scientific status of aromatherapy. Perspectives in Biology and Medicine. 37(3) 409-415.

Kolata G, Eichenwald K. 1999. Business thrives on unproven care, leaving science behind. The New York Times, Oct 3, 664.

Kyle L. 2000. World sensorium. National Association for Holistic Aromatherapy Aromatherapy Journal. 10(3) 41-42.

Mathers P. 1991. Learning to cope with the stress of palliative care. In Penson J, Fraser R. (eds.), Palliative Care for People with Cancer. London: Edward Arnold, 260-261.

McNeil D. 2002. Scientist at work: confronting cancer. The New York Times. Tuesday April 9, 202. F7.

Mundy A. 2001. Dispensing with the Truth. New York: St. Martins Press.

Nightingale F. 1859. Notes on Nursing: What It Is and What It Is Not. London: Harrison & Sons.

Okie S. 2001. Report faults priorities of cancer care in the US. Albany, NY Times Union. June 20th. A5.

Oz M. 1998. Healing from the Heart. Dutton: New York.

Pear R. 1999. Medical mistakes kills tens of thousands annually. Albany, NY Times Union. Nov 30th. A1.

Ryman D. 1991. Aromatherapy. London: Piatkus.

Shames K. 1993. The Nightingale Conspiracy. Montclair, NJ: Enlightenment Press.

Schultz N. 2002. Personal communication.

Smith R. 1992. The ethics of ignorance. Journal of Medical Ethics. Reprinted in Newsletter of People's Medical Society 12, 4-51.

Thompson C. 2001. Oil on troubled waters. Nursing Times 97(15) 24-26.

Vickers A. 1996. Massage and aromatherapy: a guide for health professionals. London: Chapman and Hall.

Weil A. 2001. Personal communication.

2

The Nature
of Aromatherapy

When, from a long-distant past nothing subsists, after the people are dead, after the things are broken and scattered; taste and smell alone, more fragile but more enduring, more insubstantial, more persistent, more faithful, remain poised a long time, like souls, remembering, waiting, hoping, amid the ruins of all the rest; and bear unflinchingly, in the tiny and almost impalpable drop of their essence, the vast structure of recollection.

Marcel Proust
Remembrance of Things Past

The Nature of Aromatherapy

CONTRARY TO popular opinion, aromatherapy is not just about smelling things. The true definition of aromatherapy is much more specific: the use of essential oils for therapeutic or medical purposes. However, the way in which those essential oils are used is not specified. English aromatherapist Shirley Price defines aromatherapy as "the use of essential oils, all of which are derived from plants" (Price & Price 1999). American aromatherapist Jeanne Rose classifies aromatherapy as "the healing of essential oils through the sense of smell by inhalation, and through other application of these therapeutic volatile substances" (Rose 1992). An aromatherapy school in the United Kingdom defines aromatherapy as "a natural treatment which uses the concentrated essential oils from plants in association with massage, friction, inhalation, compresses and baths" (Kusmerik 1992). French physician Valnet (1990) writes that aromatherapy involves essences obtained from plants that are generally given "in the form of drops, or capsules."

There are four different types of aromatherapy: clinical, stress management, beauty therapy, and environmental fragrancing (Gilt 1992). British aromatherapy pioneer Robert Tisserand classifies them as psychotherapeutic, esthetic, holistic, and nursing and medical aromatherapy (Tisserand 1993a).

Without doubt, "nice smells" added to a massage in a beauty salon are something akin to flowers on the table at a restaurant; they are not specific ingredients of the meal, but they certainly enhance it. This is a form of esthetic aromatherapy. Beauty therapists do not usually treat disease. However, at the other end of the aromatherapy spectrum, medical aromatherapy suggests that specific medical conditions can be treated with essential oils. French medical aromatherapists Franchomme, Penoel, Gattefosse, and Belaiche have each written books dedicated to this subject. These two types of aromatherapy—esthetic and medical—are very distinct. The misunderstandings that arise often concern the types of aromatherapy that fall in between and what they entail.

Holistic aromatherapy suggests the therapist is involved with all parts of the patient—in other words, with mind, body, and spirit. Holistic aromatherapy involves "supporting" a patient; this is consistent with Tisserand's diagrammatic outlines. It is a procedure often carried out by body workers who may or may not know much about the chemistry of the essential oils or the pathologic conditions for which they are appropriate. These therapists are not "treating" the patient so much as supporting other treatments the patient may be receiving, which can be either orthodox or alternative.

Esthetic aromatherapy is about pleasure. Choosing a smell because it is pleasing is similar to studying a beautiful picture. The picture is treasured for the pleasure it gives, not for its intrinsic molecular structure. To put it another way, the use of perfumes, scented bath soaps, and incense sticks are the use of esthetic aromatherapy, and the world would be a sadder place without them. When patients are nearing the end of their lives, the focus is on keeping them comfortable, not prolonging life. At that stage, esthetic aromatherapy can give both pleasure and comfort.

Psychoaromatherapy concerns the ways smells or odors affect our brains by influencing the production of endorphins and noradrenaline. Whether we realize it or not, our entire life is affected by smell. All forms of aromatherapy have been around for hundreds of years. They are definitely not "New Age." Despite the explosion of products on the market that include the word *aromatherapy* on their labels, the use of essential oils in products is not new. Only the use of their synthetic copies is a recent development.

History of Aromatherapy: An Outline

Ancient History

The use of aromatic plants (and thus aromatherapy) was originally part of herbal medicine. Herbal medicine dates back thousands of years and is not confined to any one geographical area. Almost every part of the world has some history of the use of aromatics in its health care system.

Iraq

Perhaps the earliest use of aromatics was discovered only recently. In 1975, during investigation of an archaeologic dig in Iraq, concentrated extracts of yarrow, knapweed, grape hyacinth, mallow, and other plants were found near a Neanderthal skeleton dating back 60,000 years (Erichsen-Brown 1979). Of the eight species of herbs discovered there, seven are still being used today in medicine (Griggs 1981). Yarrow is an aromatic herb that produces an essential oil often used in aromatherapy.

France

One of the earliest records of plant medicine is in the form of paintings drawn on the walls of caves in Lascaux, Dordogne, in southern France (Ryman 1991). These drawings show the use of medicinal plants and date back to 18,000 BC. Much later, in the thirteenth century, a medieval religious sect called the Cathars lived in the area around Languedoc and Montaillou in southern France (Le Roy Ladurie 1984). Vegetarian and deeply spiritual, their priests (called *parfaits*) were also highly skilled in herbal and aromatic medicine. Regarded as heretics by the Catholic Church, they were tortured and murdered during the Inquisition. One night, more than 100 Cathar men, women, and children were tied to stakes and burned alive (Guirdham 1990).

Mesopotamia

The Sumerians, who lived in Mesopotamia around 5500 BC, were sophisticated herbalists. In their matriarchal society women were the healers. They were either shamans called *Ashipu* or herbalists called *Asu* (Lawless 1994). They left as their legacy clay tablets bearing prescriptions, names of plants, methods of preparation, and dosages for their treatments (Erichsen-Brown 1979). Aromatic medicine figured strongly in this early culture, and pots have been found that could have been used in plant distillation. In the *Epic of Gilgamesh,* a Sumerian poet writes, "There is a plant whose thorns will prick your hand like a rose. If your hands reach that plant you will become a young man again" (Swerdlow 2000).

Egypt

One of the most famous manuscripts listing aromatic medicines is the Egyptian Papyrus Ebers manuscript, found near Thebes in 1872. This document, written during the reign of Khufu (around 2800 BC), was followed by another document, written about 2000 BC, that mentions "fine oils and choice perfumes." These manuscripts, written while the Great Pyramid was still being built, reveal that during the time of Moses, frankincense, myrtle, galbanum, and eaglewood were used as medicines to cure symptoms of disease. There is also mention of myrrh being used to treat hay fever.

When Tutankhamun's tomb was opened in 1922, the boy-king's floral collars were still faintly aromatic. Thirty-five alabaster jars of perfume were found in his burial chamber, but all of them were broken or empty. Many had contained frank-incense and myrrh, highly valued commodities and likely the first items to be stolen from the tomb (Steele 1991). The ancient Egyptians also used aromatics in their embalming process. They removed most of the internal body parts and re-placed them with fragrant preparations such as cedar and myrrh. In the seven-teenth century some of these mummies were sold and distilled to be used in med-icines themselves (Levabre 1990).

China

The earliest known text containing written instructions on how to use herbs as medicines was written by the Chinese in approximately 2800 BC. *The Great Herbal (Pen Ts'ao)* is believed to have been written by Shen Nung. In it he lists some 350 plants, many of which are still being used today. One of them is the herb *Ephedra sinica,* which was among those found in the Neanderthal grave in Iraq. *The Great Herbal* dates back to around 2800 BC. Another emperor, Huang Ti, sometimes called the Yellow Emperor, wrote the *Huang Ti Nei Ching Su Wen.* The English translation is called *The Yellow Emperor's Classic of Internal Medicine* (Rose 1992a). Today, a huge concrete statue of ginseng presides over the state-run herbal market in Anguo, China (3 hours south of Beijing), indicating how im-portant herbal medicine remains. The Chinese method of soaking a cloth in herbs and resting it on the skin indicates how the Chinese have always accepted the ef-ficacy of transdermal delivery—something Western medicine denied for many years. There is a great similarity between Ayurvedic and Chinese medicine, prob-ably dating back to when India and China first traded. As early as 1000 BC, the Chinese were exchanging herbs with India (Swerdlow 2000).

India

Vedic medicine (the precursor to Ayurvedic medicine) has at its core the *Vedas,* a series of texts that refer to plants as "supreme, a remedy for need and a bless-ing for the heart." The first Sanskrit medical treatises, *Caraka Samhita* and *Sushrata Sambita,* date back to 2000 BC and describe the use of 700 plants, many of them aromatics such as ginger, coriander, myrrh, cinnamon, and sandalwood (Swerdlow 2000). Ayurvedic medicine was pushed underground by the Muslim invasion of India in the eleventh and twelfth centuries and later by the British occupation. The British prohibited the funding of Ayurvedic colleges and clin-ics. India fought back in 1921 with a document presented to the British gov-ernment in Madras, India, stating that no Western scientist should think of criticizing Ayurveda until he had learned the Sanskrit language (Swerdlow 2000).

In the last few decades Ayurveda has become popular again, in part because of the influence of Deepak Chopra, MD (Chopra 1991). Preparing an Ayurvedic medicine can take many days of following the Sanskrit instructions. Ayurveda has a strong spiritual base, and in northern India, Ayurvedic physicians are known as holy men. Traditional Indian shamans were known as *perfumeros* and were healers who used the scents of aromatic plants (Steele 1991). Today, aromatics remain an important part of Ayurvedic medicine.

Tibet

Tibetan medicine is thought to date back to pre-Buddhist times and is based on the *Four Tantras of Tibetan Medicine,* written in the eighth century. This is a whole medical system and is similar to Chinese medicine in that it focuses on the person (or the society in which the person lives), rather than the disease. Tibetan medicine has traditionally used aromatic herbs, often as inhalations. These herbs are usually prescribed in complex remedies such as Aquilaria A, which contains aromatics including clove, cardamom, sandalwood, and myrrh (Lawless 1992).

Greece

Theophrastus was a pupil of Aristotle and inherited the botanical garden at Athens that Aristotle had planted (Stearn 1998). In 300 BC, Theophrastus wrote *Enquiry into Plants,* in which he described specific uses for aromatics. At that time doctors who used aromatic unctions were called latralyptes. One aromatic formula, called *Kyphi,* contained 16 different ingredients. Kyphi was used as an antiseptic and an antidote to poison; it was soothing to the skin and would also "lull one to sleep, allay anxiety and brighten dreams." It was Theophrastus, later called the "father of botany" (Ryman 1991), who discovered the perfume of jasmine was stronger at night. Hippocrates (who lived around 460 BC) is recognized as the father of medicine. He wrote "aromatic baths are useful in the treatment of female disorders, and would often be useful for the other conditions too" (Chadwick & Mann 1983). He understood the principles of psychosomatic disorders, and his was possibly the first statement on holism: "In order to cure the human body it is necessary to have knowledge of the whole" (Lawless 1994). Hippocrates also knew aromatics could have important antibacterial properties, and when an epidemic of plague broke out he urged the people to use aromatic plants to protect themselves and stop the spread of the disease. He also wrote, "the growth of plants forms an excellent parallel to the study of medicine" (Chadwick & Mann 1983).

Greek army doctors traveled with large supplies of herbal remedies, and, in a manual written for the Emperor Claudius in 43 AD, detailed instructions were given on how to recognize plants abroad and how to pick and pack them. Everyone seemed to be using aromatic medicine in some form. Even audiences watching competitive sports in the stadium at Daphne were sprinkled with rose water to keep up their spirits and urge on the games. Helen of Troy was famed for her use of aromatics in mood-enhancing potions.

The legendary Greek Pedanios Dioskurides (often spelled Dioscorides) lived around 100 AD and wrote the famous *De Materia Medica.* This foundation of Western herbal medicine lists and illustrates some 700 plants that were in use at the time (Holmes 1993). Included are aromatics such as basil, verbena, cardamom, rose, rosemary, and garlic. Each section of *De Materia Medica* begins with a drawing and description of a plant and the contraindications are carefully listed (Griggs 1981). Dioscorides suggests that one of them, tarragon *(Artemesia dracunculus)* might be useful in four different treatments: for cancer, for gangrene, to produce abortions, and as protection against viper bites. Tarragon was later used by Native Americans during difficult labor and to induce menstruation. Native Americans believed tarragon was such an important herb it was classified a "chief medicine," requiring the collector to pull it (pick it) and not dig it up out of respect for its power.

When Claudios Galenos (known in English as Galen) was appointed personal physician to Emperor Marcus (130-200 AD) he continued the use of fragrant oils and referred to the fragrance of narcissus as the "food of the soul." Galen also introduced a system for identifying plants (Griggs 1981). In his famous work *Peri,* he listed not only different herbs but different grades of herbs like cinnamon (Holmes 1993). Unfortunately, many of the 500 works he compiled were destroyed when his clinic in Rome burned down. However the system introduced in his largest work (which consisted of 11 books) survived. By describing a disease process in terms of temperature and moisture, Galen laid the cornerstone of modern physiology (Lawless 1994). He also described a plant's energetic profile, which is similar to both Chinese and Ayurvedic approaches. This approach is continued today with contemporary writers (Holmes 1993; Mojay 2000). During the immediate pre-Christian era, Jewish women spiked wine with myrrh and frankincense, which have anesthetic effects, and gave it to those being tortured. The early Christian era considered aromatics to be pagan because they could heighten sensual pleasure. In 529 AD, Pope Gregory the Great passed a law banning all Materia Medica. This was the first hiccup in the history of aromatherapy. The school of philosophy at Athens closed down, and the works of Galen and Hippocrates were smuggled to Syria. There the works of Galen, Hippocrates, and Dioscorides were translated into Arabic by Hunayn ibn Ishaq al'Ibadi who was paid for his efforts with an amount of gold equal to his weight.

Arabia

In the prologue to *The Canterbury Tales,* Chaucer describes four Arabic physicians. Arabic doctors were regarded as the greatest medical authorities in the fourteenth century. One of Chaucer's physicians is an historical figure known as Ibn Sina—later called Avicenna (Tschanz 1997). Arabia added a whole host of new aromatics such as senna, camphor, tamarind, nutmeg, and cloves to the list of medicinal plants, and began to play an important part in the development of herbal and aromatic medicine. Arabs suggested rose and orange-blossom water to make medicines taste more palatable, and they were familiar with the anesthetic effect of inhaled henbane. Arabic physicians also used topical sugar to staunch bleeding. Sugar promotes new cell growth by drying the bed of the wound and dehydrating the bacteria there. This practice is still used today by some physicians (Swerdlow 2000).

By the third century AD, the city of Alexandria had become a center for medicine, continuing the Greek tradition of the science of aromatics. At the start of the ninth century, the first private apothecary shops opened in Baghdad. Medicines were manufactured and distributed commercially to physicians and pharmacists who dispensed them to the public as pills, tinctures, suppositories, and inhalants.

Abd Allah ibn Sina (980-1037) was born in what is now called Bukhara (present-day Uzbekistan). His name was later westernized into Avicenna. Ibn Sina was to the Arabic world what Aristotle was to the Greeks. He was a child prodigy: a scholar who at the age of 10 could recite the entire Koran and who went on to excel in medicine, poetry, math, physics, and philosophy. At the age of 20 ibn Sina was appointed court physician and during his life he wrote more than 20 medical texts including the *Canon of Medicine,* which remained a standard medical textbook until the sixteenth century (Lawless 1994). The *Canon* lists 760 medicinal plants and the drugs that can be derived from them. Ibn Sina also laid out the basic rules of clinical drug trials, principles that are still followed today (Tschanz 1997).

Ibn Sina is also credited with inventing a new kind of apparatus for distilling essential oils, called an *alembic.* During the tenth century many classic texts were translated from Arabic to Latin, and ibn Sina's *Canon of Medicine* first appeared in Europe in the twelfth century. It is interesting that Constantinus Africus and Gerard of Cremorna, the two translators of this classical text, lived in different towns and came from two different worlds—one Arabic and one Christian. This joint project was possible because the two scholars lived in towns close to the border dividing the Arabic and Christian worlds at that time. Ibn Sina's portrait still hangs in the great hall of the School of Medicine at the University of Paris, and Dante Alighieri held him in the same regard as Hippocrates and Galen.

Europe

By the thirteenth century, "the perfumes of Arabia" mentioned by Shakespeare had spread to Europe. Bad odors were thought to harbor disease (interestingly *malaria* literally translated means bad air), and being surrounded by pleasant odors was supposed to give protection against disease, especially the plague. Physicians wore birdlike masks containing aromatics to protect themselves. They also carried plague torches, fragrant herbs burned in a tiny brazier at the top of a long stick, containing aromatic resins and sprinkled houses affected by disease with aromatic waters like eau de cologne (Stoddart 1990).

Glovemakers in London became licensed to impregnate their wares with essential oils, and legend has it this is why so many glovemakers and perfumers survived the Great Plague. Scent boxes and pomanders containing solid perfumes (which originated in the East) became popular among the aristocracy. During this time the Abbess of Bingen, St. Hildegarde, wrote four books on medicinal plants.

By the sixteenth century, many Europeans had written their own collective works on herbs and aromatics. With the Renaissance and subsequent world exploration, many spices were added to Europe's knowledge of herbs. Cocoa *(Theobroma cacao)* was discovered in South America and tea tree was found in Australia. During one expedition in the winter of 1535, French explorer Jacques Cartier discovered a cure for scurvy from the Native Americans. Cartier's ship was frozen in the St. Lawrence River at St. Croix in Quebec, Canada. Most of the ship's company had fallen ill and had purple blotches on their skin, swollen legs, joint pain, and putrid gums. Several were dying. Cartier's friend, a Native American called Agaya, who had been very sick, suddenly appeared to be completely well. Intrigued, Cartier investigated and discovered Agaya had drunk an extract made from the tree Native Americans called Annedda.

Native Americans

Annedda is now thought to have been white spruce *(Picea glauca),* and this was the first documentation of successful scurvy treatment (Erichsen-Brown 1979). Native Americans were also adept at treating wounds, often with a tree gum like *Abies balsamea.* They treated dysentery with cedar leaves, and they used sweat lodges to promote healing. Native Americans also used narcotic plants such as water hemlock in topical applications, vigorously scratching the skin until it bled before applying the herb. Native-American medicine has produced many plant remedies such as Black cohosh root *(Cimicifuga racemosa)* for musculoskeletal pain and as an aid for labor and hormonal imbalances (Low Dog & Riley 2001) and May apple resin *(Podophyllum peltatum),* originally used for warts and today used to treat skin cancer. Only recently has Native American medicine become respected for its depth, history, and sophistication (Erichsen-Brown 1979). One of its advocates, Tieraona Low Dog, MD, is an eminent physician herself.

Fourteenth Century to Present

Paracelsus was born Philippus Aureolus Theophrastus Bombast von Hohenheim in 1493 near Zurich, Switzerland. Although his father was a physician, it is unclear whether Paracelsus ever completed his medical training. He wandered from university to university and was something of a rebel. His wanderings took him to live with the Tartars in Asia from whom he learned herbal medicine. He also learned anatomy from executioners. While he was on his travels he took the name Paracelsus.

Paracelsus was the subject of many legends, some suggesting he had magic powers and could conjure a hurricane with a twirl of his hat (Swerdlow 2000). He was a controversial figure and angered the orthodox medical community of the day by burning volumes of Avicenna's work at a public bonfire in the marketplace in Basel, Switzerland. Paracelsus was frustrated by what he felt were old principles and wanted to experience something innovative and new. He questioned Galen's work and thought the plethora of herbal manuals in circulation were written by "quacks" who abused sick people's lack of knowledge and were only after quick money.

Paracelsus believed the way forward was to isolate an active ingredient from a plant. "What the eye perceives in herbs or stone or trees is not yet a remedy; the eye sees only the dross. The remedy must be cleansed from the dross, then it is there. This is alchemy" (Griggs 1981). Paracelsus believed isolating the active ingredient would enhance the medicine's strength and increase its safeness. He was associated with the revolution supporting mineral preparations, and he used mercury, iron, sulfur, and antimony as well as herbs. Although Paracelsus remained fascinated by alchemy all his life (Griggs 1981), he was also a strong believer in the doctrine of signatures: that plants indicate the organ of the body they can help either by their shape or by the place where they grow. It is obvious from his copious writings (14 large volumes) that Paracelsus used herbs knowledgeably, and he was very successful.

Although a specific action of a plant may appear to depend on a single chemical constituent, isolating it may not make the effect more active or safer. Nature is not a fool; plants have their own synergistic action that is irreplaceable. In the plant world, the sum of the parts really does add up to more than the total (Mills 1991). If the most active constituent is removed and applied in isolation, it may have a different effect or negative side effects. The ability of one part of a plant to "switch off" negative properties of another part is sometimes called *quenching* (Watt 1991). For example, isolated citral (an aldehyde found in lemongrass) produces a more severe sensitization reaction at a lower concentration than does the complete essential oil, which contains a higher percentage of citral.

This concept is further demonstrated by extracting and separating all the active ingredients of an essential oil, then recombining them. They will not necessarily produce the same effect as the complete essential oil (or herb). However, this is how drug companies usually approach research of herbs: they isolate and synthesize. To this day Paracelsus is regarded as the first medical pharmacologist, the "patron saint" of drug companies.

When Rene Descartes (1596-1650) declared that man was a machine, the next hiccup occurred for aromatherapy. Descartes' philosophy, the basis of Cartesian thinking, is summed up in his own words, "*cognito, ergo sum,*" or "I think, therefore I am" (Cook 1978). Descartes went on to say mind and body bore no relationship to one another, and the concept of soul faded. The idea that an aromatic compound could have an effect on the body via the brain fell into disrepute. Not until the eighteenth century when a physician named Gaub suggested that "bodily diseases may often be more readily alleviated or cured by the mind, that is by the emotions, than by corporeal remedies" did the idea of a connection between mind and body return (Lawless 1994). In 1763 Julien La Mettries wrote an essay that said man was a machine. Gaub disagreed and wrote a response, suggesting doctors should search for substances that affect the mind. Today it is gradually becoming accepted that smell affects the mind. The mind is not an isolated, single organ, but is connected to every cell of our body. The way each cell feels intimately affects the way a person feels overall (Pert 1997).

United Kingdom

William Turner (1520-1568) was one of the earliest English herbalists. A Cambridge graduate, he believed in the doctrine of signatures and gave many plants, such as lungwort and liverwort, their common names to indicate their use. At this time, qualifying to become a physician took up to 10 years. Interestingly, Shakespeare's son-in-law John Hall called himself a physician, although he had only a Master of Arts degree. However, this did not stop him from purchasing 300 plants, "practicing" medicine, and leaving notes from 178 different cases. One of his patients was the Earl of Compton who lived some 40 miles away, several days' journey by horseback (Swerdlow 2000).

During Shakespeare's time the apothecaries, from whom physicians purchased their medicines, were also prescribing. In 1512, in an attempt to control the situation, the British Parliament introduced the first laws controlling the prescription and sale of medicines. Six years later, the Royal College of Physicians of London was established.

However, the seventeenth century is mainly remembered as the golden era for herbal medicine. Nicholas Culpeper, who posthumously became one of the more famous herbalists, published his *Complete Herbal* in 1660. During the 1700s essential oils were widely used in "mainstream" medicine. In William Salmon's *The Compleat English Physician* oils of cinnamon, lavender, lemon, clove, and rue are listed with others in a recipe to "cheer and comfort all the spirits, natural, vital and animal"(Tisserand 1979). In 1770 the British Parliament passed an act to protect men from the "guiles of perfumed women" who might trick them into matrimony as the "witchcraft of scent could manipulate their mind" (Watson 2000). The United States followed with a paper published in the *New York Medical Journal* on the "connections of the sexual apparatus with the ear, nose and throat" that suggested perfume was a conscious attempt to "stimulate lecherous thoughts" (Dabney 1913).

The first scientific evaluation of essential oils occurred in the nineteenth century, and many of the results were published in William Whitla's *Materia Medica and Therapeutics* in 1882. The industrial and scientific revolutions followed. During the next two centuries scores of essential oils were analyzed. It was thought important to identify and isolate therapeutic components of plants (just as Paracelsus had advocated). In the late 1890s specific components such as geraniol and citronellol were identified, and in 1868 William Henry Perkin announced the synthesis of coumarin.

Modern Drug Development

Synthetic copies of perfumes and aromatics began to be appear, and the era of modern drug development dawned—the third hiccup for aromatherapy.

Willow bark became aspirin, and foxglove became digitalis. Despite important research on the therapeutic effects of many essential oils by Cadeac and Meunier in France and Gatti and Cajola in Italy, essential oils and herbal medicine lost out to the profits of synthetic drugs. With the 1930 partnership of Rockefeller in the United States and Faben in Germany, the petrochemical pharmaceutical industry became a major economic and political force.

Following the Flexner report on the nation's medical schools in 1910 (which was paid for by the Carnegie Foundation), almost all homeopathic and naturopathic medical schools in the United States were squeezed out. Herbal medicine, including the use of aromatics, was excluded from medical school curricula. Petrochemical drug companies became the major underwriters of all medical colleges in the United States. More importantly they also became the major funders of the American Medical Association and therefore 90% of all medical research (Buckle 2001).

Renaissance of Aromatherapy

The modern renaissance of aromatherapy began in France with the work of a chemist, a physician, and a nurse: Gattefosse, Valnet, and Maury.

Rene-Maurice Gattefosse, a chemist, lived in France from 1881 to 1950. He was interested in both the psychologic and physiologic effects of aromatics and mainly used topical application of essential oils. It was because of an accident that Gattefosse was first drawn to aromatherapy. In 1910, while he was working in his laboratory, an explosion occurred, covering him with burning substance. He rolled on the grass to extinguish the flames. A few days later the wounds became infected with gas gangrene but "one rinse of essential oil of [English] lavender (Lavandula angustifolia) stopped the gassification of the tissue"(Tisserand 1993). Impressed by the way his wounds had healed, Gattefosse dedicated his life to researching essential oils. Many of his patients were soldiers wounded in the trenches of World War I. Among the essential oils Gattefosse used were thyme, chamomile, clove, and lemon. Until World War II, those essential oils were used both as natural disinfectants for wounds, and to sterilize surgical instruments (Ryman 1991).

Gattefosse was one of the first people to use the word *aromatherapy*. He discovered essential oils take between 30 minutes and 12 hours to be absorbed completely by the body after being applied topically. His work *Aromatherapie: The Essential Oils — Vegetable Hormones* (giving detailed medical case studies performed by various physicians) was published in France in 1937. The manuscript was discovered by Jeanne Rose, translated into English, edited by Robert Tisserand, and published in English in 1993 (Tisserand 3).

Throughout World War II, French physicians used essential oils on infected wounds and as a treatment for gangrene. Perhaps the course of aromatic medicine would have been different if Alexander Fleming had not discovered a piece of moldy bread that led to the manufacture of penicillin. With the emergence of manufactured antibiotics—full of promise, profit, and easy availability—came the fourth hiccup in the history of aromatherapy, and its demise seemed certain. However, during World War II, American nurses stationed at Pearl Harbor used handkerchiefs infused with perfume to help cope with the nauseating aroma of burned flesh (Sarnecky 2001). They also offered the scented handkerchiefs to their patients. Fessler (1996) suggests this was an early example of modern aromatherapy.

Jean Valnet, MD, was born in the early 1900s and died only a few years ago. A French army physician, he spent much of his life researching aromatherapy and was interviewed in 1993 by Christine Scott for the *International Journal of Aromatherapy* (Scott 1993-1994). His publication *Aromatherapie* (Valnet 1937) was the first "medical" publication on aromatherapy, full of case studies and citing numerous references. Valnet wrote it "is not necessary to be a doctor to use aromatherapy. But one has to know the power of essential oils in order to avoid accidents and incidents" (Scott 1993-1994).

During his time in Indochina, when he was commander of an advanced surgical unit, Valnet used essential oils with the full approval of his superiors. However, despite impressive results, when he returned to France he found the orthodox medical community unhappy with his use of unconventional medicine and they tried to strike him from the general medical list. Fortunately for aromatherapy, some of his patients were high-ranking government officials, including the Minister of Health, so this did not happen (Scott 1993-1994). Valnet's book, *The Practice of Aromatherapy*, possibly *the* classic on aromatherapy, has been translated into German, Italian, Spanish, and Japanese, as well as English.

Marguerite Maury's life was initially one of tragedy. Born in Austria, she married very early and had her first child while still a teenager. Sadly her son died from meningitis when he was only 2 years old. Shortly afterward, her husband was killed in action, and his death was closely followed by her father's suicide. Keen to make a new start, Marguerite decided to move to France and train as a nurse. While working in France as a surgical assistant, she met and married Dr. Maury. He shared her love of the arts and her fascination with alternative approaches to medicine, and together they formed a cohesive and inspirational team.

Marguerite Maury classified the use of essential oils into various clinical departments: surgery, radiology, dermatology, gynecology, general medicine, psychiatry, spa treatment, physiotherapy, sports, and cosmetics. She won two international prizes for her research on essential oils and the skin, and her book, *Le Capital Jeunesse,* was published in 1961 and translated into English 3 years later. She left a dedicated and now famous pupil, Daniele Ryman, to continue her work (Maury 1964).

Gattefosse, Valnet, and Maury may have been the first pioneers of modern aromatherapy, but there were plenty of now-famous names waiting in the wings. Tisserand and Price made aromatherapy a household word in England and sparked the interest of the medical and nursing community. Many researchers—too many to list—followed. Of particular note are Gildemeister in Germany, Guenther and Lawrence in the United States, Leclerc and Belaiche in France, and Dodd, Deans, and Svoboda in the United Kingdom, all of whom wrote extensively about the clinical use of essential oils. Today, there is a wealth of information and sufficient evidence to suggest the medicine of the future could be a sweet-smelling one.

How Essential Oils Work

The study of where essential oils go when they are absorbed and how they are absorbed and eliminated by the body is called *pharmacokinetics*. Essential oils are absorbed into the body through digestion, through the "internal skin" lining of orifices (mouth, vagina, and anus), by olfaction, and through the external skin (Jager et al 1992).

There is fairly heated debate as to how aromatherapy should be used. Some people believe the term *aromatherapy* means just that: inhalation. But, in many parts of the world, aromatherapy is often combined with touch, as the absorption of essential oils through the skin coupled with soothing touch (or warmth) may enhance and prolong their therapeutic effects. Some believe the sublingual, rectal, and vaginal routes of absorption are the most effective. Others believe essential oils are most useful when taken orally and digested. Clearly there is a difference in metabolism between a substance that is ingested and one that is applied topically (to internal or external skin) or inhaled. Ingestion of essential oils is more akin to Western medicine.

There is a substantial body of knowledge about the absorption of essential oils through the shaved skin of animals or by injection into their peritoneal cavities, but published research on the absorption of essential oils through human skin or by ingestion is limited. There is published research to show inhaled essential oils affect the human brain, but clearly the use of aromatherapy in a clinical setting is in its infancy. Patients say aromatherapy works, and the whole movement of aromatherapy in health care appears to be led by patients as much as practitioners.

Using aromatherapy in a clinical setting is still a bit like pioneer work. Nurses using aromatherapy say they feel a little like modern-day Florence Nightingales. Although it is impossible to provide evidence of efficacy without research, a pattern of efficacy is emerging. Health professionals believe there is sufficient anecdotal evidence to show clinical aromatherapy is efficacious, cost effective, and safe, but the information is scattered. A major collaborative effort is needed to bring together all that information so the "pattern" becomes clear. That pattern will be the basis for future research.

Routes of Absorption of Essential Oils

Essential oils contain many different components, and these components are absorbed by the body. Thus lavender is not found in the bloodstream, but linalyl acetate and linalol, two of the major components found in lavender, are found in the bloodstream after inhalation, topical (internal or external) application, or ingestion of lavender essential oil.

There are four methods by which the components within essential oils can be absorbed.

1. Topical: using external skin via touch, compress, or bath
2. Internal: using internal skin via mouthwashes, douches, pessaries, or suppositories
3. Oral: via gelatin capsules or diluted in honey, alcohol, or a dispersant (purchasable from most good essential-oil companies)
4. Inhaled: directly or indirectly, with or without steam

Each method of application has its own physiologic process, advantages, and disadvantages.

Topical Application

"A good name is like a precious ointment; it filleth all around about, and will not easily away; for the odors of ointments are more durable than those of flowers."
Francis Bacon, 1561-1626

The skin is a complex, multifaceted membrane, varying from a fraction of a millimeter thick on the eyelid to approximately 3-mm thick on the back. The skin is the largest organ in the body. For many years the skin was thought to be a barrier, and it was believed drugs could not be absorbed through the skin. Women were ridiculed for putting creams and lotions on their faces in an effort to preserve their youthfulness. Now it is acknowledged that cosmetics not only penetrate the stratum corneum but are also absorbed into the viable epidermis (Zatz 1993). Autoradiography can be used to demonstrate the absorption of lipid-soluble substances through the skin (Fig. 2-1) (Suzuki et al 1978).

Nicotine patches are common since the advent of patch therapy, and many conventional drugs are now administered transdermally on a continuous basis. Examples of such drugs are antianginals such as nitroglycerine, the female hormones estradiol and progesterone, antihypertensives such as clonidine, narcotics such as fentanyl, and antispasmodics and antiemetics such as scopolamine (Cleary 1993). Topical anesthetic lidocaine and cortisone dexamethasone have also been introduced using a transdermal patch in combination with an electric current (Zetzer et al 1991). Tests are currently in progress to establish how commercially viable it will be to deliver beta-blockers timolol and bupranolol, antihistamines tripolidine and azatadine, and testosterone via this method. Furthermore, the *New York Times* reported that scientists may have found a way to avoid the sting of vaccinations by spreading the vaccine on the skin. The vaccinations tested on the mice were diphtheria, tetanus, and cholera (Associated Press 1998).

Not every substance is absorbed through the skin in the same amount. Hotchkiss (1994) demonstrated that only 1% of Cypermethrin (a pesticide) was absorbed, but 65% of benzoic acid (a fungicide) was absorbed through human skin. Two processes are involved in topical absorption: penetration and permeation (Reiger 1993). Penetration is the actual entry of a substance into and through the skin, whereas permeation is the subsequent absorption of a substance

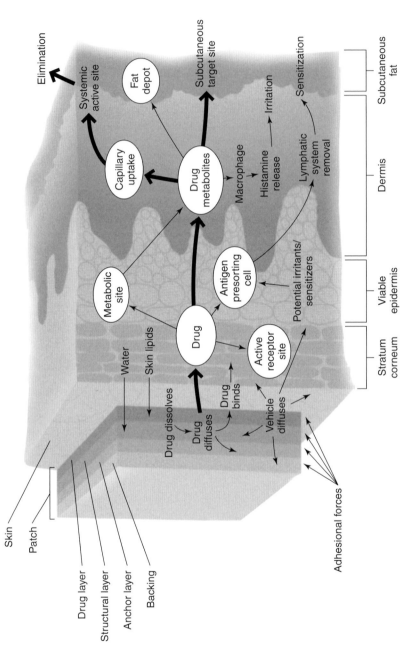

FIGURE 2-1   Diagram to show drug absorption through skin.   (From Zatz J. 1993. Factors affecting absorption of topically applied substances. In Zatz J (ed.), Skin Permeation: Fundamentals and Applications. Wheaton, IL. Allured.)

into the body. Obviously the former is more important if the skin is being treated and the latter if a systemic treatment is sought.

The process of diffusion and permeation are in part described by Fick's laws (Rieger 1993). These are a series of mathematical descriptions of diffusion through membranes. More important than the actual concentration of the substance (in this case the essential oil), is its chemical activity or potency. Therefore if an essential oil contains a small amount of a potent component (a phenol), its chemical potential is greater than that of an essential oil containing a larger amount of a less potent chemical (an alcohol).

If the essential oil is diluted in a substance with lower permeability, its progress, or pharmacokinetics, are adversely influenced. In other words, essential oils diluted in a fixed oil (carrier oil) are absorbed more slowly than undiluted essential oils. The actual carrier medium can also affect (and to a certain extent inhibit) the concentration of the active ingredients of essential oils. For example, in one study, the germicidal effects of phenol (a common constituent of essential oils) could not be exerted when it was applied to the skin in a fatty base (Zatz 1993a). Heat appears to enhance penetration, and hot water may speed up the absorption of essential oils into the skin. Studies have shown that penetration of the dermis is increased 100-fold if essential oils are dispersed in a bath (Buchbauer 1993a).

Essential oils are lipid soluble, and they can be absorbed through the skin rapidly. Fuchs et al (1997) reported that carvone, a ketone component found in essential oils, was found in the bloodstream of a human subject within 10 minutes of a massage. Carvone was also found in the subject's urine. The subject, a 25-year-old woman, wore a mask to avoid inhaling the aroma. The exact time required for absorption depends on the weight of the molecule and certain physio-chemical properties, such as polarity and optical activity (Jager et al 1992). In simple terms, polarity refers to polar molecules, so called because they have a negative and positive "pole" which attract opposite charges (Bowles 2000). Optical properties refers to the ability of molecules to rotate in polarized light (Williams 1996). In the case of lavender, most of the two main constituents, linalol and linalyl acetate, were absorbed within 20 minutes and eliminated within 90 minutes. The disadvantage of applying essential oils topically is not all of the essential oil is absorbed unless an occlusive dressing is applied. Otherwise, much of the essential oil evaporates because of its high volatility. Straehli, who researched the kinetics of essential oils in 1940, found that all the essential oils appear in the breath following absorption through the skin, although the time interval differs with each essential oil (Tisserand 1985).

The greater the percentage of skin covered, the greater the penetration by an essential oil (Balacs 1993). Friction, caused by stroking or massage, encourages dilation of blood vessels in the dermis, which increases absorption of the essential oils (Pratt & Mason 1981). Because the stratum corneum (the outer layer of the epithelium) is partly hydrophilic and partly lipophilic, some water-based and some oil-based components can pass through it (Riviere 1993). Essential oils are lipid soluble so they gain rapid access to lipid-rich areas of the body (Buchbauer 1993), such as the myelin covering of medullated nerve fibers. This lipid solubility also enables the relatively small molecules of components within the essential oils to cross the blood-brain barrier: the separation of neurons from capillary walls by astrocytes (Anthony & Thibodeau 1983).

Although some areas of skin are more accessible, all areas of the skin are permeable. Clearly this indicates that it is not necessary, or sometimes even advisable, to give a patient a full-body treatment. Patients' feet are usually easily accessible, and they rarely have intravenous infusions attached to them. Treatment of feet requires no removal of clothes apart from shoes and socks, and therefore the feet are possibly the least embarrassing body part to have touched (except for the hands). Another advantage of using the feet is they are not highly innervated areas like the face, nor are they areas of low innervation like the back (Weiss 1979).

Caution should be taken when applying essential oils to damaged skin, because damaged skin is more absorbent of outside chemicals. Moore et al (1980) found twice as much lead was absorbed by abraded skin as undamaged skin. In a clinical setting, damaged skin includes skin affected by systemic disease; dermatology problems; or dehydration caused by a cold, dry environment or the daily use of strong detergents. Stress (either physical or emotional) results in vascular shut-down, which produces cold hands and feet. Psychologic stress also perturbs the epidermal permeability-barrier homeostasis (Garg et al 2001); in the case of essential oils this means that less is absorbed. However, when a patient is sweating, the body is trying to get rid of heat and the blood vessels are dilated. But dilated blood vessels can increase penetration of essential oils. Older skin, because it is thinner and its barrier function is diminished, tends to absorb essential oils faster.

Topical absorption can be enhanced with an occlusive dressing (Fuchs et al 1997). This reduces the potential for evaporation. Fuchs et al (1997) found that with an inclusive wrap, substantially more of the essential oil components were absorbed. Bronaugh's study (1990) showed that 75% of a fragrance was absorbed when the skin was covered, and only 4% was absorbed when the skin was not covered. Covering the skin also increases its temperature and hydration and therefore enhances penetration. Topically applying essential oils has several advantages: they do not need to be digested, they are simple to use, and the essential oils are excreted slowly. This is also the most direct way to treat topical issues such as skin problems or muscle complaints. There are a few disadvantages. One disadvantage is that the skin contains certain enzymes that can activate (or inactivate) toxic chemicals (Tisserand & Balacs 1995). Another disadvantage of applying essential oils topically is that some essential oils (those containing phenols) can be epidermal irritants and others (containing furocoumarins) may cause photosensitivity.

Epidermal absorption is still not fully understood, and pharmacokinetics is a relatively new field. What is safe to put on the skin and in what concentration is an ongoing dialogue between cosmetic manufacturers. For many years the most commonly used hospital bactericide for hand washing and consumer products was hexachlorophane. At the time, it was thought to be completely safe. However, hexachlorophane was later demonstrated to be a potential neurotoxin (Sherman & Leech 1973). Because of a manufacturing error in the 1970s, a baby powder was manufactured that contained 10 times the intended concentration of hexachlorophane. This resulted in the deaths of several babies in France. It is thought that because the diapers acted as an occlusive dressing, the drug's absorption was enhanced (Jackson 1993). The use of hexachlorophane in medical products such as Ster-Zac and Dermalex was halted in 1973 because of the toxic effects it might produce when absorbed into the body (McFerran 1996).

Finally, a serious disadvantage is that many essential oils plants are still grown with pesticides. While gas chromatography might indicate this, because it analyzes the different compounds in an essential oil, pesticides are not beneficial to human skin and can also cause a reaction that has nothing to do with the essential oil. Expressed essential oils are most likely to have high levels of pesticides.

Topical application of essential oils can be used for the following:
   Relieving localized trauma such as bruising, sprains, stings, or burns
   Relaxing and warming specific muscles
   Cooling specific areas
   Relieving neuralgic conditions
   As an antiinflammatory
   As an antispasmodic
   As a specific antiviral, antifungal, or antibacterial agent for skin infections
   For systemic treatments including hormonal imbalance
   As a general body relaxant

Topical applications can be given as follows:
   In a carrier oil (cold-pressed vegetable oils)
   In an ointment
   In a gel
   Undiluted (see Chapter 4)
   In a bath (sitz, hand, foot, or full)
   As a compress
   In a wound irrigation

The amount of an essential oil absorbed through the skin depends (not in any specific order) on the following:
   Dilution used
   Amount used
   Amount of skin surface covered
   Choice of essential oil
   Choice of carrier (lotion, oil, cream, alcohol, water)
   Part of the body used
   Temperature of the skin
   Integrity of the skin
   Heat of the environment
   Age of the skin

In an aromatherapy massage, or when the essential oil is applied using the "m" technique, much of the essential oil evaporates into the room and is inhaled by the patient. Therefore the benefit is likely to be a synergy of the topically applied and inhaled essential oils together. Both, mixed with gentle touch, allows the patient to relax and breathe deeply. It is difficult to separate the two means of entry, and it is suggested they could work synergistically. Currently there is no body of comparative knowledge on the gastrointestinal and cutaneous absorption of the same test material (Jackson 1993).

Oral and Internal Administration

The oral route for administering essential oils is important and can be an excellent way to treat gastrointestinal problems. Almost all other problems can be helped using other methods. For those who have a license to prescribe, the oral route (aromatic medicine) is very powerful. Aromatic medicine can produce impressive results, especially with chronic or acute infections. In the United Kingdom the Aromatherapy Organization Council, the lead body for aromatherapy, advises against the oral use of essential oils. The Royal College of Nursing accepts all methods of aromatherapy as part of nursing care except the oral use of essential oils. However, the internal skin route (using the inner skin of the mouth, rectum, and vagina) is an extension of the external skin route (Schultz 2002) and is very relevant to nursing care.

Essential oils can be used in a mouthwash, which is excellent for mouth infections, and are very important in dental care. Gargles can be very effective in treating tracheitis. Essential oils can also be diluted in a douche or on a tampon and are very effective for some vaginal infections. Essential oils can also be used in both vaginal and rectal pessaries to treat infection and inflammation. Both rectal and vaginal routes have a distinct advantage in the treatment of reproductive or urinary conditions because the essential oils are absorbed directly into the surrounding tissue. Recurrent cystitis responds well to this method of treatment.

In aromatic medicine, essential oils can be administered orally either in a gelatin capsule, honey water, or alcohol (Valnet 1990). For more information, please see Chapter 7. This is a highly specialized field that requires proper training and, in the United States, probably a license to prescribe. Despite the fact that many essential oils are used in small amounts as flavoring agents in our food, pure essential oils are concentrated and are not to be experimented with casually. Just as a whole bottle of Tylenol can be lethal (although this drug is still sold over the counter because the public is expected to take only one or two tablets at a time), so a few essential oils can be lethal if several milliliters are ingested at once. Price and Price (1999) suggest the maximum number of essential oil drops taken internally should be limited to 3 drops 3 times a day for a period of 3 weeks maximum. Brinker (2000) suggests up to $2^1/_2$ ml a day. (If there are 20 drops per milliliter, this works out to be 50 drops a day, which does seem a little high.) However, much depends on the essential oils and its chemical constituents.

A safer option is to offer herbal teas. These are gentle and are sold over the counter. Common herbal teas are chamomile, peppermint, ginger, and fennel. **Warning: Encouraging patients to take essential oils by mouth is not advised unless the person advocating it is trained in this method.**

Inhalation

"Smells are surer than sounds and sights to make your heartstrings crack." Rudyard Kipling (Birchall 1990)

Of all the methods for introducing essential oils into the human body, inhalation is the simplest and fastest. It is also the oldest method, and the use of aromatics in rituals is well documented. Perfume, as the name implies, began its existence as a ritual source of odor spread by heat and smoke (Watson 2000). The Oxford Dictionary defines perfume as "odorous fumes of burning substance," and the word is derived from the Latin *fume,* meaning smoke (Oxford Dictionaries 1964). Inhalation may be the oldest method of drug use, but it is also turning out to be one of the most current. The latest drug to be used via olfaction is insulin. In this revolutionary method of treating diabetes, powdered or liquid insulin is inhaled once a day (Epstein 2001). Inhalation takes the essential oils from the outside of the body to deep inside the body in one easy step. The lungs have a huge surface area that is intimately connected to the blood system via the alveoli. Jori et al (1969) showed that inhaled cineole (an oxide found in eucalyptus and several other essential oils) can have a measurable effect at very low concentrations.

Olfaction

The nose has two distinct functions: to warm and filter incoming air and to act as the first part of the olfactory system. If inhalation was the same as olfaction, then olfactory stimuli would be obvious each time a breath was taken, which is not the case; taking a normal breath is different than sniffing an essential oil (Alexander 2001). However, aromas can have instant effects, and sometimes just thinking about a smell can be as powerful as actually smelling it (Betts 1996). Odors have psychologic and physiologic effects. Until very recently smelling salts were the standard method for reviving someone who had fainted. A person knows immediately if a smell is pleasant or unpleasant and what memories it evokes. Smell is a chemical reaction; receptors in the brain respond to chemicals within the essential oil. As a person breathes in, these chemicals move up behind the bridge of the nose, just beneath the brain, where they attach themselves to millions of hair-like receptors connected to the olfactory bulb. These receptors are extremely sensitive and can be stimulated by very subtle scents. Different odors bind to distinct arrays of receptors. This allows people to discriminate between more than 10,000 odors, even though there are only about 1000 odor receptors.

Because olfactory receptors are so sensitive, they are easily fatigued, which explains why smells seem less obvious as the body tires or adapts to them (Anthony

& Thibodeau 1983). Air flows through the nostrils at different rates because of turbinate swelling. Every few hours, the nostril taking in more air switches from left to right. In one study, odors breathed through one or the other nostril produced different effects; 17 out of 20 participants identified l-carvone differently, depending on which nostril was dominant. However, there are no differences with regard to the electrical changes in the brain between the left and right nostrils (Walter et al 1964). Essential oils are highly complex and are made up of many different chemical components, or odor molecules. These molecules travel via the nose to the olfactory bulb and on to the limbic system of the brain.

The limbic system (LS) is vital for normal human functioning and is the oldest part of the human brain, supposedly having evolved first. (In lower vertebrates it is called the *smell brain*, because these animals depend on their sense of smell for survival.) The LS is a complex inner ring of brain structures below the cerebral cortex, arranged into 53 regions and 35 associated tracts (Watts 1975). The main structures in the limbic system are the amygdala, septum, hippocampus, anterior thalamus, and hypothalamus. These structures are connected by a number of complicated pathways (Anthony & Thibodeau 1983). Of these regions, the amygdala and hippocampus are of particular importance in processing aromas.

The amygdala is an almond-shaped group of subcortical nuclei located under the surface of the front medial portion of the temporal lobe. It is thought to play a pivotal role in processing emotion and in the formation of emotional memory, and it governs emotional response. The amygdala is known to affect survival behavior and is intimately responsible for the sensation of fear. It is also thought to play an important role in controlling aggression. Autism has been linked to a change in the cells of the amygdala (Edelson 2001). Diazepam (Valium) is thought to reduce the effect of external emotional stimuli by increasing gamma aminobutyric acid (GABA)-containing inhibitory neurons in the amygdala (LeDoux 1996). True lavender *(Lavandula angustifolia)* is thought to have a similar effect on the amygdala, producing a sedative effect similar to diazepam (Tisserand 1988). This is interesting because tricyclics or benzodiazepines, which were commonly used by orthodox medicine to treat chronic pain, also inhibit the action of nociceptor neurotransmitters. True lavender is a common essential oil used topically for pain relief that also appears to enhance the effect of orthodox pain medication.

The hippocampus is where the memory of smell is triggered, so this part of the limbic system is concerned with the formation and retrieval of explicit memories (LeDoux 1996). It is also closely involved with the three types of memory: semantic (facts and concepts), episodic (recollection of events), and spatial (recognition). The hippocampus is thought to be the storage area for new experiences before they become permanent memories that are then believed to be stored in the cerebral cortex. The hippocampus is particularly vulnerable to ischemia, Alzheimer's disease, and epilepsy (Healing Arts 2001). A stroke can affect memory, but only if it causes bilateral damage to the hippocampus.

As well as influencing the expression of emotions, instinctive behaviors, drives, and motivations, the limbic system plays an essential role in learning and memory (Kirk-Smith 1993). Buchbauer (1993a) states the limbic system is responsible for sexual desires and feelings of wellness and harmony. The posterior, superior part of the cingulate gyrus is related to sexual behavior and is linked to obsessive-compulsive behavior (Diamond et al 1985).

The limbic system also receives most sensory input and passes it on to the voluntary and involuntary motor centers. Gatti and Cajola (1923) noted that odors produced an immediate effect on respiration, pulse, and blood pressure, and therefore concluded that odors had produced, by a reflex action, a dramatic effect on the functioning of the central nervous system. Singewald et al (2000), nearly 80 years later, found that the locus coeruleus played a pivotal role in conditioned fear and inescapable shock.

The effect of odors on the brain has been "mapped" using computer-generated tomographics. These brain electrical activity maps indicate how subjects linked to an electroencephalogram psychometrically rate odors presented to them (Van Toller et al 1992). Smells can have a psychologic effect even when the aroma is below the level of human awareness. Lorig et al (1990) reported the effects of subliminal (below consciousness) smelling of vanilla. The scent of vanilla was found to elicit positive mood change. Aromas can also have an effect while a person is sleeping (Bardia et al 1990).

An electrical phenomenon discovered by Grey in 1964 called contingent negative variation (CNV) showed the sedative effects of diazepam decreased CNV, and the stimulant effect of caffeine increased CNV. When fragrances were tested, these also caused different effects. Lavender produced a similar reaction to diazepam, decreasing CNV, and jasmine had the reverse effect, increasing CNV (Torii et al 1991). Rovesti and Columbo's research (1973) showed that olfactory receptors are also affected by nonvolatile molecules in aerosols. This was confirmed with research conducted by Vellmair et al in 1998.

Anosmia   Certain genetic conditions, such as Kallman's syndrome, produce anosmia (Bartoshuk & Beauchamp 1994), the lack of a sense of smell. Sometimes there is specific anosmia, which means a certain aroma, such as androstenone, is not smelled or is perceived differently. When the olfactory nerve has been severed by trauma, aromas are unable to connect to the limbic part of the brain. However essential oils can still enter the body through the lungs, skin, or ingestion. When a person has a sinus infection or a heavy cold, some aromas may get through; they tend to be the most penetrating, such as peppermint and eucalyptus. Temporary loss of smell can also follow a severe shock or infection. Smell is closely aligned to the sense of taste. Taste is divided into four categories: salty, sour, sweet, and bitter. Salty and sour tastes involve ion channels in the cells of receptor membranes, whereas sweet and bitter tastes bind to receptor proteins (Bartoshuk & Beauchamp 1994).

Administration Via the Olfactory System   Inhalation can be targeted directly to a single patient, in which case it is called direct inhalation, or it can be used in a more general way, for example in a room of people. This second method is called indirect inhalation. Indirect inhalation can use a selection of apparatus: electrical, heat, or battery operated.

Direct Inhalation

1. Tissue or cotton ball: Put one to five drops of essential oil(s) on a facial tissue or cotton ball and inhale for 5 to 10 minutes. Alternately, aroma ribbons can be attached to the bedclothes of children or adults for an easily applied sleeping or comfort aroma. Cut off a 1-inch piece of ribbon and attach it to the mattress or pillow with a diaper pin. **Caution: Ensure that the pin is secure and that a child cannot put the ribbon in his or her mouth.**

2. Steam: Add one to five drops of essential oil to a bowl of steaming water. Place a towel over the patient's head and ask him or her to inhale for 10 minutes. Remember to ask the patient to close his or her eyes and remove spectacles. Because soft contact lenses can absorb some of the essential oil and cause stinging, it is a good idea to remove lenses before steam inhalation. **Caution: Avoid this procedure with the elderly, confused, very young, or infirm.**

3. Hood: The hood is a new method of delivery, initially designed for a laboratory experiments, that uses a controlled and measured supply of essential oil and involves a stream of vaporized aroma combined with air and pumped at a constant rate into an oxygen-therapy hood (Palmer et al 1999).

Indirect Inhalation

1. Room fresheners: Add one to five drops of essential oil to a bowl of hot water and place in a safe space. The warmth of the water gradually allows the essential oils to evaporate with the water. This is excellent in air-conditioned facilities where the atmosphere may be dry.

2. Burners: Burners usually have a small candle that heats a container suspended above. Float one to five drops of essential oil on top of water in the container. The water stops the essential oil from burning and leaving a yellow, sticky residue. **Caution: Keep away from children and pets.**

3. Fans: Fans can be battery or electrically operated and come with a number of small, absorbent pads. Add one to five drops to the pad, place in the fan, and switch on. Inexpensive spare pads can be made by cutting incontinence pads or pantyliners into the correct small, square size.

4. Humidifiers: Humidifiers can be purchased in most drug stores. Fill the container with water. Place essential oils on a tissue and put the tissue in the direct pathway of the exiting steam. Do not float the essential oil on top of the water inside the humidifier because it will not come out with the steam, but will remain floating on the water. This is an excellent method for treating croup and asthma.

5. Diffusers: Diffusers can be multifaceted, with different compartments timed for different hours, or a more simple apparatus. Gentle heat causes the essential oil to evaporate.

6. Nebulizers: Nebulizers are electrical units with small, glass attachments into which drops of undiluted essential oil are placed. Microdroplets of the essential oil are atomized into the air, often at timed intervals, ionizing the air. Most nebulizers use no heat. They can be expensive and fragile, but they are most effective for large areas. **Caution: Avoid overdosing with essential oils.**

7. Spritzer sprays (essential oils in water): Sprays are excellent for hot flashes or fatigue. **Caution: Avoid spraying on plants or flowers by mistake.**

Benefits of Inhalation: Inhalation is effective for both physical and psychologic complaints. It is a simple method, is fast acting, and is empowering for the patient. Inhaled essential oils can be particularly useful for treating the following:

Upper and lower respiratory tract infections

Hay fever, sinusitis, and headache

Asthma

People who cannot be touched, for physical or psychologic reasons

Prevention of cross-infection

Depression or fatigue

Insomnia

Finally, the nose, as well as governing the smell system, contains a touch system, which is often (wrongly) thought to be part of the smell system. This touch system is the trigeminal system and forms part of the fifth cranial nerve. It can detect aggressive odors such as acetic acid and ammonia and causes the head-swiveling reflex (Van Toller & Dodd 1991).

REFERENCES

Alexander M. 2001. How Aromatherapy Works: Vol. I, Principle Mechanisms in Olfaction. Odessa, FL: Whole Spectrum Arts and Publications.

Anthony C, Thibodeau G. 1983. Nervous System Cells in Anatomy and Physiology. St. Louis: Mosby.

Associated Press. 1998. Scientists see vaccinations without sting. New York Times. Feb 26 A15.

Balacs T. 1993. Essential oils in the body. In Aroma 93 Conference Proceedings. Brighton, UK: Aromatherapy Publications, 12-20.

Bardia P, Boecker M, Lammers W. 1990. Some effects of different olfactory stimuli on sleep. Sleep Research. 19, 145.

Bartoshuk L, Beauchamp G. 1994. Chemical senses. Annual Review of Psychology. 45 419-449.

Betts T. 1996. The fragrant breeze: The role of aromatherapy in treating epilepsy. Aromatherapy Quarterly. 51(Winter) 25-27.

Birchall A. 1990. A whiff of happiness. New Scientist. 25(August) 44-47.

Brinker F. 2000. The Toxicology of Botanical Medicines, 3rd ed. Sandy, OR: Eclectic Medical Publications.

Bowles J. 2000. The Basic Chemistry of Aromatherapeutic Essential Oils. Sydney, Australia: Pirie Printers.

Bronaugh R. 1990. In vivo percutaneous absorption of fragrance ingredients in rhesus monkeys and humans. Food and Chemical Toxicology. 28(5) 369-373.

Buchbauer G. 1993. Molecular interaction. International Journal of Aromatherapy. 5(1) 11-14.

Buchbauer G. 1993a. Biological effects of fragrances and essential oils. Perfumer and Flavorist. 18(19) 19-24.

Buckle J. 2001. The ethic of plant v petrochemical medicine. International Journal of Aromatherapy. 11(1) 8-17.

Chadwick J, Mann W (eds.). 1983. Hippocratic Writings. Harmondsworth, UK: Penguin Books.

Chopra D. 1991. Perfect Health: The Complete Mind/Body Guide. New York: Harmony Books.

Cleary G. 1993. Transdermal drug delivery. In Zatz J (ed.), Skin Permeation: Fundamentals and Applications. Wheaton, IL: Allured Publishing, 207-238.

Cook C (ed). 1978. Pears Cyclopedia, 87th ed. London: Pelham, B19.

Dabney V. 1913. Connections of the sexual apparatus with the ear, nose and throat. New York Journal of Medicine. 97, 533.

Diamond M, Schreibel B, Elson L. 1985. The Human Brain Coloring Book. New York: Harper.

Edelson S. 2001. Autism and the limbic system. Retrieved January 2002 from http://www.autism.org.

Epstein R. 2001. For some, insulin without needles. New York Times. July 17, F5.

Erichsen-Brown C. 1979. Medicinal and Other Uses of North American Plants. New York: Dover Publications.

Fessler D. 1996. No Time For Fear: Voices of American Military Nurses in World War II. Lansing, MI: Michigan State University Press.

Franchomme P, Penoel D. 1990. Phytoguide: Aromatherapy Advanced Therapy for Infectious Illnesses. International Phytomedical Foundation. Limoges, France: Jollois.

Fuchs N, Jager W, Lenhardt A et al. 1997. Systemic absorption of topically applied carvone: Influence of massage technique. Journal of the Society of Cosmetic Chemists. 48(6) 277-282.

Garg A, Chren M, Sands L et al. 2001. Psychological stress perturbs the epidermal permeability barrier homeostasis. Archives of Dermatology. 137(1) 53-59.

Gattefosse R. 1937. (Translated in 1993 by R. Tisserand.) Aromatherapie: Les Huile Essentielles-Hormones Vegetales (Gattefosse's Aromatherapy.) Saffron Walden, UK: CW Daniels, 89.

Gatti G, Cajola R. 1923. L'Azione delle essenze sul sistema nervosa. Rivista Italiana delle Essenze e Profumi. 5, 133-135.

Gilt A. 1992. Aromatherapy 2000 and beyond. Journal of Alternative and Complementary Medicine. 9, 19-20.

Griggs B. 1981. Green Pharmacy. London: Jill Norman & Hobhouse.

Guirdham A. 1990. The Cathars and Reincarnation. Saffron Walden, UK: CW Daniels.

Healing Arts. 2001. Medial temporal lobe (the limbic system). Retrieved January 2002 from http://www.healing-arts.org.

Holmes P. 1993. The Energetics of Western Herbs, Vols. 1 and 2. Berkley, CA: Nattrop Publishing.

Hotchkiss S. 1994. How thin is your skin? New Scientist. Jan 29, 24-27.

Jackson E. 1993. Toxicological aspects of percutaneous absorption. In Zatz J (ed.), Skin Permeation: Fundamentals and Applications. Wheaton, IL: Allured Publishing, 177-193.

Jager W, Buchbauer G, Jirovetz L et al. 1992. Percutaneous absorption of lavender oil from a massage oil. Journal of the Society of Cosmetic Chemists. 43(1) 49-54.

Jori A, Bianchelli A, Prestini P. 1969. Effects of essential oils on drug metabolism. Biochemical Pharmacology. 18(9) 2081-2095.

Kirk-Smith M. 1993. Human olfactory communication. In Aroma 93 Conference Proceedings. Brighton, UK: Aromatherapy Publications, 86-103.

Komori T, Fujiwara R, Tanida M et al. 1995. Effects of citrus fragrance on immune function and depressive states. Neuroimmunomodulation. 2:174-180.

Kusmerik J. 1992. Aromatherapy for the Family. London: Institute of Classical Aromatherapy, Wigmore Publications.

Lawless J. 1992. The Encyclopedia of Essential Oils. Shaftesbury, UK: Element Books.

Lawless J. 1994. Aromatherapy and the Mind. London: Thorsons.

LeDoux J. 1996. The Emotional Brain. New York: Simon & Schuster, 170, 264.

LeRoy Ladurie E. Bray B, translator. 1984. Montaillou. London: Penguin Books.

Levabre M. 1990. Aromatherapy Workbook. Vermont: Healing Arts Press.

Lorig T, Herman K, Schwartz G et al. 1990. EEG activity during administration of low concentration odors. Bulletin of the Psychonomic Society. 28, 405-408.

Low Dog T, Riley D. 2001. An integrative approach to menopause. Alternative Therapies in Health and Medicine. 7(4) 45-55.

Maury M. Ryman D, translator. 1964. Le Capital Jeunesse (The Secrets of Life and Youth). London: Macdonald.

McFerran T (ed.). 1996. A Dictionary of Nursing, 2nd ed. Oxford UK: Oxford University Press.

Mills S. 1991. Out of the Earth. London: Viking Arkana.

Moore M, Meredith P, Watson W et al.1980. The percutaneous absorption of lead-203 in humans from cosmetic preparations containing lead acetate, as assessed by whole-body counting and other techniques. Cosmetic Toxiocology. 18:399-405.

Mojay G. 1996. Aromatherapy for Healing the Spirit. London: Giai Books, Ltd.

Oxford Dictionaries. 1964. Concise English Dictionary. Oxford, UK: Oxford University Press.

Palmer B, Stough C, Patterson J. 1999. A delivery system for olfactory stimuli. Behavior Research Methods, Instruments, & Computers. 31(4) 674-678.

Pert C. 1997. Molecules of Emotion. New York: Scribner, 304.

Pratt J, Mason A. 1981. The Caring Touch. London: Heyden.

Price S, Price L. 1999. Aromatherapy for Health Professionals. London: Churchill Livingstone, 93.

Proust M. 1981. Remembrance of Things Past, Vol 1. New York: Random House.

Reiger M. 1993. Factors affecting sorption of topically applied substances. In Zatz J (ed.), Skin Permeation: Fundamentals and Applications. Wheaton, IL: Allured Publishing, 33-72.

Riviere J. 1993. Biological factors in absorption and permeation. In Zatz J (ed.), Skin Permeation: Fundamentals and Applications. Wheaton, IL: Allured Publishing, 113-125.

Rose J. 1992. The Aromatherapy Book. San Francisco: North Atlantic Books.

Rose J. 1992a. A history of herbs and herbalism. In Tierra M (ed.), American Herbalism. Freedom, CA: Crossing Press, 3-32.

Rovesti P, Columbo E. 1973. Aromatherapy and aerosols. Soaps, Perfumery and Cosmetics. 46:475-477.

Ryman D. 1991. Aromatherapy. London: Piatkus.

Sarnecky M. 2001. Nurses at Pearl Harbor: the real story. Reflections of Nursing Leadership. 17-20, 51.

Schultz N. 2002. Personal communication.

Scott C. 1993-1994. In profile with Valnet. International Journal of Aromatherapy. 5(4) 10-13.

Sherman R, Leech R. 1973. Neuropathology in newborn infants bathed in hexachlorophene. Morbidity and Mortality. 22, 93.

Singewald N, Kaehler S, Sinner C et al. 2000. Serotonin and amino acid release in the locus coeruleus by conditioned fear and inescapable shock. 6th Internet World Congress for Biomedical Sciences. Presentation #27.

Stearn W. 1998. Botanical Latin, 4th ed. Portland, OR: Timber Press.

Steele J. 1992. Anthropology of smell and scent in fragrance. In Van Toller S, Dodd G (eds.), Fragrance: The Psychology and Biology of Perfume. London: Elsevier Applied Science, 287-302.

Stoddart D. 1990. The Scented Ape. Cambridge, UK: Cambridge University Press, 5.

Suzuki M, Asaba K, Komatsu H et al. 1978. Autoradiographic study on percutaneous absorption of oils useful in cosmetics. Journal of Society of Cosmetic Chemists. 29, 265-282.

Swerdlow J. 2000. Nature's Medicine: Plants That Heal. Washington, DC: National Geographic Society.

Tisserand R. 1979. The Art of Aromatherapy. Saffron Walden, UK: CW Daniels.

Tisserand R. 1985. The Essential Oil Safety Data Manual. Brighton, UK: Tisserand Aromatherapy Institute.

Tisserand R. 1988. Lavender beats benzodiazepines. International Journal of Aromatherapy. 1(2) 1-2.

Tisserand R. 1993a. Aspects of aromatherapy. In Aroma 93 Conference Proceedings. Brighton, UK: Aromatherapy Publications, 1-9.

Tisserand R, Balacs T. 1995. Essential Oil Safety. London: Churchill Livingstone, 30.

Torii S, Fukuda H, Kanemoto H et al. 1991. Contingent negative variation and the psychological effects of odor. In Van Toller S, Dodd G (eds.), Perfumery: The Psychology and Biology of Fragrance. London: Chapman and Hall, 107-118.

Tschanz D.1997. The Arab Roots of European Medicine. Aramco World. May/June 20-31.

Valnet J. 1937. Aromatherapie: Les huiles essentielles hormones vegetales. Paris: Girardot.

Valnet J.1990. The Practice of Aromatherapy. Saffron Walden, UK: CW Daniels.

Van Toller S, Hotson S, Kendal-Reed M. 1992. The brain and the sense of smell. In Van Toller S, Dodd G (eds.), Fragrance: The Psychology and Biology of Perfume. London: Elsevier Applied Science, 195-217.

Van Toller S, Dodd G. 1991. Preface. In Van Toller S, Dodd G (eds.), Perfumery: The Psychology and Biology of Fragrance. London: Chapman and Hall, xii-xv.

Vellmair D, Byrne M, Hotchkiss S et al. 1998. An experimental study of the dermal penetration of aerosol particles. Journal of Aerosol Sciences. 28(supplement 1) 297-298.

Walter R, Cooper R, Aldridge V et al. 1964. Contingent negative variation: an electric sign of sensorimotor association and expectancy in the human brain. Nature. 203, 380-384.

Watson L. 2000. Jacobson's Organ. New York: Norton.

Watt M. 1991. Plant Aromatics. Witham, UK: Watt.

Watts G. 1975. Dynamic Neuroscience: Its Application to Brain Disorders. New York: Harper and Row.

Weiss S. 1979. The language of touch. Nursing Research. 28, 76-79.

Williams D. 1996. The Chemistry of Essential Oils. Weymouth, Dorset, England: Michelle Press.

Zatz J. 1993. Factors affecting sorption of topically applied substances. In Zatz J (ed.), Skin Permeation: Fundamentals and Applications. Wheaton, IL: Allured Publishing, 11-32.

Zatz J. 1993a. Modification of skin permeation by solvents. In Zatz J (ed.), Skin Permeation: Fundamentals and Applications. Wheaton, IL: Allured Publishing, 127-162.

Zetzer L, Regalado M, Nichter L et al. 1991. Iontophoresis versus subcutaneous injection: a comparison of two methods of local anesthesia delivery in children. Pain. 44(91) 73.

3

BASIC PLANT TAXONOMY, CHEMISTRY, EXTRACTION, BIOSYNTHESIS, AND ANALYSIS

The problem with wonder drugs is that they breed in the public mind a sense that medicine can and always should work miracles, even with benign problems. What gets forgotten is the price we always pay by tampering so totally with Mother Nature

McTaggart (1996)

Learning how and why a plant manufactures an essential oil is relevant to understanding aromatherapy. The way plants make essential oils gives some insight into their complexity. Traditionally, biochemists have studied primary metabolism and organic chemists have studied secondary metabolism. In aromatherapy, it is of interest to have an overall picture of both metabolic processes. Why some plants make essential oils is the subject of ongoing scientific debate and is relevant to the therapeutic potential of the essential oil in humans.

The process of extraction clarifies the need for unadulterated essential oils. Unadulterated essential oils are required for clinical use, and the process of steam distillation or expression can produce an essential oil with no residue. However, there are new and exciting methods of obtaining extracts that may become part of aromatherapy in the future. How essential oils are absorbed into the body is a subject of heated discussion and is a topic I attempt to cover. There is no doubt that new evidence will emerge after this book is published.

I am very appreciative of the help and advice given by the expert reviewers of this section: James Duke, PhD; Howard Freund, PhD; Bob and Rhi Harris; Tom Numark; Keith Shawe, PhD; and Neal Schultz, MD. I am also appreciative of the published work of John Mann, PhD.

Part I: Basic Plant Taxonomy and Chemistry

The lovesick, the betrayed and the jealous all smell alike.

Colette

The Latin names of plants can seem a bit intimidating initially, but they are the best way to be sure of what is in that bottle of essential oil, and they are recognized the world over, from China to Peru. Latin has been used for thousands of years in botany and was first used in this context by Pliny in 23 AD. However, it was Carl Linnaeus (1707-1778) who established the basis for naming plants in Latin (Stearn 1998).

A plant only has one Latin name, but it may have many common names, and those common names may also be used for completely different plants. Take for example bergamot. In aromatherapy, bergamot refers to the oil extracted from the peel of the citrus fruit, *Citrus bergamia*. This should not be confused with the medicinal plant *Monarda didyma*, which is also known as bergamot. Similarly, the word *geranium* refers to the species *geranium* for gardeners, but in the world of aromatherapy it refers to *Pelargonium graveolens*.

Every plant has a unique name in Latin composed of two words. The first word is the name of the genus, and the second is the name of the species—rather like our first name and surname. Classification of plants is called *taxonomy*. All plants can be grouped into categories. For plants to be properly identified they are divided into division, class, order, family, genus, and species. This process takes into account the number, shape, and position of leaves on the stem; the shape and position of the flowers; the number and shape of the petals; whether the plant is hairy, prickly, or smooth; whether the stem is ridged; and so on.

Life on earth began about 4 billion years ago with a single-celled organism that did not have a nucleus. Many of these basic organisms, including algae and bacteria, are still living in our world today. Through gradual evolution a vast range of aromatic plants evolved that presently produces 30,000 known volatile oils (Elpel 1998).

Lavender

Lavender belongs to a plant family called Lamiaceae or Labiatae: the mint family. This family includes many species used in aromatherapy. Plants in this family usually have five united petals with two lobes on the top and three on the bottom forming lips (labia). The leaves are usually directly opposite each other on the stem, and often the stem is square. The Latin name for the lavender genus is *Lavandula*. The most commonly used lavender is a hybrid, *lavandin*, which is a widely used cross between two *Lavandula* species: *L. angustifolia* and *L. latifolia*.

There is also another species of lavender, *L. stoechas,* which can be used clinically. See Table 3-1. However, as frequently happens in the plant kingdom, two of the species also have other names. *Lavandula angustifolia* is sometimes called *L. vera* or *L. officinalis,* although the correct name is *L. angustifolia* (Lawrence 1989). This plant also has several common names: English lavender, French lavender, and true lavender. *Lavandula latifolia* is sometimes called *L. spica,* and its common name is spike lavender or spike. Spike is completely different from spikenard *(Nardostachys jatamansi),* which is closely related to valerian and belongs to the family Valerianaceae.

Lavandula angustifolia and Lavandula latifolia were listed in the *British Pharmacopoeia* and supplied to hospitals in vats labeled simply "lavender." However, the two plants have very different therapeutic properties. *L. angustifolia* is a sedative, relaxant, and hypotensor. *L. latifolia* is a stimulant and expectorant.

CHAMOMILE

Chamomile can cause confusion to the newcomer, too. There are three main types of chamomile used in aromatherapy: German, Roman, and Moroccan (Table 3-2). They are quite different and produce different-colored essential oils that

Table 3-1 🐦 *Lavenders and Some of Their Properties*

Latin Name	Common Name	Properties
Lavandula angustifolia *Lavandula vera* *Lavandula officinalis*	True lavender	Calming, sedative, good for burns, analgesic, antibacterial, immune-system enhancer
Lavandula latifolia *Lavandula spica*	Spike lavender	Expectorant, mycolytic, possible stimulant
Lavandula stoechas	Stoechas	Useful against Pseudomonas spp., high in ketones

Table 3-2 🐦 *Chamomiles and Some of Their Properties*

Latin Name	Common Name	Properties
Matricaria recutita	German chamomile	Dark blue, useful for skin complaints and inflammation
Chamaemelum nobile	Roman chamomile	Pale blue or yellow, sedative, useful for spasms
Ormenis mixta	Moroccan chamomile	Mainly used by perfume industry, some antibacterial activity

have different properties, but they all belong to the same family: Asteraceae or Compositae—the daisy family.

German chamomile *(Matricaria recutita)* is a smoky smelling, dark-blue oil that contains chamazulene. The oil's color depends directly on the amount of chamazulene present and the method of extraction. It should be noted that chamazulene is not present in the fresh flower (or in its CO_2 extract) but is produced during distillation (Lawless 1992). It is possible to obtain a green or yellow German chamomile oil that has less than 3% chamazulene, but the dark-blue variety always has more than 7% (Svab & Sarkany 1975). The price of German chamomile oil is usually related to the amount of chamazulene it contains.

Chamazulene is an antiinflammatory with a history of use in the treatment of skin problems (Jakovlev et al 1983). German chamomile also contains a second antiinflammatory compound called alpha-bisabolol, which is a monoterpenol (Carle & Gomaa 1992). In addition, this species has antibiotic properties and is effective against *Staphylococcus aureus*, hemolytic *Streptococcus*, and *Proteus vulgaris*. Valnet, a French MD, claims that wound infections bathed with a solution of 1 part German chamomile in 100,000 parts water have been healed (Valnet 1990). German chamomile is also thought to "stimulate liver regeneration and subcutaneous treatments will initiate formation of new liver tissue"(Rose 1992). CO_2-extracted German chamomile is brown and almost solid at room temperature. It smells of sweet apples with an earthy undertone.

Roman chamomile *(Chamaemelum nobile)* is a colorless to pale blue oil that turns yellow with storage. Listed in the *British Herbal Pharmacopoeia*, it contains up to 80% esters. Esters have antispasmodic properties, and essential oil of Roman chamomile is traditionally used as an antispasmodic and relaxant whereas the herb is used as a carminative. Roman chamomile also has mild antiinflammatory properties (Franchomme & Penoel 1990), particularly if the oil is collected from white-headed flowers instead of the classic yellow-headed flowers (Rossi et al 1988).

Moroccan chamomile *(Ormenis multicaulis or O. mixta)* is a relative newcomer to the aromatherapy field and is mainly used in the perfume industry. Little is known about its clinical effects. In all respects it is different from the other chamomiles and cannot be regarded as a substitute for either of them.

DIFFERENT PARTS

Occasionally, different parts of the same plant can produce different essential oils. In the case of the bitter orange plant (*Citrus x aurantium* var. *amara*), three different types of essential oils can be obtained: Petitgrain from the stems and leaves, Neroli from the petals, and bitter orange from the fruit. Neroli and petitgrain-type essential oils can also be obtained from other citrus species. Bergamot essential oil is obtained from the rind of a fruit that is a subspecies of the bittersweet orange. The shorthand for *Citrus aurantium* subspp. *bergamia* (bergamot) is *Citrus bergamia* (Guenther 1976).

Sometimes just the part of the plant is listed (for example, cinnamon bark or cinnamon leaf). Cinnamon bark contains approximately 50% eugenol (a phenol). Cinnamon leaf contains 80 to 96% eugenol. Eugenol is strongly antimicrobial; it can inhibit bacterial growth on food for 30 days (Moleyar & Narasimham 1992). However, it is also dermacaustic and can dissolve metal, false teeth, and pearls (Ryman 1991). Small amounts of cinnamon bark and cinnamon leaf are used by the fragrance and pharmaceutical industries. Cinnamon is also one of the flavorants of Coca-Cola (Lawless 1992).

CLONES AND CHEMOTYPES

To complicate the situation still further, some plants have been cloned or cultivated to produce different chemotypes (Table 3-3). This means the essential oil has a specific chemical profile that might make it more suitable for treating a particular ailment or safer to use. Common thyme *(Thymus vulgaris)* has several chemotypes: linalol, geraniol, a-terpineol, thujanol-4, carvacrol, and thymol (Vernet & Gouyon 1976). The first four are all safe to use on the skin, because they are high in alcohols. However, thymol and carvacrol are phenols and can cause skin irritation. Red thyme, which commonly grows in garden lawns, is a phenol type.

Tea tree, eucalyptus, rosemary, and German chamomile are other essential oils that have commercial chemotypes. Chemotypes will become more common as aromatic plants are grown on a more global level as cash crops (Franz 1993).

Table 3-3 ✖ *Some Examples of Essential Oil Chemotypes*

Latin Name	Chemical Constituents	Research Paper
Achillea millifolium	Caryophyllene, farnasene, azulene-free	Hethelyi et al 1988 Oswiecimska 1974
Artemesia dracunculus	Methyl chavicol, sabinene	Tucker & Maciarello 1987
Ocimum basilicum	Linalool, methyl chavicol, eugenol	Sobti et al 1978
Matricaria recutita	Bisabolone oxide, bisabolol, chamazulene, chamazulene-free	Frantz 1993
Salvia officinalis	α- & β-thujone, cineole, thujone-free	Tucker & Maciarello 1990

CHEMISTRY OF ESSENTIAL OILS*

The chemical components that make up essential oils are produced during the second stage of biosynthesis and are called secondary metabolites (Fig. 3-1). Terpenes make up the largest group of secondary metabolites with some 1000 monoterpenes and 3000 sesquiterpenes known (Harborne 1988). However, the

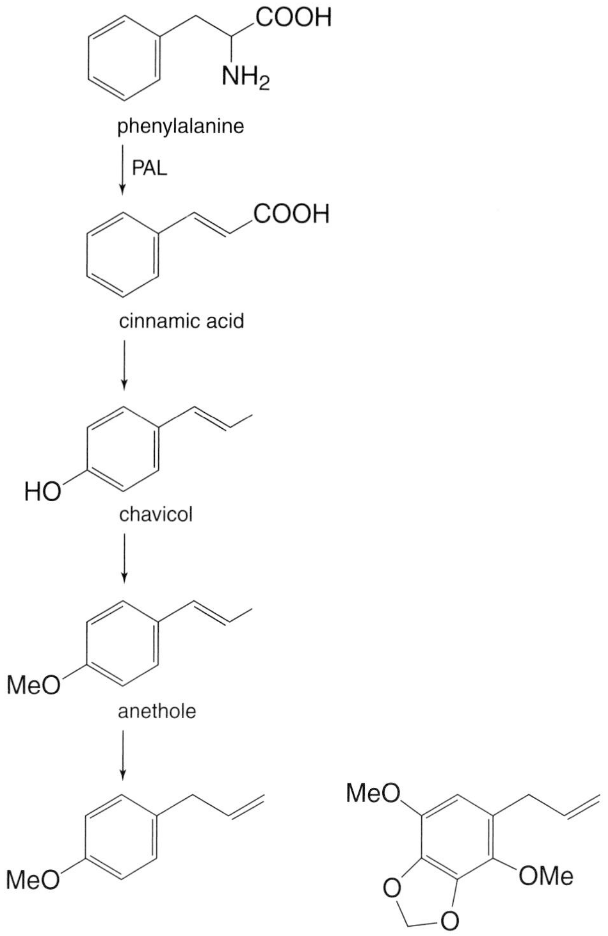

FIGURE 3-1   Biosynthesis of phenylpropanes.   (Adapted from Waterman P. 1993. The Chemistry of volatile oils. In Hay R, Waterman P (eds.), Volatile Oil Crops: Their Biology, Biochemistry and Production. Essex, UK: Longman Scientific and Technical, 47-61.)

*I was greatly helped with revising this section by the following books: *The Chemistry of Essential Oils* (Williams 1996), *The Basic Chemistry of Aromatherapeutic Essential Oils* (Bowles 2000), and *Volatile Oil Crops* (Hay & Waterman 1993). These books are highly recommended for additional reading.

number of phenylpropanes (which contain benzene rings) is much smaller—approximately 50. Terpenes arise from the mevalonic pathway. Phenylpropanes come from the shikimic pathway.

Mevalonic Pathway

This pathway depends on mevalonic acid, a chemical intermediate containing six carbon atoms made by the plant and vital to its life (Waterman 1993). The plant converts mevalonic acid to a 5-carbon structure (with the isoprene arrangement) typical of all terpenes. This is then converted to geranyl pyrophosphate (GPP)—the first recognizable 10-carbon molecule. This process can continue with another enzyme catalyst to result in the first 15-carbon molecule, sesquiterpene compound, farnesyl pyrophosphate (FPP). Once the plant has formed GPP, the substance can be converted into alcohols or aldehydes.

Shikimic Pathway

This pathway utilizes an enzyme called phenylalanine ammonia lyase (PAL) to produce phenolic compounds that include benzene rings (Waterman 1993). This pathway also produces alkaloids such as morphine.

Terpenes, Isoprene Units

Terpenes make up the largest single class of compounds, although phenylpropenes tend to have the largest impact on the aroma (Waterman 1993). Terpenes found in essential oils are made up of the isoprene units (building blocks) referred to previously. Each isoprene unit contains 5 carbon atoms, and some people believe the shape resembles the skeletal profile of a dog in flight (Table 3-4) (Williams 1996). One of the carbon atoms is attached by a double bond. Monoterpenes have two isoprene units, sesquiterpenes have three, and diterpenes have four. Because each isoprene unit has five carbon atoms, it is simple math to work out the number of carbon atoms per molecule (Table 3-5).

Monoterpenes make up the largest number of terpenes and can be subdivided into groups that indicate their structure. All terpenes end in -*ene*. They are light molecules and evaporate quickly. Monoterpenes are often referred to as top notes. They oxidize easily and combine with oxygen over time to become alcohols.

In aromatherapy, the term *terpenoid* is given to terpene molecules that include oxygen (Tisserand & Balacs 1995). Terpenoid is not a chemical term in a

Table 3-4 ✖ *Structure of Terpenes*

Molecular Structure	Name	Chemical Constituent
Chain, no ring	acyclic	α-myrcene
One ring	cyclic	Δ-limonene
Two rings	bicyclic	

Table 3-5 ⚘ *Number of Carbon Atoms in Terpenes*

Chemical Constituent	Number of Isoprene Units	Number of Carbon Atoms
Monoterpene	2 isoprene units	10 carbon atoms
Sesquiterpene	3 isoprene units	15 carbon atoms
Diterpene	4 isoprene units	20 carbon atoms

strict sense, but it can be useful to distinguish between molecules that do not have oxygen and those that do. All terpenes have antiseptic properties (Table 3-6). Camphene, phellandrene, pinene, myrcene, and limonene are common examples of monoterpenes. Limonene is thought to be antitumoral (Zheng et al 1992; Gould 1997) and occurs in most citrus oils and in dill *(Anethum graveolens)*. Myrcene, found in lemongrass *(Cymbopogon citratus)*, has analgesic properties (Lorenzetti et al 1991)). Monoterpenes in general have a stimulating effect, but they can become skin-sensitizing if used over time. Because they are insoluble in water, the perfume industry frequently removes terpenes from an essential oil so the oil can be used in toilet water. In this case the essential oil is said to be "terpeneless" (Guenther 1972).

Sesquiterpenes are less volatile but because they are larger structures, they have a greater potential for stereochemical diversity (Waterman 1993). Sesquiterpenes have stronger odors, are antiinflammatory and have bactericidal properties (Table 3-7). As terpenes, they still oxidize over time into alcohols. In patchouli

Table 3-6 ⚘ *Some Terpenes and Their Properties*

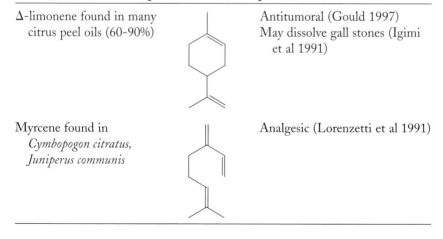

Δ-limonene found in many citrus peel oils (60-90%)

Antitumoral (Gould 1997)
May dissolve gall stones (Igimi et al 1991)

Myrcene found in *Cymbopogon citratus, Juniperus communis*

Analgesic (Lorenzetti et al 1991)

Table 3-7 🦋 *Some Sesquiterpenes and Their Properties*

Chamazulene found in *Matricaria recutita*	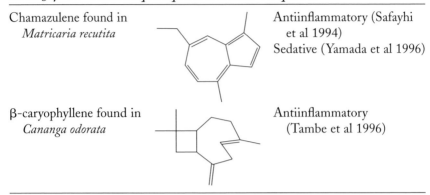	Antiinflammatory (Safayhi et al 1994) Sedative (Yamada et al 1996)
β-caryophyllene found in *Cananga odorata*		Antiinflammatory (Tambe et al 1996)

oil this oxidation is thought to improve the odor. Chamazulene actually has 14 carbon atoms but is often included with sesquiterpenes. Chamazulene and caryophyllene have antitumor activity (Mills 1991). Chamazulene is found in German chamomile, bisabolene is found in black pepper, and caryophyllene is found in ylang ylang *(Cananga odorata).*

The very few diterpenes found in essential oils tend to oxidize into alcohols. This process produces sclareol in clary sage and viridiflorol in niaouli. However, diterpenes may occur in solvent extracts. Taxol is a diterpene (Lewinsohn 2001).

Alcohols

Terpenic alcohols are found in many essential oils. Their names all end in *-ol.* Structurally, they have a hydroxyl group attached to one of their carbon atoms (Table 3-8). Monoterpenic alcohols (monoterpenols) are thought to be good antiseptics with some antibacterial and antifungal properties. Isoborneol inhibits the herpes virus (Armaka et al 1999). Some alcohols, such as terpinen-4-ol, are uplifting; others like linalool are thought to be sedatives. Usually essential oils with a high percentage of monoterpenols are safe to use undiluted on the skin. Examples include geraniol in palmarosa *(Cymbopogon martini)* and citronellol in *Eucalyptus citriodora* (Lewis Walter & Elvin-Lewis Memory 1977). Isoborneol has antiviral properties and is a potent inhibitor of herpes simplex virus type (Amarka et al. 1999). Perillyl alcohol has been shown to regress pancreatic, mammary, and liver tumors in animal studies and to revert tumor cells to a differentiated state (Belanger 1998). However, in human studies, oral doses did not regress these tumors. There have been no studies to date on topically applied or inhaled perillyl alcohol that I could find.

Sesquiterpenols have 15 carbon atoms and a variety of therapeutic effects (Table 3-9). When α-eudesmol was injected directly into the spinal cords of rats, it significantly reduced edematous effusion following brain injury (Asakura et al

Table 3-8 ❧ *Some Alcohols and Their Properties*

Linalool in *Lavandula angustifolia*		Sedative (Buchbauer et al 1991; Re et al 2000) Antispasmodic (Lis-Balchin & Hart 1999)
Geraniol in *Cymbopogon martini*		Antifungal (Carson & Riley 1995) Potentiates antiherpetic activity of SON (Shoji et al 1998)
Terpinen-4-ol in *Melaleuca alternifolia*		Effective against *Pseudomonas aeruginosa* (Budhiraja et al 1999; Jedlickova et al 1992)

Table 3-9 ❧ *Some Sesquiterpenols and Their Properties*

Farnesol found in		Effective against *Trichomonas vaginalis* (Viollon et al 1996) Hypotensor (Luft et al 1999)
α-bisabolol found in *Matricaria recutita*		Antiinflammatory (Jakovlev et al 1979)
Patchoulol found in *patchouli cablin*		Effective against bacteria that cause foot odor (Yang et al 1996)

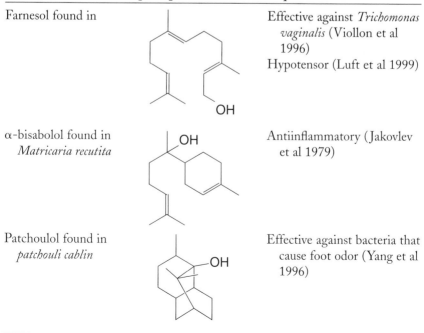

2000). It also appeared to reduce potassium- and electric shock-induced seizures (Chio et al 1997). The anticonvulsant properties of α-eudesmol were compared to phenobarbitone in another study by Santos et al (1997). α-eudesmol is found in West Indian Sandalwood *(Amyris balsamifera)* and *Psidium guyanensis.*

Nerolidol, found in *Melaleuca quinquenervia* (a special chemotype of niaouli), completely inhibited development of the malaria-bearing mosquito (Lopez et al 1999). The Amazonian Waiapi tribe treat malaria by inhaling the essential oil from the leaf of *Virola surinamensis* (a rainforest tree that contains nerolidol). Santalol found in sandalwood is an effective antiviral agent against early-stage cold sores (Benencia & Courreges 1999) and was also found to work as a sedative in mice (Okegawa et al 1995). Sclareol kills tumor cells in vitro (Dimas et al 1999) and is used extensively for ambergris fragrance (Bauer et al 1990).

Phenols

A phenol is a hydroxyl group attached to a benzene ring (Table 3-10). Like alcohols, phenol names end in *-ol,* but this is where the similarity ends. There are only four common phenols found in essential oils: thymol, carvacrol, eugenol, and chavicol. There are two ethers from phenols: one from eugenol and one from

Table 3-10   *Some Phenols and Their Properties*

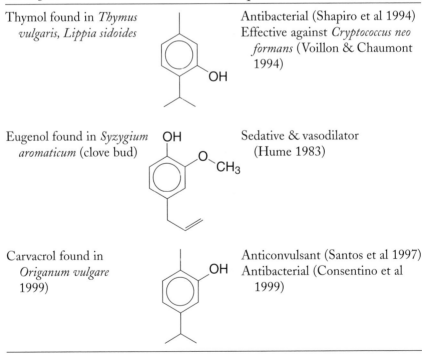

Thymol found in *Thymus vulgaris, Lippia sidoides*		Antibacterial (Shapiro et al 1994) Effective against *Cryptococcus neo formans* (Voillon & Chaumont 1994)
Eugenol found in *Syzygium aromaticum* (clove bud)		Sedative & vasodilator (Hume 1983)
Carvacrol found in *Origanum vulgare* 1999)		Anticonvulsant (Santos et al 1997) Antibacterial (Consentino et al 1999)

chavicol. Benzene (aromatic) rings can easily be formed from aliphatic (nonbenzene) rings, but the reverse reaction rarely occurs (Guenther 1972). Phenols need to be treated with care because many of them are skin irritants. Most have very strong antibacterial properties, and some have a stimulatory effect on both the nervous system and the immune system. Thymol (from *Thymus vulgaris*) also has anthelmintic properties. Eugenol is a powerful antiinflammatory (Sharma et al 1994) and decreases gut motility in diarrhea. It also inhibits prostaglandin synthesis (Bennett et al 1988).

Aldehydes

An aldehyde has an oxygen atom double bonded to a carbon atom at the end of a carbon chain (Table 3-11). The fourth bond is always a hydrogen atom (Bowles 2000). Aldehydes usually end in *-al* and often have sedative, calming effects, as well as being important to the aroma of the plant. Examples include citral in lemon balm *(Melissa officinalis)*, citronellal in lemongrass *(Cymbopogon citratus)*, geranial in lemon eucalyptus *(Eucalyptus citriodora)*, and neral in lemon verbena *(Aloysia triphylla)*. Geranial and neral are isomers, meaning they have the same molecular make-up but the carboxyl molecule is in a different place. For a long time they were thought to be so similar they were combined and called citral.

Table 3-11 ❦ *Some Aldehydes and Their Properties*

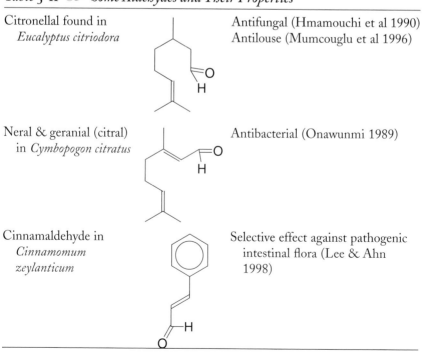

Citronellal found in *Eucalyptus citriodora*	Antifungal (Hmamouchi et al 1990) Antilouse (Mumcouglu et al 1996)
Neral & geranial (citral) in *Cymbopogon citratus*	Antibacterial (Onawunmi 1989)
Cinnamaldehyde in *Cinnamomum zeylanticum*	Selective effect against pathogenic intestinal flora (Lee & Ahn 1998)

Citral has strong antiseptic and antibacterial properties (Onawunmi & Oguniana 1981). Citronellal possesses antifungal properties (Hmamouchi et al 1990).

Esters

Esters are a combination of an acid and an alcohol and take their name from the acid and alcohol (Table 3-12). Hence, acetic acid and linalool produce Linalyl acetate. Acids do not occur in essential oils but can be found in floral waters. Esters end in *-ate*, and have antispasmodic and calming properties. Some are also antifungal. They often smell very fruity. Examples include Linalyl acetate found in lavender *(Lavandula angustifolia)*, clary sage *(Salvia sclarea)*, bergamot *(Citrus aurantium subsp. bergamia)*, and genaryl acetate found in sweet marjoram *(Origanum majorana)*. One essential oil with a very high ester content (85%) is Roman chamomile *(Chamaemelum/Anthemis nobilis)*, which includes angelic and tiglic esters (Bauer et al 1990).

Ketones

A ketone is derived from an alcohol by oxygenation and has an oxygen atom double bonded to a carbon atom, which is also bonded to two other carbon atoms (Table 3-13) (Bowles 2000). Ketones end in *-one* with a single exception: camphor. This substance has no relation to the plant camphor. Ketones should always be treated with respect because certain ketones can produce convulsant effects (usually when taken orally). Because ketones are resistant to metabolism, they can build up in the liver. An easy way to remember that they are a potential problem is to think of ketosis. Potentially toxic ketones include d-pulegone (found in pennyroyal), which caused the death of a 23-year-old woman in 1897. It must be stressed that this lady did drink a tablespoonful (15 ml) of undiluted essential oil (Allen 1897). Pennyroyal tea caused the death of two infants. A child who

Table 3-12 ✖ *Some Esters and Their Properties*

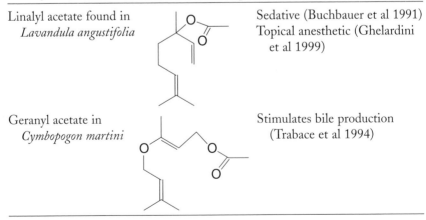

Linalyl acetate found in *Lavandula angustifolia*		Sedative (Buchbauer et al 1991) Topical anesthetic (Ghelardini et al 1999)
Geranyl acetate in *Cymbopogon martini*		Stimulates bile production (Trabace et al 1994)

Table 3-13 & *A Ketone and Its Properties*

Menthone in *Mentha piperita*		Inhibition of platelet aggregation in decompression sickness (Murauama & Kumaroo 1986)

developed hepatic malfunction and presented with severe epileptic encephalopathy was tested for pulegone; results were positive (Bakerink et al 1996). Once again large amounts of the essential oil had been ingested.

There are some nontoxic ketones. Most of these are good for the skin and for scars, a view supported by Lavabre (1990). Safe ketones include jasmone in jasmine *(Jasminum officinale)* (International School of Aromatherapy 1993), fenchone in fennel *(Foeniculum vulgare var. dulce)*, and isomenthone in geranium *(Pelargonium graveolens)*. A special diketone found in everlasting *(Helicrysum italicum)* has antihematoma properties and reduces contusions with great speed.

Oxides

Oxides in organic chemistry typically involve an oxygen bridge between two neighboring carbon atoms (Table 3-14). The use of the term *oxide* in aromatherapy is a little more general because the carbons are not neighbors. In chemical terminology, an oxide is called an ether or a peroxide. However, the term *ether* might be confusing because there is another group of phenolic ethers that have different properties. An oxide has an oxygen atom in a chain of carbons, which forms a ring (but not a benzene ring). The most common oxide is cineole—a strong expectorant. Both 1,4-cineole and 1,8-cineole occur in essential oils (Tisserand & Balacs 1995). Sometimes called eucalyptol, 1,8-cineole is found in blue gum *(Eucalyptus globulus)*, rosemary *(Rosmarinus officinalis CT cineole)*, and bay laurel *(Lauris nobilis)*. Other oxides are ascaridole found in wormseed *(Chenopodium ambrosioides var. anthelminticum)* and rose oxide found in geranium *(Pelargonium graveolens)* and rose *(Rosa damascena)*. The freshly baked smell

Table 3-14 & *An Oxide and Its Properties*

1,8 cineole found in *Eucalyptus globulus*		Antiinflammatory (Juergens et al 1998) Enhances pentobarbitol effects (Santos & Rao 2000) Expectorant (Duke 1992)

that wafts around bread counters in supermarkets is often due to an oxide called 2-furaldehyde (Bauer et al 1990).

Lactones

Lactones always have an oxygen atom double bonded to a carbon atom. The carbon atom is attached to another oxygen atom that is part of a closed ring (Table 3-15). Lactones are present in most expressed oils and tend to end in -*lactone* or -*ine.* The percentage of lactones present may be low, but they play an important role as expectorants and mucolytics. However, lactones tend to have the same potential neurotoxic effects as ketones. Many essential oils belonging to the Asteraceae family contain lactones that can also cause skin sensitivities (Gordon 1999).

Alantolactone is present in elecampane *(Inula helenium)* and is used to treat purulent bronchitis (Rose 1994). Isolantolactone is found in sweet inule *(Inula graveolens)* and is effective in treating bronchial congestion. Lactones that contain 15 carbon atoms seem to have distinctive antiinflammatory properties (Bowles 2000). Nepetalactone, found in catnip *(Nepeta cataria),* showed sedative and analgesic effects in rats (Aydin et al 1998). A bicyclic lactone (a phthalide) is responsible for the odor of celery root (Bauer et al 1990).

Coumarins

Coumarins are a type, or subgroup, of lactones. They have an oxygen atom double-bonded to a carbon atom. That carbon atom is attached to another oxygen, which is part of a closed ring, and they also have a benzene ring attached (Table 3-16). Coumarins usually end in -*one* (pronounced *own*), as in umbelliferone, or with -*in*, as in coumarin. Coumarins may be present in small amounts, in essential oils but they are very potent. Franchomme states that coumarins augment the antispasmodic effect of esters. Coumarins include khellin and visnagin, which are

Table 3-15   *Some Lactones and Their Properties*

Nepetalactone found in *Nepata caesarea* (catnip)		Analgesic & sedative (Aydin et al 1998)
Alantolactone found in *Inula graveolens*		Respiratory antiinflammatory (Mazor 2000)

Table 3-16 ❧ *Structural Similarities between Coumarin and Warfarin*

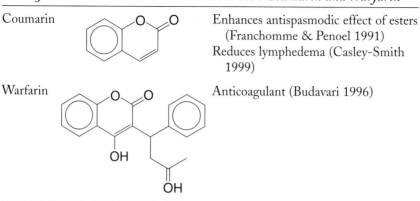

Coumarin		Enhances antispasmodic effect of esters (Franchomme & Penoel 1991) Reduces lymphedema (Casley-Smith 1999)
Warfarin		Anticoagulant (Budavari 1996)

strong vasodilators found in khella *(Ammi visnaga)* essential oil (Lewis Walter & Elvin-Lewis Memory 1977). Khella is also a bronchodilator (Budavari et al 1996). Reconstituted compounds from Khella form the ingredients of the pharmaceutical product Intal, an inhaled asthma medication (Rose 1992).

There is sometimes confusion regarding the chemical dicoumarol, which forms the basis of warfarin, an anticoagulant drug (Mills 1991). Dicoumarol is created naturally by the breakdown of sweet clover plant, but it is created synthetically by drug companies (Budavari 1996). However, if you look at the chemical drawing, you will find a coumarin group within it (see Table 3-16) (Bowles 2000), although coumarin-rich essential oils have *not* yet been shown to have a measurable anticoagulant effect.

Small amounts of furanocoumarins (up to 2%) are present in citrus-peel oils and a few other essential oils such as angelica *(Angelica archangelica)* root, cumin *(Cuminum cyminum),* and rue *(Ruta graveolens)* (Tisserand & Balacs 1995). Virginian cedarwood *(Juniperus virginiana)* and lemon verbena *(Lippia citriodora)* are also phototoxic (Price & Price 1999).

Furanocoumarins react in the presence of ultraviolet light and can have a phototoxic effect, resulting in burns or erythema. Higher percentages are needed to have a phototoxic effect on darker skin (Zaynoun et al 1977). A phototoxic effect was produced with a 2.4% concentration on pale skin and an average of a 15% concentration on dark brown or black skin. On some skin the resulting pigmentation can remain for life. Bergamottin, a furanocoumarin, was found to be anti-tumoral in vitro (Miyake et al 1999).

Ethers

Ethers occur when a methyl or ethyl group is attached to a benzene ring via an oxygen molecule (Table 3-17). Ethers are thought to be responsible for some of the hallucinogenic properties of certain essential oils when taken orally. The hypothesis is that estragole and anethole could be metabolized into 4-methoxy-

Table 3-17   ❧   *An Ether and Its Property*

Transanethole in *Foeniculum vulgare* (fennel)	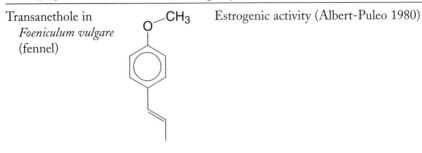	Estrogenic activity (Albert-Puleo 1980)

amphetamine or the corresponding ketone (Benoni et al 1996). Unlike phenols, ethers are not aggressive on the skin.

APART FROM CHEMISTRY

Some people believe there is more to an essential oil than the sum of its parts: there is a synergy of all those parts working together. Many people also believe there is an energy or vibration to an essential oil, and it may be this part that plays the major role in healing. Some people think of essential oils as having yin- and yang-like qualities. Oils with yanglike qualities are thought to tone the whole body, stimulate immune growth, support the metabolic response, raise internal temperature, and stimulate the nervous system. Oils with yinlike qualities are thought to reduce temperature, decrease activity in the nervous system, and have a calming effect. This process of attributing yin- and yang-like properties to essential oils is key to the work of Peter Holmes (1989) and Gabriel Mojay (1996).

REFERENCES

Albert-Puleo M. 1980. Fennel and anise as estrogenic agents. Journal of Ethnopharmacology. 2(4) 337-344.

Allen W. 1897. Note on a case of supposed poisoning by pennyroyal. Lancet. 1:1022-1023.

Amarka M, Papanikolaou E, Sivropoulou A et al. 1999. Antiviral properties of isoborneol, a potent inhibitor of herpes simplex virus type 1. Antiviral Research. 43(2) 79-92.

Asakura K, Matsuo Y, Oshima T et al. 2000. Omega-Agatoxin IVA sensitive Ca(2+) channel blocker, alpha-eudesmol, protects against brain injury after focal ischemia in rats. European Journal of Pharmacology. 394(1) 57-65.

Aydin S, Beis R, Ozturk Y et al. 1998. Nepetalactone: A new opioid analgesic from *Nepeta caesarea Boiss.* Journal of Pharmacy and Pharmacology. 50(7) 813-817.

Bakerink J, Gospe S, Dimand R et al. 1996. Multiple organ failure after ingestion of pennyroyal oil from herbal tea in two infants. Pediatrics. 98(5) 944-947.

Bauer K, Garbe D, Surburg H. 1990. Common Fragrance and Flavor Materials. Weinheim, Germany: VCH Publishing.

Belanger J. 1998. Perillyl alcohol: Applications in oncology. Alternative Medicine Review. 3(6) 448-457.

Benencia F, Courreges M. 1999. Antiviral activity of sandalwood oil against herpes simplex virus 1 and 2. Phytomedicine. 6(2) 119-123.

Bennett A, Stamford P, Tavares I. 1988. The biological activity of eugenol, a major constituent of nutmeg *(Myristica fragrans):* Studies on prostaglandins, the intestine and other tissues. Phytotherapy Research. 2:124-130.

Benoni H, Dallakian P, Taraz K. 1996. Studies of the essential oil from guarana. Zeitschrift Lebensmittel-Untersuching und-forshung. 203(1) 95-98.

Bowles J. 2000. The Basic Chemistry of Chemotherapeutic Essential Oils. Sydney, Australia: Pirie Printers.

Buchbauer G, Jirovetz L, Jager W et al. 1991. Aromatherapy: Evidence for sedative effects of the essential oil of lavender after inhalation. Zeitschrift fur Naturforschung. 46(11-12) 1067-1072.

Budavari, S, et al (eds.). 1996. The Merck Index, 12th ed. Whitehouse Station, NJ: Merck & Co. Inc.

Budhiraja S, Cullum M, Sioutis S et al. 1999. Biological activity of *Melaleuca alternifolia* (teatree) oil components, terpinen-4-ol in human hyelocytic cell line HL-60. Journal of Manipulative Physiological Therapeutics. 22 (7) 47-53.

Carle R, Gomaa K. 1992. The medicinal use of *Matricaria flos.* British Journal of Phytotherapy. 2:147-153.

Carson C, Riley T. 1995. Antimicrobial activity of the major components of the essential oil of *Melaleuca alternifolia.* Journal of Applied Bacteriology. 78(3) 264-269.

Casley-Smith J. 1999. Benzo-pyrones in the treatment of lymphedema. International Journal of Angiology. 18(1) 31-41.

Chio L, Ling J, Chang C. 1997. Chinese herb constituent beta-eudesmol alleviated the electroshock seizures in mice and electrographic seizures in rat hippocampal slices. Neuroscience Letters. 231(1) 171-174.

Colette. 1975. "Break of Day." Reprinted in *Earthly Paradise,* Robert Phelps Ed. New York: Noonday Press.

Consentino S, Tuberoso C, Pisano B et al. 1999. In vitro antimicrobial activity and chemical activity of Sardinian Thymus essential oils. Letters in Applied Microbiology. 29(2) 130-135.

Dimas K, Kokkinopoulos D, Demetzos C et al. 1999. The effect of schlareol on growth and cell cycle progression of human leukemic cell lines. Leukemia Research. 23(3) 217-234.

Duke J. 1992. Handbook of Biologically Active Phytochemicals and Their Activities. Boca Raton: CRC Press.

Elpel T. 1998. Botany in a Day. Pony, MT: Hollowtop Outdoor Primitive School, LLC.

Franchomme P, Penoel D. 1991. Aromatherapie Exactement. Limoges, France: Jollois.

Franz C. 1993. Genetics. In Hay R, Waterman P (eds.), Volatile Oil Crops: Their Biology, Biochemistry and Production. Essex, UK: Longman Scientific and Technical, 63-96.

Ghelardini C, Galeotti N, Salvatore G et al. 1999. Local anesthetic activity of the essential oil of *Lavandula angustifolia.* Planta Medica. 65(8) 700-703.

Gordon L. 1999. Compositae dermatitis. Australasian Journal of Dermatology. 40(3) 123-128.

Gould M. 1997. Cancer chemoprevention and therapy by monoterpenes. Environmental Health Perspectives. 105 (Suppl 4) 977-979.

Guenther E. 1972. The Essential Oils, Vol. I. Malabar, FL: Krieger.

Guenther E. 1976. The Essential Oils, Vol. III. Malaber, FL: Krieger.

Harborne J. 1988. Introduction to Ecological Biochemistry. London: Academic Press.

Hay R, Waterman P (eds.). 1993. Volatile Oil Crops: Their Biology, Biochemistry and Production. Essex, UK: Longman Scientific and Technical.

Hethelyi E, Danos B, Tetenyi P. 1988. Investigation of the essential oils of the *Achillea* genus. I. The essential oil composition of *Achillea distans*. Herba Hungarica. 27:35-42.

Hmamouchi M, Tantaoui EA, Es-Safi N et al. 1990. Elucidation of antibacterial and antifungal properties of *Eucalyptus* essential oils. Plantes Medicale Phytotherapie. 24(4) 278-279.

Hume W. 1983. Effect of eugenol on constrictor response in blood vessels of rabbit ear. Journal of Dental Research. 62(9) 1013-1015.

Igimi H, Tamura R, Yamamoto F et al. 1991. Medical dissolution of gallstones: Clinical experience of d-limonene as a simple, safe and effective solvent. Digestive Diseases and Sciences. 36(2) 200-208.

International School of Aromatherapy. 1993. A Safety Guide on the Use of Essential Oils. London: Nature By Nature Oils.

Jakovlev V, Isaac O, Thiener K et al. 1979. Pharmacological investigations with compounds of chamomile: New investigations on the antiphlogistic effects of (-)a-bisabolol and bisabolol oxides. Planta Medica. 35:125-140.

Jakovlev V, Isaac C, Flaskamp E. 1983. Pharmacological investigations with compounds of chamomile. VI. Investigations on the antiphlogistic effects of chamazulene and matricin. Planta Medica. 49(2) 67-73.

Jedlickova Z, Mottl O, Sery V. 1992. Antibacterial properties of the Vietnamese Cajeput oil and Ocimum oil in combination with antibacterial agents. Journal of Hygiene, Epidemiology, Microbiology, and Immunology. 36(3) 303-309.

Juergens U, Stober M, Schmidt-Schilling L et al. 1998. Anti-inflammatory effects of eucalyptol (1,8-cineole) in bronchial asthma: inhibition of arachidonic acid metabolism in human blood monocytes ex vivo. European Journal of Medical Research. 3(9) 407-412.

Lavabre M. 1990. Aromatherapy Workbook. Vermont: Healing Arts Press.

Lawless J. 1992. Encyclopedia of Essential Oils. Shaftesbury, UK: Element Books.

Lawrence B. 1989. Essential Oils: 1981-1987. Wheaton, IL: Allured Publishing.

Lee HS, Ahn YJ. 1998. Growth-inhibiting effects of *Cinnamomum cassia* bark-derived materials on human intestinal bacteria. Journal of Agriculture, Food, and Chemistry. 46:8-12.

Lewinsohn E. 2001. The biosynthesis of essential oils. Notes from Essential Oils Course, Rutgers University. August 12-16.

Lewis Walter H, Elvin-Lewis Memory R. 1977. Medical Botany. New York: John Wiley.

Lis-Balchin M, Hart S. 1999. Studies on the mode of action of the essential oil of lavender *(Lavandula angustifolia)*. Physiotherapy Research 13(6) 540-542.

Lopez N, Kato M, Andrade E et al. 1999. Antimalarial use of volatile oil from the leaves of *Virola surinamensis* by Waiapi Amazon Indians. Journal of Ethnopharmacology. 67(3) 313-319.

Lorenzetti, Souza G, Sarti S et al. 1991. Myrcene mimics the peripheral analgesic activity of lemongrass tea. Journal of Ethnopharmacology. 34(1) 43-48.

Luft U, Bychkov R, Gollasch M et al. 1999. Farnseol blocks the L-types Ca2+ channel by targeting the alpha 1C subunit. Arteriosclerosis, Thrombosis & Vascular Biology. 19(4) 959-966.

Miyake Y, Murakami A, Sugiyama Y et al. 1999. Identification of coumarins from lemon fruit *(Citrus limon)* as inhibitors of in vitro tumor promotion. Journal of Agriculture and Food Chemistry. 47(8) 3151-3157.

Mills S. 1991. Out of the Earth. London: Viking Arkana, 295.

Moleyar V, Narasimham P. 1992. Antibacterial activity of essential oil components. International Journal of Food Microbiology. 16:337-342.

Mumcuoglu K, Galun R, Bach U et al. 1996. Repellency of essential oils and their components to the human body louse, *Pediculus humanus.* Entomologia Experimentale et Applicata. 78(3) 309-314.

Okegawa H, Ueda R, Matsumoto K et al. 1995. Effect of a-santalol and b-santalol from sandalwood on the central nervous system of rats. Phytomedicine. 2(2) 119-126.

Onawunmi G, Oguniana E. 1981. Antibacterial constituents in the essential oil of *Cymbopogon citratus.* Ethnopharmacology. 24:64-68.

Onawunmi G. 1989. Evaluation of the antimicrobial activity of citral. Letters in Applied Microbiology. 9:105-108.

Oswiecimska M. 1974. Korrelation zwischen Chromosomenzahl und Prochamazulenen in Achillea von osteuropa. Translated. Correlation between number of chromatosomes and prochamazulene in Easteurapean Achillea. Planta Medica. 25(4) 389-395.

Price S, Price L. 1999. Aromatherapy for Health Professionals, 2nd ed. London: Churchill Livingstone, 51.

Re L, Barocci S, Sonnino S et al. 2000. Linalool modifies the nicotinic receptor-ion channel kinetics at the mouse neuromuscular junction. Pharmacological Research. 42(2) 177-182.

Rose J. 1992. The Aromatherapy Book. San Francisco: North Atlantic Books.

Rose J. 1994. Guide to Essential Oils. San Francisco: Jeanne Rose Aromatherapy.

Rossi T, Melegari M, Bianchi A et al. 1988. Sedative, anti-inflammatory and anti-diuretic effects induced in rats by essential oils of varieties of *Anthemis nobilis:* a comparative study. Pharmacological Research Communications. 20(Suppl 5) 71-74.

Ryman D. 1991. Aromatherapy. London: Piatkus.

Safayhi H, Sabieraj J, Sailer E et al. 1994. Chamazulene an antioxidant type inhibitor of leukotriene B4 formation. Planta Medica 60(5) 410-413.

Santos F, Rao V, Silveira E. 1997. The leaf essential oil of *Psidium guyanensis* offers protection against pentylenetetrazole-induced seizures. Planta Medica. 63:133-135.

Santos F, Rao V. 2000. Anti-inflammatory and antinociceptive effects of 1,8 cineole, a terpenoid oxide present in many plant essential oils. Physiotherapy Research. 14(4) 240-241.

Shapiro S, Meir A, Guggenheim B. 1994. The antimicrobial activity of essential oil components towards oral bacteria. Oral Microbiology and Immunology. 9:202-208.

Sharma J, Srivastava K, Gan E. 1994. Suppressive effects of eugenol and ginger oil on arthritic rats. Pharmacology. 49:314-318.

Shoji Y, Ishige H, Tamura N et al. 1998. Enhancement of anti-herpetic activity of anti-sense phosphorothioate oligonucleotides 5 with geraniol. Journal of Drug Targeting. 5(4) 261-273.

Sobti S, Pushpangadan P, Thapa R et al. 1978. Chemical and genetic investigations in essential oils of some Ocimum species, their FI hybrids and synthesized allopolyploids. Lloydia 4:50-55.

Stearn W. 1998. Botanical Latin, 4th ed. Portland, OR: Timber Press.

Svab J, El-Din-Awaad C, Fahmy T. 1967. The influence of highly different ecological effects on the volatile oil content and composition in the chamomile. Herba Hungarica. 6(2) 177-188.

Tambe Y, Ysujiuchi H, Honda G et al. 1996. Gastric cytoprotection of the non-steroidal anti-inflammatory sesquiterpene, beta-carylophyllene. Planta Medica. 62(5) 469-470.

Tisserand R, Balacs T. 1995. Essential Oil Safety. London: Churchill Livingstone.

Trabace L, Avato P, Nazzoccoli M et al. 1994. Choleretic activity of Phapsia Chem 1, 11, 111 in rats: Comparison with terpenoid constituents and peppermint oil. Phytotherapy Research. 8(5) 305-307.

Tucker A, Maciarello M. 1987. Plant identification. In Simon J, Grant L (eds.), Proceedings of the First National Herb Growing and Marketing Conference. West Lafayette, IN: Purdue University Press, 341-372.

Tucker A, Maciarello M. 1990. Essential oils of cultivars of Dalmation sage *(Salvia officinalis)*. Journal of Essential Oil Research. 2:139-144.

Valnet J. 1990. The Practice of Aromatherapy. Saffron Walden, UK: CW Daniels.

Vernet P, Gouyon D. 1976. Le polymorphisme chimique de *Thymus vulgaris.* Parfums, Cosmetiques, Aromes. 30:31-45.

Viollon C, Mandin D, Chaumont J. 1996. Antagonistic activities, in vitro, of some essential oils and natural volatile compounds in relation to the growth of *Trichomonas vaginalis.* Fitoterapia. 67(3) 279-281.

Waterman P. 1993. The chemistry of volatile oils. In Hay R, Waterman P (eds.), Volatile Oil Crops: Their Biology, Biochemistry and Production. Essex, UK: Longman Scientific and Technical, 47-61.

Williams D. 1996. The Chemistry of Essential Oils. Dorset, UK: Michelle Press, 40.

Yamada K, Miura T, Mimaki Y et al. 1996. Effect of inhalation of chamomile oil vapor on plasma ACTH level in ovariectomized rat under restriction stress. Biological & Pharmaceutical Bulletin. 19(9) 1244-1246.

Yang D, Michel D, Mandin D et al. 1996. Antifungal and antibacterial properties in vitro of three Patchouli essential oils from different origins. Acta Botanica Gallica. 143(1) 29-35.

Zaynoun S, Johnson B, Frain-Bell W. 1977. A study of bergamot and its importance as a phototoxic agent. Contact Dermatitis. 3:225-239.

Zheng GQ, Kenney P, Luke T. 1992. Anethofuran, carvone and limonene: potential cancer chemopreventive agents from dill weed oil and caraway oil. Planta Medica. 58: 338-341.

Part II: Extraction, Biosynthesis, and Analysis

"It looked totally innocent, like a light tea—and yet contained, in addition to the four-fifths alcohol, one fifth of a mysterious mixture that could set a whole city trembling with excitement."

Suskind P. 1986.
Perfume: The Story of a Murderer. London: Penguin Books, 62.

Essential Oils and Extracts from Aromatic Plants

There are several ways of extracting the volatile components from plants. Some methods produce essential oils, and other methods produce extracts rather than essential oils. See Figure 3-2 and Table 3-18 for comparisons of the extraction procedures used for aromatic extracts and essential oils. Traditionally aromatherapy has specified the use of essential oils, but some other methods of extraction and the products they yield are becoming more acceptable.

Extraction of Essential Oils

Essential oils are either distilled or expressed (Arctander 1960). Distillation can mean water distillation, water-and-steam distillation, steam distillation, or steam-and-vacuum distillation (Arctander 1960).

Water distillation

Material from the plant is in direct contact with boiling water. Arctander (1960) suggests that such direct heating methods may produce a burnt note to the essential oil. Most water distillation stills have a grid. This protects the plant material from the heating elements, and the process is similar to that of water-and-steam distillation.

Water-and-steam distillation

In water-and-steam distillation, steam is blown into the mixture of water and plant material.

Steam distillation

This method formerly involved a copper still, but now the still is more likely to be made of stainless steel. The aromatic plant material is placed on a grid through which steam passes, usually at a temperature not above 100°C (Bowles 2000). See

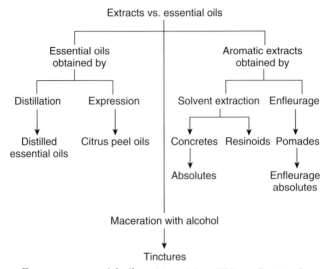

FIGURE 3-2   Extracts vs. essential oils.   Adapted from Williams D. 1989. Lecture Notes on Essential Oils. With kind permission of Eve Taylor, London.

Table 3-18 ❧ *Advantages and Disadvantages of Various Extraction Processes*

Extraction Process	Advantages	Disadvantages
Distillation	Economical Large quantities can be processed Simple apparatus Little labor needed	Changing constituents Depending on time/temp
Expression	No heat required Simple apparatus	Some flavoring left Only citrus peel oils Oxidize quickly
Enfleurage	Low temperature needed Possible problem with solvent	Time consuming Labor intensive
CO_2 extraction	Constant product No heat used	Expensive
Solvent extraction	Constant product	Solvent residues

Fig. 3-3 for more details. The water boils at temperatures between 88° C and 930° C depending on the altitude at the distillation site. Altitude can be particularly relevant when essential oils are distilled locally. A decrease in boiling point has significant influence on the hydrolytic effect of the steam on the essential oil (Arctander 1960).

Most American or European stills use high-pressure steam. This is the fastest way of distilling essential oils with high-boiling constituents such as vetiver, sandalwood, and clove. The steam loosens the volatile nonpolar constituents of the plant and they pass, with the steam, into a condenser that cools the mixture. Steam also alters some of the components within an essential oil, for example turning matricin to chamazulene. Some of the polar components from the plant dissolve in the water producing floral water. The mixture of floral water and essential oil come out together, but as essential oils and floral water do not mix, they quickly separate. The majority of essential oils float above the floral water, but some sink, depending on their specific gravity.

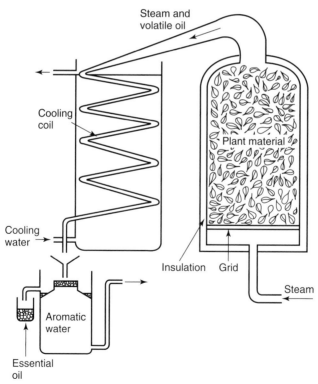

FIGURE 3-3   Steam distillation.   Reproduced from Price S. 1983. Practical Aromatherapy, with the kind permission of Harper Collins, London.

The degree of heat and the amount of time are vital parts of the distillation process as some components of plants are very sensitive to heat and others take much longer to distill (Guenther 1974). The distillation process for *Lavandula angustifolia* is approximately one hour, but it is considerably longer for sandalwood or vetiver. The length of the distillation process will affect the chemical composition of the essential oil (Guenther 1976). Steam distillation is suitable for the highly volatile components such as the terpenes. The heavier the molecule (sesquiterpenoids), the longer the process will take. Until fairly recently the side product, the floral water (otherwise called hydrolat) was thrown away, but now, hydrolats (or hydrosols) are becoming known for their own therapeutic actions, especially for babies, children, and the elderly.

Steam-and-vacuum distillation

This method uses steam distillation with partial vacuum (Arctander 1960). The pressure used is typically 100-200 mmHg. The advantage of this method is the speed with which the essential oil is extracted. The disadvantage is that a very effective and fast method of cooling is required.

Portable distillation Portable distillation equipment is simple to make and can be used for small quantities of plants when essential oils must be distilled on site (Alkaire & Simon 1992). Otherwise, small cooker-top stills can be purchased for home use.

Subdivisions of steam distillation

Cohobation means the water used in the distillation process is reused many times (Guenther 1974).

Fractional distillation means the essential oil is distilled at specific temperatures for specific lengths of time to collect different factions (or functional groups) within the essential oil. For example, peppermint contains terpenes that become volatile at approximately 150° C and menthone and menthol that boil at 200°-230° C (Guenther 1974).

Rectification aims to separate the volatile and nonvolatile components of an essential oil. If an essential oil is thought to contain impurities, it can be purified by redistillation. This process is called rectification. Sometimes peppermint and caraway seed oils can take on an unpleasant odor if they have been in contact with the wall of a hot still. This aroma can be removed through rectification (Guenther 1974). To give some idea of yield, 200 kg of *Lavandula angustifolia* flowers will produce 1 kg of essential oil. However, between 2 and 5 metric tons of rose petals are needed to produce the same amount of rose oil.

Expression

Only involves the peel of citrus plants such as grapefruit. The peel of the fruit is racked or abraded by mechanical scrapers, and the essence collected by centrifugal separation. Sometimes the whole fruit is crushed prior to the essential oil being separated from the juice and peel. Expressed oils will naturally contain a proportion of waxes and other nonsoluble components that may cause phototoxicity.

Methods for Producing Extracts (not essential oils)

There are other methods of extraction that produce compounds mainly used by the fragrance and cosmetics industry. One such compound is called an absolute. An absolute is not a true essential oil but an extract obtained using petrol-based chemicals. It is impossible to remove all of the chemical solvent. In 1989, the International Fragrance Research Association issued guidelines as to the recommended level of benzene in an absolute: it should not exceed 10 parts per million (ppm) (International School of Aromatherapy 1993). Residual solvent found in extracts could provoke an adverse reaction.

Solvent extraction

This three-stage method was first used on flowers by French chemist and pharmacist Pierre Jean Robiquet in 1835 and rapidly became a popular method (Guenther 1974). The advantage was extraction could occur at room temperature. However, this is a complicated process requiring an expensive apparatus.

1st stage: Solvents such as benzene, petroleum ether, and, more recently, hexane have been used to extract the volatile parts from plants. This first stage produces a waxy mixture called a concrete (often approximately 50% essential oil and 50% wax). Hexane is believed to be safe and is used in several food-extraction processes. However, it is impossible to remove all the solvent following extraction.

2nd stage: A solvent, usually ethanol, is used to dissolve the wax. This step is repeated several times.

3rd stage: The alcohol/wax mixture is evaporated by vacuum.

Enfleurage

This method was mainly used on fragile blossoms such as jasmine and tuberose and is rarely used today. I watched this process in Grasse, France in 2000, and it was very labor intensive. Animal fat is pounded until it is soft, and then glass plates are coated with the fat. Each fat-covered glass plate is called a chassis. Fresh blossoms are placed close together on the chassis and left until the fat becomes saturated with essential oil. The chassis are constantly replenished with fresh blossoms, and the old blossoms discarded. The resulting oil/fat mixture is called a pomade. The pomade is mixed with alcohol to remove the fat, and the remaining extract is called an absolute. However, 99% of jasmine and tuberose extract is now produced by solvent extraction.

Carbon dioxide

Supercritical carbon dioxide (CO_2) extraction, an innovative method using "fluidized" CO_2, has been available since the 1980s and is making significant inroads in the flavor, perfume, and aromatherapy worlds. Brew masters in Germany were looking for a hops flavor extract that had no heat or chemical "off" notes, and German scientists found an extraction technique that did not involve heat or chemical solvents. When the temperature of CO_2 is maintained at approximately 31° C, under pressure it acts like a fluid and dissolves the CO_2-soluble part of an herb. The advantages are no heat or chemical solvents are used and the process produces a gentle, "unstressed" extraction. However, the chemistry of the resulting extract differs from that of essential oils extracted via steam distillation. For example, steam-distilled German chamomile (*Matricaria recutita*) essential oil is dark blue because heat and water create chamazulene, a sesquiterpene. Matricine, the colorless precursor to chamazulene, occurs naturally in the plant and is thought to be a superior antiinflammatory. Matricine is present in the German chamomile extract yielded by the CO_2 method.

CO_2 supercritical extraction is an expensive and technologically sophisticated process, but it is well accepted in creating pure flavors and perfume oils. As there is a great deal more published research on the therapeutic properties of plants, and this method produces a concentrated and undistorted plant extract (with volatile oils in it), this is a method to watch. It may become a more accepted part of aromatherapy within the next few years.

Florasol

A fairly new chemical process has been developed and patented in England by rose-grower and scientist Dr. Peter Wilde (Tisserand 1994). His method involves extracting essential oils by means of a new solvent. The unique character of this solvent is that its boiling point is around 30° C. Plant material can be extracted at room temperature and the solvent removed without boiling. This ensures the plant material is not damaged by high temperatures. The solvent residue is 1000 times less than the hexane content in a concrete or absolute obtained using traditional methods. The extract is neither acid nor alkaline. (When using liquid CO_2, some dissolves, which lowers the pH and produces a slightly acidic product.) Florasol oils are used routinely by the flavor and food industry and have the approval of the European Commission on Foods for Human Consumption. The United States Food and Drug Administration has accepted Florasol extracts as generally regarded as safe. Of particular note is the fact that these products do not produce concretes that require further refining with alcohol (Wilde 1995).

Aroma Intensities

The aromas of essential oils have different intensities, and these may last for differing periods of time. The perfume industry refers to these properties as notes and divides them into top, middle, and base notes (Price 1983). These divisions indicate how rapidly the essential oil will lose its vitality. A top note might last, in an unstopped bottle, for a few hours before losing its odor, a middle note might last a couple of days, and a base note may last for several weeks.

In the 19th century, Septimus Piesse (1855), a chemist and perfumer, created a classification system for perfume that corresponded to a musical scale (Poucher 1993). In 1923, a man named Poucher built onto the work of Piesse and developed a classification method based on a perfume's evaporation rate scaled from 1 to 100. Scents that evaporated quickly (1-15) were called top notes, for example, mandarin (2) and nutmeg (11). Middle notes (16-69) included marjoram (18), ylang ylang (24), and rose (43). Base notes lasted the longest (70-100), for example angelica (94). Perfumes with the highest ratings last the longest and evaporate the slowest (for example, frankincense, patchouli, sandalwood, and vetiver). Poucher's classification system was updated in 1991 and is still used today by perfumers (Poucher 1993).

The odor of an essential oil deteriorates as a result of oxidation. Some essential oils evaporate more quickly than others. As an essential oil evaporates, certain components within it combine with oxygen in the air. This process is called oxidization. For example, alcohols combine with oxygen to become aldehydes (Bowles 2000). The rate of evaporation depends on the volatility of the essential oil, and volatility depends on the components within the essential oil. Citrus oils such as bergamot or grapefruit will evaporate faster than flower oils such as rose. Therefore they will oxidize more quickly. The least volatile oils are the resins and woods. Heat and sunlight can speed up oxidation. The oxidization of an essential oil will affect the odor of an essential oil and its therapeutic potential (Tisserand & Balacs 1995).

Resinoids are obtained from resins such as amber and mastic, balsams such as benzoin, or gum-like substances such as frankincense and myrrh. Frequently the method used to obtain resinoids is extraction by hydrocarbon solvents. Frankincense and myrrh can also be obtained by straight steam distillation. Resins are soluble in alcohol but not in water; gums are soluble in water but not in alcohol (International School of Aromatherapy 1993).

BIOSYNTHESIS: HOW AND WHY PLANTS MAKE ESSENTIAL OILS

Essential oils come from aromatic plants. Green plants are capable of synthesizing complex carbohydrates from hydrogen, carbon, and oxygen. Life, as we know it, would not continue if there was not an independent mechanism that synthesized complex molecules from simple ones. The huge task of providing "energy for life" is the sole responsibility of green plants, but this chemical process requires energy. The energy required by plants to change hydrogen, carbon, and oxygen to complex carbohydrates comes from the sun. This process is called photosynthesis.

Until the late 1950s, essential oils and all other secondary metabolites were thought to be the waste products of a plant. This was because human energy had been focused on the structure of compounds found in plants (and essential oils) rather than on their function. Essential oils occurred in such small amounts in plants that they were thought to be unimportant. However, some scientists suspected that essential oils were relevant to the plant and began to explore their therapeutic potential.

Not every plant produces essential oils; aromatic plants tend to congregate in specific families like Asteraceae (chamomiles), Rutaceae (citrus oils), or

Lamiaceae (lavender and mints). Overall, only 1% of flowering plants produce essential oils in any significant amount. However, plants produce more than 100,000 different chemical compounds, and the vast majority of these are not essential to the physiology of the plant or its reproduction. Interestingly, some chemical components found in plants, particularly some of the essential oils, can actually be harmful to the plant and are stored in special cellular compartments to prevent injury to the plant. Leakage of these essential oils can impair the process of photosynthesis on which the plant depends for its life.

There are hundreds of aromatic plants, but not all of them produce essential oils in sufficient quantity for distillation to be viable. For example, hyacinth is usually obtained by solvent extraction, and then the solvent is distilled (Lawless 1992). The same is true for lily of the valley and lilac (International School of Aromatherapy 1993). Some plants produce essential oils that can be toxic, such as thuja, wintergreen (Tisserand 1988), and arnica (Lawless 1992). (Arnica, the herb but not the essential oil, is traditionally used in very small amounts in homeopathic treatments.) The amount of essential oil contained in a plant varies tremendously and so do the components within essential oil. Sometimes the smallest quantity of a chemical in an essential oil has a major part to play. For example, the smell of a rose (*Rosa damascena*) originates from a component found in rose that is only 0.1 parts per million.

Photosynthesis

Photosynthesis is the process by which a plant, under the influence of sunlight, can make, in its chlorophyll-containing cells, carbohydrates from the carbon dioxide of the atmosphere and hydrogen from the water in the soil. Photosynthesis is vital to the survival of the plant because carbohydrates are essential for life. The main function of carbohydrates is to store energy. This includes sugars, starch, and cellulose. Cellulose is used for the structure of the plant.

Carbohydrates have the general formula $(CH_2O)n$, when n represents the number of CH_2O "units" present. The name of the carbohydrate is determined by the number of carbons it contains (Tables 3-19 and 3-20).

The last two, di- and polysaccharides, are known as complex carbohydrates and are the types that occur in plants. When plants convert carbon dioxide and water into complex organic molecules, oxygen is released back into the atmosphere. Ultimately these complex organic molecules made by the plant will be degraded by plant-eating animals back into carbon dioxide and water, along with the release of energy required for further synthesis of compounds or metabolic processes.

$$CO_2 + H_2O + \text{light, energy, chlorophyll} = CH_2O + O_2$$

Plant metabolism has two distinct stages. The first occurs in light and is called photosynthesis. The second takes place without sunlight and is sometimes called the "dark reaction" (Mann 2001b). During this stage carbon dioxide is reduced to produce carbon sugars. Photosynthesis takes place in the green leaves of

Table 3-19 🌿 *Sugars Occuring in Plants*

Six carbon atoms	$C_6H_{12}O_6$	Hexose sugar (glucose)
Five carbon atoms	$C_5H_{10}O_5$	Pentose sugar
Three carbon atoms	$C_3H_6O_3$	Triose sugar

Table 3-20 🌿 *Sugars and Their Names*

Sugar molecules in isolation	Monosaccharides
Sugar molecules in pairs	Disaccharides
Sugar molecules in chains	Polysaccharides

plants in tiny organs called *chloroplasts,*which are where the green pigment *chlorophyll* is stored. Chlorophyll is responsible for capturing sunlight's energy and converting it to chemical energy. The quantity of essential oil in aromatic plants in dry, hot, Mediterranean countries peaks in the summer months. For example, common sage (*Salvia officinalis*) produces three times the amount of essential oil in the summer as it does in the winter.

The light stage: photosynthesis

There are two stages to the light-mediated process (photosynthesis). The first part of the light stage involves light absorption by chlorophyll. The second stage involves splitting of water molecules. Water from the soil enters the plant via the roots and is transported to the leaves by a specialized system called the *xylem.* From there it diffuses into the chloroplasts where photolysis splits the hydrogen and oxygen bonds, producing high-energy electrons, then adenosine triphosphate (ATP) and more water. ATP is a form of chemical energy.

The dark stage

In the dark stage, CO_2 from the atmosphere is converted into carbohydrates, the main product being monosaccharide sugar. This process, when hydrogen is added to the molecule, is called *reduction.* CO_2 enters the plant's leaves from the air through tiny pores on the underside of the leaf, called *stomata.* The CO_2 then travels via large, air-filled spaces to the cells containing the chloroplasts. The reduction of CO_2 and the subsequent synthesis of carbohydrates is achieved by a number of enzyme-controlled reactions, all of which require energy. The energy is supplied by ATP, which is created in the light stage of photosynthesis and also in another metabolic process known as *respiration.* Written chemically, photosynthesis looks like this:

$$6CO_2 + 12H_2O \quad\longrightarrow\quad C_6H_{12}O_6 + 6H2O + 6O_2$$

Natural Products

There are two major classes of natural products: primary and secondary metabolites (Mann 2001a). However the dividing line between primary and secondary metabolism is rather blurred (Mann 2001b) as the two types of metabolism are interconnected. Primary metabolism involves the synthesis and utilization of specific chemicals essential for the survival and health of the organism. Such chemicals are sugars, amino acids, fatty acids, nucleotides, and the polymers obtained from them. Secondary metabolism uses a different metabolic pathway and involves the production of chemicals that have no apparent importance to the organism (Mann 2001a). Secondary metabolism produces alkaloids, bitters, glycosides, gums, saponins, steroids, and essential oils. Secondary metabolism is further discussed in the section titled "Chemistry of Essential Oils" (see page 43).

Storage of Essential Oils in Plants

Essential oils are stored in specific parts of a plant (Table 3-21). For example, rose essential oil is found in the petals of the flowers, not the roots, leaves, or stem. However, sometimes an essential oil is found in different parts of the same plant, as in the case of angelica root and angelica seed. In this particular case the chemistry of each essential oil is different. The essential oil from the root of angelica is phototoxic (can cause a skin reaction when ultraviolet light is used on the skin within 24 hours of applying), but essential oil from the seed is not phototoxic.

Table 3-21 ❧ *Parts of Plant Where Essential Oils Are Stored*

Rose	Flower
Angelica	Root, seed
Eucalyptus	Leaf
Juniper	Berry
Sandalwood	Wood
Cinnamon	Bark, leaf
Clove	Leaf, bud
Myrrh	Resin
Black pepper	Seed
Rosemary	Whole herb
Mandarin	Fruit peel
Pine	Needles

Table 3-22 ❧ *Types of Storage for Essential Oils*

Part	Plant
Single secretion cells	Ginger, black pepper, cardamom, valerian, lemongrass
Secretory cavities	Citrus fruits, clove, myrrh, frankincense
Secretory ducts	Tarragon, angelica, aniseed, pine
Secretory hairs	Many plants in the Lamiaceae and Geraniaceae families

Secretory and Storage Structures of Essential Oils in Plants

For additional reading, Svoboda and Svoboda's excellent, illustrated book, *Secretory Structures of Aromatic and Medicinal Plants* (2001), is a must, and the information in this section is based on it. Essential oils are stored in special secretory structures (Table 3-22), either on the surface of the plant or within the plant tissue, and are found in many different types of plant: perennial, annual, biennial, evergreen, and deciduous (Svoboda & Svoboda 2001). Secretory structures vary and include single, secretion-containing cells that are similar to the surrounding cells, secretory ducts, secretory cavities, osmophores, glandular trichomes, and epidermal cells. Often the family or genus of a plant will have a similar secretory system. This can be useful in plant identification.

Single, secretion-containing cells are common in many aromatic plants such as the leaves of lemongrass, rhizome of ginger, seed coat of cardamom, fruit wall of black pepper, bark of cinnamon, and root of valerian. Secretory ducts are elongated cavities found in plants such as coriander, cumin, angelica, dill, anise, and fennel (all members of the Umbelliferae family). Secretory cavities are prevalent in the fruit and leaves of lemon, orange, and bergamot in the Citrus family. They are also found in the bark of myrrh and frankincense and in clove buds. Osmophores are found in orchids and are areas of tissue with secretory cells different structurally from the surrounding cells. Glandular trichomes are modified epidermal hairs found on leaves and stems of plants such as basil, lavender, and marjoram in the Lamiaceae family. Epidermal cells diffuse essential oil directly through the cytoplasm and cell wall to the outside, and the amount of essential oil diffused is very low. Examples of aromatics with epidermal cells are rose and jasmine.

There are various theories as to why some plants produce secondary metabolites such as essential oils. They could be a defense. Secondary metabolites appear to protect the plant from being eaten by herbivores (plant-eating animals or insects), by repelling them. For example, wild tobacco (*Nicotiania sylvestris*) can increase its production of nicotine by three or four times when it is under attack, and the bitter taste deters predators (Mann 2001b). Often a secondary metabolite can reduce the growth or maturation of an insect eating the aromatic plant. Grasshoppers eating *Cyperus iria* become sterile, and tenulin (a sesquiterpene lactone) in *Helenium amarum* disrupts the growth and development of insect larvae (Mann 2001b). Although mammals can cope with terpenes in their diet, many mammals and rodents find the aroma (and taste) of terpenes repellent and will not feed from aromatic plants. Voles, (a small rodent common in Europe) for example, will not eat pine needles. However, there are obvious exceptions. Australian possums and kangaroos are two mammals that have adapted and live off a diet of Eucalyptus leaves.

Certain plants exude aromas that deter insects. The Lamiaceae family has two well-known plants, pennyroyal and peppermint, that deter insects. The mosquito that carries yellow fever is repelled by mugwort (*Artemisia vulgaris*), and recent clinical studies have found that the mosquito carrying malaria is repelled by *Artemisia annua*. Artemisinin (called *qinghaosu* in Chinese medicine) is a sesquiterpene found in *Artemisia annua* and is responsible for repelling mosquitoes. This plant has been used in Chinese medicine for that purpose for 2000 years!

Another possibility for the purpose of essential oils is to increase pollination by attracting insects. Many chemical compounds found in the odor glands of insects are also found in flower fragrances. Usually it is a mixture of compounds that generates the aroma the insect is seeking. Each part of the fragrant area of the plant may present a different volatile profile. The rose, for example, produces different aromas in its petals than in the sepals and stamens.

Odor is thought to be more important to a pollinating insect than color. This is obvious with night-flying creatures. Some flowers are pollinated by bats and others are pollinated by moths. Insects are so sensitive to smell they can pick up a scent at 1/100 the level discernible to a human. Floral fragrances such as monoterpenes are important insect attractants. Some plants, such as *Datura innoxia* produce a narcotic, so the hawkmoth becomes addicted and returns regularly for "fixes" (Mann 2001a). Insects live in a world where actions are triggered by smell rather than noise or light.

Another theory as to why plants produce secondary metabolites is to prevent attack by bacteria, viruses, and fungi. Plants respond to attack from bacteria, fungi, or viruses by producing stress metabolites called phytoalexins. Some phytoalexins are used by pharmaceutical companies to protect foodstuffs from infection or spoiling (Guenther 1972).

Allelopathy is the ability of a plant to prevent other plants from growing too close to it. Bracken and ferns leach germinating inhibitors (usually phenols) into the ground to deter other species from germinating or growing too close. Aromatic plants can use essential oils such as camphor to protect the land around them from other plants. Terpenes are the largest group of chemical components found in aromatic plants, and many terpenes can inhibit the respiration of other plants (Mann 2001b). The sage bush (*Salvia leucophylla*), which is prolific in the near-desert terrain of southern California, contains chemical compounds 1,8-cineole and camphor that deter other plants' germinating.

Yet a further hypothesis for the production of essential oils is their antitranspirant activity. Essential oils aid survival in difficult climatic conditions when a haze of volatile oils may influence stomatal closure and prevent excess water loss from the leaves.

Quality of Essential Oils

Finally, there are many factors that can affect the quality of the essential oil (Table 3-23). The chemical makeup of all living plants depends on climate and environmental conditions (such as rainfall, sunlight, soil acidity, altitude) and pollution (Guenther 1972). The chemistry of the same species of rose grown in Bulgaria will be subtly different from one grown in England. Similarly, *Lavandula angustifolia* grown high in the mountains will contain more esters, which are thought to have a greater antispasmodic effect, than *Lavandula angustifolia* grown closer to sea level. If *Lavandula angustifolia* is distilled at a high altitude this will also increase the amount of esters. *Lavandula angustifolia* essential oil with a higher percentage of esters will have an aroma that is softer and fruitier. There are so many variables that the simplest way to be sure of the composition of the essential oil is to use modern analytical methods as well as the nose. This will be covered in the next section.

WHAT ARE ESSENTIAL OILS USED FOR?

Of the hundreds of essential oils produced, there are classics in common, everyday use the world over. These essential oils have research-based therapeutic properties and a long history of use. Many aromatic herbs are used in cooking, such as basil, thyme, coriander, rosemary, dill, oregano, and bay. Some are drunk in tisanes, including peppermint, lime flower, and chamomile. Several names of plants that produce essential oil will already be familiar. Some have been used in orthodox medicines for centuries, for example peppermint in mouthwashes and eucalyptus in Vicks VapoRub. Essential oils continue to play an important part in our lives. You may be surprised at the uses for some of them, as illustrated in Table 3-24 (Guenther 1972).

Table 3-23   *Factors affecting quality of essential oil.*

Soil type

Climate

Geography

Altitude

Use of fertilizers and pesticides

Time of harvest (including both time of year and time of day)

Genetics

Age of plant

Temperature at which essential oil is distilled

Length of time essential oil is distilled

Number of times essential oil is distilled

Table 3-24 ⚜ *Uses for Essential Oils*

Adhesives, alcoholic beverages, animal feed, automobile industry

Baked goods

Candle makers, canning industry, ceramics, chewing gum, confectionery, contact lenses

Dental preparations

Food industry (especially prepared foods)

Household goods (including furniture polish, lavatory cleaner, air-freshener, and washing powder)

Ice cream, insecticides

Meat-packing

Paint, paper, perfume, pharmaceuticals, printing

Rubber manufacturing

Soap, soft drinks

Textile production, tobacco

Veterinary supplies (including meats)

ANALYSIS TESTS FOR PURITY IN ESSENTIAL OILS

Gas chromatography linked to mass spectrometry (GCMS) is one of the most important tests to ascertain purity. The GC part separates the essential oil into individual constituents (like linalyl acetate) and shows their relative concentrations in a computerized printout showing a succession of peaks. The lighter molecules will peak first, and the MS part will identify those peaks. Although a GCMS will identify and quantify the chemical components, it may not always detect additional synthetic chemicals that have been added to extend or alter the essential oil.

To begin the test, a minute amount (about 1 microliter) of essential oil is injected into a tubular column temperature controlled to vaporize the sample. The constituents are separated by the differences in their solubilities in a nonvolatile absorbent that coats the inner walls of the tube. The vaporized sample is carried through the tube in a slow stream of helium or nitrogen, and all constituents are kept in the vaporous state by means of hot air circulating in the column. The results of the analysis are recorded as a series of peaks drawn by a pen recorder that plots a trace of each of the components of the essential oil as it exits the column. As the components exit, they are bombarded with high-energy electrons that fragment them. The characteristic fragmentation pattern for each molecule is identified by comparing it with a computerized pattern in a database.

A second important method of analysis is through optical rotation. The molecules within essential oils have the ability to rotate a plane of polarized light. This activity is measured by a polarimeter. Molecules that rotate counterclockwise are called laevorotatory, or l for short. Those that rotate clockwise are called dextrorotatory, or d. This designation is indicated in the name of the molecule, as in d-limonene. The angle at which the light is rotated is an important physical characteristic by which an essential oil can be recognized. Almost all essential oils show optical activity. This test can reveal synthetic compounds that alter the optical rotation.

Another method of analysis is the refractive index. When light passes through a liquid it is refracted. This refraction can be measured and is consistent for a given essential oil. In scientific terms, it is the ratio of the speed of light of a given frequency in a vacuum to the speed of light in a medium of some kind, at a specified temperature. It is important that the test be carried out at the same temperature as the reference (the standard).

A fourth analysis is the infrared test. Electromagnetic radiation can be passed through an essential oil and produces a spectrum that is like the fingerprint of the essential oil. Adulteration of the oil will show up clearly with this method.

The fifth and most important tool of analysis is the nose. When first experimenting with essential oils, you may find it hard to notice differences between synthetic and real essential oils and pure oils and adulterated ones. However with patience the nose learns. To sample an essential oil correctly, do not smell directly from the bottle. Put one or two drops on to a special smell strip (made from paper a little like blotting paper). Recap the bottle. Holding the smell strip approximately 6 inches in front of your face, move it slowly from one side to the other and back again. The sense of smell may be different from one nostril to the other as the aroma reaches different parts in the brain. One nostril may detect a sweeter smell than the other. Move the strip back and forth several times. Closing your eyes might aid concentration. It can be useful to rate the aroma on a scale of 0 to 10: 0 means disliking the odor intensely, and 10 means the odor is very pleasant. Write down a word or sentence that describes the aroma. When testing essential oils from an unknown source, first try one known to be authentic to "fix" the smell imprint in the mind. Then try the new one. The trained human nose is the most important piece of equipment in finding out whether the essential oil has been adulterated.

BUYING ESSENTIAL OILS

In the last few years there has been a rapid increase in the number of essential-oil companies. Many operate by direct mail. The commercial sections of healthcare journals include advertisements for many essential oil distributors. In the USA, most health-food shops, some drugstores, and certain department stores also carry a range of essential oils. Many essential oil mail-order companies have been set up quickly and with little knowledge of the oils. Customers believe they are buying essential oils of the highest grade (Scholes 2001).

Although many companies appear to provide true essential oils, this is not always the case. Some dealers openly state in their literature or on the bottles that their oils are diluted. Other companies are not so honest, and customers are led to believe that they are purchasing 100% pure essential oil. The phrase "pure essential oil" can mean many things. Essential oils are extremely easy to dilute or adulterate (Guenther 1972). The most common method of dilution is the addition of a vegetable oil. When this occurs, the essential oil leaves a ring as it evaporates. If alcohol is added to dilute the oil, it is sometimes discernible in the aroma. Adulteration by adding a cheaper substitute, for example, putting geranium oil in rose oil or petitgrain or bergamot in neroli, is commonplace. Real melissa oil is extremely difficult to find, because it is frequently adulterated with lemongrass or citral. Sometimes particular components are added, such as citronella, geraniol, or linalol (Wagner et al 1984). Some of the best melissa is actually grown in Ireland.

When purchasing essential oils, Scholes (2001) suggests first to determine the purpose for which the essential oil is being purchased. He lists several categories:

1. Medicinal or internal use
2. Candles and soaps
3. Massage and therapeutic applications
4. Cleaning products or environmental fragrancing

The second important factor is the oil's country of origin; several countries produce the same essential oil but of varying quality. For example, rose is grown and distilled in France, Bulgaria, Turkey, China, and Morocco. Scholes notes that only a few essential oils are produced in the United States—mainly peppermint, citrus, and some lavender. However, these are not suitable for the aromatherapy market because they have been grown with pesticides. There would seem to be a huge market out there for farmers wanting to grow something different!

For safety, you should only buy an essential oil that is correctly labeled. Much more information is needed than just the generic name. Product lists and bottle labels should bear the oil's complete botanical name, the country of origin, the part of the plant from which it was derived, and should note whether the oil is wild crafted or organic. Some of the best suppliers tell the buyer whether the whole flowering plant was used, or just the flowering heads. Reputable suppliers are happy to provide gas-chromatography/mass spectrometry (GCMS) information and material safety data sheets (MSDS) for their products. The chemotype, when relevant, also needs to be specified. Also mentioned on the product list should be the type of extraction used and whether the batch number is known. Organically grown plants used for essential-oil production are certified, and the bottles carry a stamp to prove it. There are various accepted organic stamps. In the United Kingdom, most authentic distributors are members of the Essential Oils Trade Association (EOTA) or the Aromatherapy Trade Council (ATC).

In the United States, the National Association for Holistic Aromatherapy offers the certification label "true aromatherapy product" (TAP). French and German oils usually have their own stamps of authenticity.

Bottles should contain integral droppers and be made of colored glass. "Pure 100 per cent essential oil" should be clearly marked. Basic safety precautions such as "do not take by mouth," "keep away from children," and "avoid contact with eyes" should also appear on the label. Apart from the label and the price, the only reliable indicators of authentic essential oils are an experienced nose and purchasing from a reputable company that would lose too much by compromising itself. It is best to ask around. Qualified aromatherapists tend to buy from the same small group of suppliers.

REFERENCES

Arctander S. 1960. Perfume and Flavor Materials of Natural Origin. Wheaton, IL: Allured Publishing, 13.

Alkaire B, Simon J. 1992. A portable steam distillation unit for essential oil crops. HortTechnology 2(4) 473-476.

Bowles J. 2000. The Basic Chemistry of Aromatherapeutic Essential Oils. Sydney, Australia: Pirie Printers.

Guenther E. 1972. The Essential Oils, Vol. I. Melbourne, FL: Krieger Publishing.

Guenther E. 1974. The Essential Oils: Individual Essential Oils of the Plant Families. Melbourne, FL: Krieger Publishing.

Guenther E. 1976. The Essential Oils, Vol. V. Melbourne, FL: Krieger Publishing.

Lawless J. 1992. Encyclopedia of Essential Oils. Shaftesbury, UK: Element Books.

Mann J. 2001a. Chemical Aspects of Biosynthesis. Oxford, UK: Oxford Science Publications, 2.

Mann J. 2001b. Secondary Metabolism. Oxford, UK: Oxford Science Publications, 7.

Poucher W.1993. Poucher's Perfumes, Cosmetics and Soaps, Vol 2, 9th ed. Chapman & Hall.

Piesse S. 1855. The Art of Perfumery. London: Longman, Brown & Green.

Price S. 1983. Practical Aromatherapy. London: Thorsons.

Scholes M. 2001. Finding the true essential oil. Aromatherapy Journal. 11(1) 19-23.

Suskind P. 1986. Perfume: The Story of a Murderer. London: Penguin Books, 62.

Tisserand R. 1985. The Essential Oil Safety Data Manual. Brighton, UK: Tisserand Aromatherapy Institute.

Tisserand R. 1994. Profile: Peter Wilde. International Journal of Aromatherapy. 6(2) 3-7.

Tisserand R, Balacs T. 1995. Essential Oil Safety. London: Churchill Livingstone.

Svoboda K, Svoboda T. 2001. Secretory Structures of Aromatic and Medicinal Plants. Wales, UK: Microscopix Publications.

Wagner H, Bladt S, Zgainski E. 1984. Plant Drug Analysis. Berlin, Germany: Springer-Verlag.

Wilde P. 1995. Flavour, fragrances and essential oils. In 13th International Congress Proceedings, Istanbul. Eskisehir, Turkey: Anadolu University Press, 351-357.

4

Essential Oil Toxicity and Contraindications

JUST BECAUSE essential oils are natural does not mean they do not have potential risks or hazards if used inappropriately. This section addresses toxicity and contraindications. Put in context, essential oils are extremely safe and carry few of the risks of many modern medicines. However, it is pertinent to the increasingly high profile of aromatherapy that all those using essential oils must be aware of possible side effects and interactions. The author is grateful to the help and advice of the expert reviewers of this section: Tony Balazs, PhD, and Ron Guba.

Part I: Essential Oil Toxicity

A sensory problem associated with fragrances is that they become less intense with repeated sniffs.

Schiffman (1992)

There is a certain amount of controversy about the toxicity of essential oils. There are those who say essential oils are dangerous and should never be taken orally. There are those who take essential oils orally or give them to their patients to take orally and see no problem. There are those who use essential oils every day, and there are those who believe taking an essential oil for longer than three weeks could lead to liver damage. Each point of view is usually based on the kind of aromatherapy training the person has received.

Jellinek (1999) writes that because the concentrations of substances in essential oils enter the body in the vapor state, the amount is smaller than the usual pharmacologic mode of application, and the likelihood of systemic side effects are reduced. Guba (2000) believes much of the concern about toxicity of essential oils is based on myth, and he gives a very strong argument to support his case. Scare tactics are counterproductive. Essential oils have been in the public domain for hundreds of years, and the number of toxicity problems is so few common sense indicates that, when used sensibly, essential oils must be safe. Perhaps what is needed is a large dose of common sense. Everything, even water, can be toxic if taken in too large a quantity.

This is where most potential problems with essential oils lie: use of extremely large amounts. For example, tea tree oil has become very popular and appears in shampoos, gels, creams, and lotions. It has been recommended for treating ticks and fleas in pets. However, Villar et al (1994) showed that, in some circumstances, large amounts of topically applied tea tree oil can be toxic to dogs and cats. Symptoms were depression, weakness, uncoordination, and muscle tremors. When tea tree oil was withheld, these symptoms disappeared within 2 or 3 days.

TOXICITY AND APPROACHES TO AROMATHERAPY

The English approach to aromatherapy focuses on using diluted essential oils (up to 5%) applied to the skin in a massage. Essential oils are used mainly for relaxation, stress management, and sometimes for upper respiratory-tract infections. There are no reports of toxic effects from using essential oils in this way. The French approach to aromatherapy may use several milliliters of undiluted essential oil on the skin at a time, sometimes several times a day. Physicians may also give patients gelatin capsules (each containing three or four drops of essential oils diluted in a carrier oil or gel) to be taken orally three or four times a day. Essential oils given in this way are used to treat infection or chronic conditions and are rarely used for relaxation. There is more chance of toxicity from the oral route, although there have been virtually no cases recorded. The majority of French physicians who use essential oils in this way are working alongside bacteriologists and pharmacists, and are well aware of toxicity issues. A potential toxicity hazard could occur when untrained people use essential oils orally and ingest too much.

Some aromatherapists (including myself) are trained in both external and internal methods of aromatherapy. Clearly there is a need and a place for both approaches, and perhaps a compromise that uses both could be the best of both worlds. However, each approach needs to take into consideration the experience, training, and expectations of the person giving the essential oils. The internal use of essential oils clearly means using them as medicines and, in the United States at least, this might be seen as outside the license of many health professionals. However, there is no licensing process for practitioners who wish to dispense herbal medicine in the United States, and the oral method of aromatherapy could easily be integrated under herbal medicine. There is an excellent chapter in

Essential Oil Safety (Tisserand & Balacs 1995) that covers toxicity in depth. This is recommended reading. There are also useful articles on the subject by Guba (2000) and Burfield (2001).

INGESTION REACTIONS

Toxicity can be nonspecific or specific. Nonspecific toxicity covers all essential oils when used in very large amounts. Specific toxicity pertains to those essential oils that can cause toxicity at lower levels, and these are outlined here (Table 4-1). Specific toxicity is roughly divided into two types: acute (short term) and chronic (long term). In acute toxicity, the worst scenario is poisoning. The symptoms of

Table 4-1 ❧ *Reported cases of overdose with common essential oils.*

Essential oil	Amount in ml	Symptoms	Source
Cinnamon	60	Dizziness, double vision, nausea, vomiting, collapse	Pilapil 1989
Citronella	15	Vomiting, shock, frothing at the mouth, deep rapid respiration, cyanosis, convulsions, brain hemorrhage, death	Mant 1961
Clove	5-10	Severe acidosis, central nervous system depression, ketones in urine, deteriorating liver function, extremely low blood glucose, generalized seizure, deep coma	Lane et al 1991 Hartnoll et al 1993
Eucalyptus	5	Vertigo, loss of coordination, abnormal respiration, epigastric pain, cold sweats Lesser amounts: excess respiratory tract mucus Greater amounts: decreased respiratory tract mucus, pinpoint pupils, rapid drowsiness, unconsciousness	Craig 1953 Patel & Wiggins 1980
Hyssop	10-20	Convulsions	Millet 1981

poisoning with ingested essential oils are nausea, vomiting, ataxia, confusion, convulsions, and coma (Patel & Wiggins 1980). Many papers about essential-oil poisoning cite instances when essential oils were taken orally; these cases usually involve children. In most instances, the amount of essential oil taken was substantially greater than is normally used orally, topically, or in inhalation aromatherapy.

Burfield (2001) cites an analysis of more than 100 pediatric poisoning accidents involving ingested eucalyptus. The study indicates that in 74% of cases, access to eucalyptus had been gained via the home vaporizer. The popularity of aromatherapy and today's easy access to bottles of essential oils mean poisoning is a potential hazard if someone decides to drink the essential oil. However most reputable companies supply bottles with integral droppers. Symptoms of oral poisoning can occur rapidly and include a burning sensation in the mouth and throat, abdominal pain, and spontaneous vomiting, although the latter may be delayed by up to 4 hours. Dangerous respiratory depression also can occur with deep coma. Convulsions may occur in children, but are rare in adults. Some fatalities have shown nephrotoxicity (Patel & Wiggins 1980). The range of when an essential oil becomes lethal is wide. For example, the safe dose for internal use of eucalyptus is 0.006 to 0.2 ml (Martindale 1977). Death in adults has occurred after ingestion of as little as 4 or 5 ml, which seems extremely low, and is usual after ingesting 30 ml (MacPherson 1925). However, people have recovered after ingesting up to 220 ml of eucalyptus essential oil (Gurr & Scroggie 1965).

Craig (1953) discusses the case of a 3-year-old who consumed 10 ml of eucalyptus (2 teaspoons). He became deeply unconscious; his pupils constricted, muscle tone was markedly reduced, and there were no tendon reflexes. His breathing was shallow and irregular at a rate of 10 breaths per minute. Insertion of an endotracheal tube produced no gag reflex. Pulse was 70 beats per minute, and blood pressure was 75/40 mm Hg. The child's serum urea was 6.3 μmol/L (38 mg/100 ml) with normal electrolytes. He was given gastric lavage with sodium bicarbonate solution. Sodium sulphate (100 ml) was left in the stomach as a cathartic. After 2 hours, his pulse, blood pressure, and respiration were normal. He was discharged after 48 hours in hospital.

Wilkinson (1991) discusses the toxic effect of ingested essential oils on three children admitted to an emergency room in Australia. Their ages were 19 months, 23 months, and 25 months. The 19-month-old ingested an indeterminate amount of lavender. The kind of lavender was not specified because poison reports tend not to include botanical names, but the chemistry of *Lavandula angustifolia*, *L. latifolia*, and *L. stoechas* are very different and therefore their toxicities are different. *L. stoechas*, which contains ketones, would be more toxic than *L. angustifolia*, which contains mainly linalyl acetate or linalol. It was also not specified whether the lavender oil was synthetic or natural. The 25-month-old took an unknown amount of tea tree oil, and the 23-month-old ingested 40 ml of eucalyptus oil. All three children were ataxic. All three were anesthetized and given gastric lavage, and two were also intubated. Charcoal was given in all cases and sorbitol in one. All three children recovered fully in the hospital.

A fourth child who consumed 30 ml of eucalyptus became comatose after falling against a coffee table. Gastric lavage was performed, and the child recovered after 4 days of fluctuating consciousness.

Much hype surrounds pennyroyal as an abortificant. However there are very few cases reported. There are a few cases of toxicity, all of them situations in which the essential oil was ingested. Pennyroyal, although not used frequently in aromatherapy, is used in herbal remedies and teas, and some of the teas contain the essential oil. Bakerink et al (1996) reported on two infant siblings who were given home-brewed tea of pennyroyal. Serum levels of pulegone and its metabolite menthofuran were then taken. The first infant tested positive for menthofuran (10 ng/ml) and manifested fulminant liver failure with cerebral edema and necrosis, followed by death. The second infant tested positive for pulegone (25ng/ml) and menthofuran (41 ng/ml) and manifested hepatic dysfunction and several epileptic seizures. There have been no recorded instances of pennyroyal toxicity following dermal application.

Temple et al (1991) reported on five cases of citronella poisoning. All involved young children who drank varying amounts of the essential oil. Because citronella is a nonspecific toxin, a large amount must be ingested to yield toxic effects. All five children recovered. William Robertson, Medical Director of Children's Hospital and Medical Center, Seattle, Washington, comments at the end of the report that he "would judge the risk of severe poisoning to be relatively remote."

Even the ubiquitous linalol has been tested for toxicity. Following oral absorption in the gut of a mouse, 55% was rapidly excreted in the urine as urea, dihydro, and tetrahydrolinalool; 15% was eliminated in feces; and 23% was expired with carbon dioxide after a lag period of several hours (Powers & Beasley 1985). After oral administration, 3% remained in the tissues: 0.5% in the liver, 0.6% in the gut, 0.8% in the skin, and 1.2% in the skeletal muscle. Acute systemic toxicity was demonstrated with ataxia, a decrease in spontaneous motor activity, lateral recumbency, vasodilation, rapid decrease in arterial blood pressure, and respiratory disturbance leading to death.

MEASURING TOXICITY

Much of the information available on toxicity is based on animal studies. Of course, this is true of conventional drugs as well. Most essential oils have had extensive toxicologic studies carried out by the fragrance industry (for inhaled and topically applied essential oils) and the flavor industry (for ingested essential oils). Guba (2000) draws attention to the way toxicology studies are carried out. Usually a very large amount of essential oil is given to the test animal in a very short period. This is totally unlike the human situation in which small amounts of essential oils are given during a longer period. The huge amounts given in animal testing are never given all at once to humans, and rarely are such large amounts given during an extended period.

There are two ways essential-oil toxicity can be measured: oral and dermal. Both are tested on animals. Oral lethal dose is usually tested on laboratory mice or rats. The animals are force-fed essential oils until 50% of them die. The amount the test group has ingested when this occurs is the median lethal dose, which is know as LD50. This is the number of milligrams or grams of essential oil per kilogram of animal body weight it took to kill half the animals.

There is a difference between a poison and a lethal substance. Whereas a lethal substance kills the system, a poison is any substance that "irritates, damages or impairs the activity of the body's tissues" and is "harmful in relatively small amounts"(McFerran 1996). A poison is not always lethal. So although the lethal dose of an essential oil can tell us what will kill a patient, substantially less than that can have poisonous effects. Even so, the amount required to produce poisonous effects is staggeringly high, depending on the oil in question.

The LD50 dermal lethal dose is determined via a test on a shaved area of the skin of animals, usually rabbits. Human skin is less permeable than rabbit skin. When 50% of the test subjects die, that is the dermal LD50. There have been very few clinical tests on human skin. Those that have been carried out involved volunteers who were given a patch test for a 24-hour period (Watt 1991). The largest patch study to date was carried out by Japanese scientists, spanned 8 years, and involved 200 human volunteers who used 270,000 patch tests. Asian skin may be more or less sensitive than Caucasian skin (International School of Aromatherapy 1993).

Simple math can also be used to show how close to the toxic level a 5% solution of an essential oil used as topical application can come. If the dermal LD50 of eucalyptus globulus is 5 g/kg (actually it is more than 10% according to Kligman), then the following equations determine toxicity:

Average woman of 150 lbs = approximately 75 kg
$5 \times 75 = 375$ grams = approximately 400 ml (allowing for specific gravity).
If the solution is 5%, 8000 ml are required = 8 L

It is unknown exactly how much of the eucalyptus is absorbed through the skin—certainly not 100%. Much depends on the skin's integrity, its temperature, and whether it is covered after application of the oil. Let us allow for 50% absorption (which is generous). It is impossible for 4 L of essential oil to be absorbed by the skin all at once. (However, there would be considerable effects from inhaling the essential oil as well.)

Oral LD50 of eucalyptus globulus is 2.48 g/kg
Average woman of 150 lbs = approximately 75 kg
$2.48 \times 75 = 186$ g = approximately 200 ml (allowing for specific gravity)

SKIN REACTIONS

In skin tests, adverse reactions can be divided into irritation, allergic sensitivity, and phototoxicity. Sensitivity and safety are covered in Chapter 4. Some essential oils are thought to be dangerous when used undiluted on the skin. These include essential oils high in phenols or aromatic aldehydes (like cinnamaldehyde). I have also found some oxide-rich essential oils can be irritating to abraded mucosa. However, many phenol-rich essential oils are used in France at high dilutions to treat infections Tiger Balm, a popular cream for aches and sprains, contains 60% essential oils including cassia, clove, and camphor. However Tiger Balm applied to a scratched skin surface is not comfortable, and it should not be applied to a baby's skin. Guba (2000) suggests using 90% nonirritant essential oil with 10% phenolic oil if high concentrations or undiluted essential oils are required.

INHALATION TOXICITY

Inhaled essential oils are unlikely to produce a toxic reaction. Hypothetically, a toxic reaction could occur if a person was confined to a nonventilated room, the temperature was very high, and there was a constant diffusion of essential oil until the air was saturated. However, the effect of this situation would be more like suffocation than a reaction to the essential oil.

REFERENCES

Bakerink J, Gospe S, Dimand R et al. 1996. Multiple organ failure after ingestion of pennyroyal oil from herbal tea in two infants. Pedatrics. 98(5) 944-947.

Burfield T. 2001. Safety of essential oils. International Journal of Aromatherapy. 10(1/2) 16-29.

Craig J. 1953. Poisoning by the volatile oils in children. Archives of Disease in Childhood. 55(5) 475-483.

Guba R. 2000. Toxicity myths: The actual risks of essential oil use. International Journal of Aromatherapy. 10(1/2) 37-49.

Gurr F, Scroggie J. 1965. Eucalyptus poisoning treated by dialysis and mannitol infusion with an appendix on the analysis of biological fluids for alcohol and eucaluptol. Australasian Annals of Medicine. 14(3) 238-249.

Hartnoll G, Moore D, Douek D. 1993. Near fatal ingestion of oil of cloves. Archives of Disease in Childhood. 69:392-393.

International School of Aromatherapy. 1993. A safety guide on the use of essential oils. London: Nurtured by Nature Oils, Ltd.

Jellinek S. 1999. Odors and mental states. International Journal of Aromatherapy. 9(3) 115-120.

Kligman A. 1966. The identification of contact allergens by human assay. Journal of Investigative Dermatology 47(5) 393-409.

Lane B, Ellenhorn MJ, Hulbert TV et al. 1991. Clove ingestion in an infant. Human and Experimental Toxicology. 10(4) 291-294.

MacPherson J. 1925. The toxicology of eucalyptus oil. The Medical Journal of Australia. 2:108-110.

Mant A. 1961. A case of poisoning by oil of citronella. Association Proceeding VI. Medicine, Science, and the Law. 1, 170-171.

Martindale W. 1977. The Extra Pharmacopoeia, 27th ed. London: Pharmaceutical Press.

McFerran T (ed.). 1996. Oxford Dictionary of Nursing, 2nd ed. Oxford, UK: Oxford University Press.

Millet Y. 1981. Toxicity of some essential plant oils. Clinical and experimental study. Clinical Toxicology. 18(12) 1485-1498.

Patel S, Wiggins J. 1980. Eucalyptus poisoning. Archives of Disease in Childhood. 55(5) 405-406.

Pilapil V. 1989. Toxic manifestations of cinnamon oil ingestion in a child. Clinical Pediatrics. 28(6) 276.

Powers K, Beasley V. 1985. Toxicological aspects of linalool: A review. Veterinary and Human Toxicology. 27(6) 484-485.

Schiffman S. 1992. Aging and the sense of smell: Potential benefits of fragrance enhancement. In Van Toller S, Dodd G (eds.), Fragrance: The Psychology and Biology of Perfume. London: Elsevier Applied Science, 54.

Temple W, Nerida A, Beasley M, et al. 1991. Management of oil of citronella poisoning. Clinical Toxicology. 29(2) 257-262.

Tisserand R, Balacs T. 1995. Essential Oil Safety. London: Churchill Livingstone.

Villar D, Knight M, Hansen S et al. 1994. Toxicity of melaleuca oil and related essential oils applied topically on dogs and cats. Veterinary and Human Toxicology. 36(2) 139-142.

Watt M. 1991. Plant Aromatics. Essex, UK: Witham.

Wilkinson H. 1991. Childhood ingestion of volatile oils. The Medical Journal of Australia. 154:430-431.

PART II: CONTRAINDICATIONS

A good name is like a precious ointment; it filleth all around about, and will not easily away: for the odors of ointments are more durable than those of flowers.

Francis Bacon

M any adverse reactions can be avoided if pure essential oils are used. Essential oils are steam distilled, and therefore the potential for adverse reactions to something other than the essential oils (e.g., a solvent) is eradicated. It is logical to assume that essential oils that have been adulterated, or extended, are more likely to cause a problem, although this is difficult to prove. Nonetheless, the possibility of adverse reactions to pure, unadulterated essential oils cannot be ruled out totally. These reactions may happen with patients who are already on multiple drug regimens or who are allergy prone. Patch testing can do much to detect, and therefore avoid, these reactions. There are also a few essential oils that can cause dermal irritation if used undiluted.

The amount of essential oil used tends to be measured in percentages or drops. However, there is some confusion over how big a drop is! Olleveant et al (1999) investigated several suppliers of bergamot oil and showed that their drop sizes differed. However, an average measurement used by aromatherapists is 20 drops of essential oil to 1 ml. Patch tests can be used to avoid skin reactions such as irritation and sensitivity and are suggested for all potential-risk patients. Dilute the essential oil to double the concentration to be used and put it on an adhesive bandage. Place the bandage on the patient's forearm and leave in place for 24 hours to assess any adverse reactions.

POSSIBLE SKIN REACTIONS

Irritation

Skin irritation is produced by an irritant component within the essential oil and occurs immediately, usually producing a red wheal or burn. The irritant component is most often a phenol (found in clove, oregano, and thyme) or an aromatic aldehyde (found in cinnamon). The reaction sensation is one of heat and burning. Immediate dilution with a carrier oil is required, followed by washing with warm water and nonperfumed soap. Do not use water initially; that pushes the essential oil into the dermis. This kind of instant irritation from a 2% to 5% dilution of a pure, fresh essential oil is a rare event and is more likely to occur with much higher concentrations. Essential oils with high percentages of phenols or aromatic aldehydes should not be used undiluted on the skin.

Skin irritation caused by a chemical used in the extraction method may also occur. Solvent chemicals are not used in true essential oils and their presence indicates that the extract is an absolute, not an essential oil. There have also been incidences of erythema following the use of topical benzoin (Rademaker & Kirby 1987; Lesesne 1992). Benzoin is sometimes used in a proprietary spray before applying an adhesive dressing. Old citrus peel oils (e.g., mandarin, bergamot, and lemon) in which the terpene content has oxidized can also lead to irritation. Expressed oils do spoil quickly, and an opened bottle should be used within 6 months. The case is similar with pine oils. Cinnamon is thought to be responsible for an adverse reaction to trichlorophenol (TCP), a commonly used antiseptic in the United Kingdom (Calnan 1976). Cinnamon is no longer used in this product.

Sensitivity: Contact Dermatitis

Sensitization to an essential oil is an allergic reaction that occurs over time. At the first exposure nothing much may happen. However, in a similar manner to some drug sensitivities (e.g., penicillin), subsequent exposures produce stronger reactions. These reactions can occur in the form of a rash, sneezing, or shortness of breath. Sensitivity also can occur after long-term habitual use. Considering the ubiquitous use of fragrance materials in everyday products, the actual risk of side effects from a fragrance is small (De Groot & Frosch 1997). However, fragrance allergy is the most common cause of cosmetic contact dermatitis, affecting 1% of the population. Of greatest concern are the "fragrance-free" products that still contain fragrance raw materials (Scheinman 1997).

On June 20, 2001, a meeting was held at the British Fragrance Association in London to propose European Economic Council legislation requiring labeling for the fragrance product industry. The proposal stated approximately 20 chemicals thought to be allergens would need to be listed on future labels. This legislation would apply if any of the chemicals constituted 0.001% of the product or more. The chemicals are common, occurring in essential oils such as linalol and geraniol. There was no differentiation between synthetic and natural chemicals. The label was to state "Can cause an allergic reaction." This kind of labeling could be enforced in the United States. Although it is laudable to try to curb the onslaught of synthetic aromas that bombard shoppers in every mall, labeling an essential oil as a potential sensitizer because it contains something on a list gives the wrong impression. Rose and lavender soaps have been used for hundreds of years without incident. However, now that synthetic fragrances are introduced into almost every product, sensitivity may well increase.

Some reactions may build up throughout many years. Juniper took 25 years to produce sensitivity in the case of a lady who sold food smoked and spiced in juniper oils. Eventually she developed a dry cough and asthma. Skin tests showed sensitivity to juniper, although it was not established whether the wood resin or the berries were to blame (Roethe et al 1973). In another instance, a 53-year-old woman who was patch tested suddenly had eczema appear on various uncovered parts of her skin: her neck, hands, and scalp (Schaller & Korting 1995). The woman had been using aroma lamps continuously for more than a year in her home, and it was presumed she had become sensitive to the scents of lavender, jasmine, and rosewood. It is not clear whether she had been using pure essential oils. However this example does underline that the same essential oils should not be used continuously or as "blanket cover."

I have found that patients taking several medications at the same time are more likely to be sensitive to essential oils than patients who are not taking several medications. Those who have an allergy-like illness such as asthma, eczema, or hay fever may also be more sensitive to potential allergenic components, such as lactones, found in essential oils. A florist who presented with an allergic reaction to Roman chamomile *(Chamaemelum nobile)* was found to have a prior sensitivity to chamomile herbal teas and ointments (Van Ketel 1982). Another florist, who had had dermatitis of the face for 1 year, was found to be allergic to the sesquiterpenes in German chamomile *(Matricaria recutita)* (Van Ketel 1987). Lavender, thought to be the safest of all essential oils, caused an allergy in a hairdresser who used lavender shampoo several times a day for several years. The allergen involved was believed to be linalol or linalyl acetate (Brandao 1986).

Sometimes the mixture of a chemical and an essential oil can trigger an allergic reaction. This was the case when an aromatherapist sprayed her roses with an insecticide, and 24 hours later developed acute, bilateral hand eczema. She had been using French marigold *(Tagetes patula)* on a patient. The oil had been obtained by solvent extraction (so it was not a true essential oil). Tests showed the allergic reaction was caused by a cross-reaction between the synthetic pyrethroid in the insecticide and the acetone-soluble extract of the marigold leaves and flowers (Bilsland & Strong 1990). French marigold is an unusual choice in aromatherapy; it smells unpleasant and always needs to be used with caution because of its high percentage of tagetone, which can cause skin reactions. Its main use is in the treatment of fungal infections, but it has been mostly replaced by tea tree oil. One wonders whether the aromatherapist believed she was using common marigold *(Calendula officinalis)*, which is a nonirritant and is used for its powerful skin-healing properties.

Citral is a potential sensitizer on its own, but essential oils of lemongrass and melissa, which contain high percentages of citral, rarely produce sensitivity reactions when used in aromatherapy. The presence of d-limonene in the essential oils may produce a quenching effect. The wide range and complexity of components in essential oils suggests that nature is offering a "balanced menu" so the receiver can take the parts of the meal the body needs and leave the rest. This may be why the effect of an isolated ingredient can be much stronger: it is no longer part of the "balanced menu".

Sandalwood, thyme, and guaiacwood oils have caused sensitivity in those sensitive to balsams (Tisserand & Balacs 1995). Sandalwood causes frequent allergic reactions, which are thought to be related to its b-santalol content (Nakayama et al 1974). Geraniol is a component of many perfumes and may cause cross-sensitivity in those who have used perfumed products for many years. Ylang ylang may cause a similar problem.

The most common allergic skin reaction is a stinging, painful wheal or generalized urticaria. These reactions are sometimes accompanied by bronchial inflammation producing asthmalike symptoms (Watt 1991). Even tea tree oil, so often recommended for its gentleness, has produced contact dermatitis when used undiluted on the skin of someone allergic to a component found within tea tree. In this particular case, the actual oil used was found to have a high eucalyptol content (De Groot & Weyland 1992). Another name for eucalyptol is 1,8-cineole, which is an oxide. However, tea tree oil is supposed to have a high content of 1-terpinen-4-ol, an alcohol, and a low proportion of 1,8-cineole.

Sieben et al (2001) investigated the effect of eight common components of fragrances on 32 fragrance-allergic patients who had previously responded with a positive skin-patch test. The eight common components studied were eugenol, isoeugenol, geraniol, oak moss, a-amyl-cinnamic aldehyde, cinnamic aldehyde, cinnamic alcohol, and hydroxycitronellal. These are the most common observed contact allergens (Marks et al 1998). Data indicated positive patch tests are a cell-mediated, antigen-specific phenomenon rather than a nonspecific irritating condition. The authors believed the increase in fragrance allergies was a response to the indiscriminate use of fragrances in food, household products, paint, and medicines. Larsen (2000) suggests cosmetic labels should include a list of common fragrance allergens so people will know to avoid those to which they are allergic.

Phototoxicity

Phototoxicity is an interaction between a component in an essential oil, the skin, and ultraviolet photons. This means exposure to sun-bed radiation or natural sunlight can produce a skin reaction. Such reactions can vary from pigmentation of the skin to severe full-thickness burns. The most common components causing phototoxicity are furanocoumarins. Lemon oil contains oxypeucedanin and bergapten, both furanocoumarins that produce phototoxic reactions. Lime and bitter orange oils also contain these components, but in smaller quantities (Naganuma et al 1985). Angelica root oil contains furanocoumarins and can also produce phototoxicity (Tisserand & Balacs 1995).

Bergamot was used in self-tanning preparations until 12 cases of skin reaction were reported after the use of this type of product. In two cases (in which skin had been exposed to the sun immediately after application of the tanning cream) symptoms of erythema as well as pigmentation were present (Meyer 1970). However, furanocoumarins can be removed from bergamot oil. The oil is then classified as bergaptene-free or furanocoumarin-free (FCF). Some therapists will not use FCF essential oils, and some distributors will not supply them, saying they will only use "whole" oils. However in areas with lots of sunshine, FCF oils might be safer. Deterpenated citrus oils contain disproportionately higher concentrations of furanocoumarins and are best avoided.

Chemical Burns

Parys (1983) reported on undiluted peppermint oil inadvertently spilled on skin that had already been traumatized by skin grafts. The area necrosed and required excision and further surgery.

Chronic Toxicity

Chronic toxicity is a term usually referring to the oral use of essential oils. Chronic toxicity is dose-dependent but also related to the length of time spent using a toxic substance. Death may eventually occur, but it is the preceding slow tissue damage that is the main problem. It is unlikely that inhaled or topically applied essential oils would cause chronic toxicity, even if large amounts were used over extended periods.

REACTIONS WITH ORTHODOX DRUGS

Drug Combinations and Pharmacokinetics

Blashke and Bjornsson (1989) define an interacting drug combination as "one that has the potential, documented in humans, to produce a clinically significant change in the pharmacologic response to its constituent drugs that is larger or smaller than the sum of the effects when the drugs are administered separately." Hansten and Horn (1989) estimate that 7.4% of all hospitalized patients experience an interacting drug combination during their hospital stay. Compounding this problem is the knowledge that individual patients respond in varying ways to the same dose of the same drug. This variation is thought to be directly related to pharmacokinetics: the mathematical description of the rate and extent of absorption, distribution, and elimination of drugs in the body (Gwilt 1994). These three processes determine the movements of drugs within the body. However, despite advances in understanding, a great deal is not yet known about drug combinations and pharmacokinetics.

Because there are documented differences between individuals with regard to the absorption of several orthodox drugs like phenytoin and digoxin, it is expected that the absorption of essential oils will also vary. Absorption depends on the mode of delivery; the transdermal route is thought to be slower and more controlled. It is thought to reduce the difference between the maximum and minimum drug concentrations attained during a dosing interval (Blaschke & Bjornsson 1995). The distribution of any drug is controlled by blood flow to the tissue or organ, as well as by the drug's ability to bind to plasma proteins. Distribution is also related to whether the drug molecules are lipid-soluble or water-soluble.

Elimination takes place at the same time as distribution and occurs primarily in the kidneys, although metabolism (which can include deactivation) occurs in the liver. Metabolism is the mechanism whereby drug action is terminated or, in the case of drugs such as aspirin, activated (Grant 1994). Some lipid-soluble, nonionized drugs can be completely reabsorbed in the liver. This metabolism includes a chemical conversion that allows the drug (or essential oil) to become more water-soluble, and therefore easier to excrete in the urine. Essential oils that are inhaled or applied topically do not go through the first stage of metabolism by the liver (Price & Price 1999).

Because they are lipid-soluble, components within essential oils gain easy access to the brain. While being transported by the bloodstream, the components travel readily to the adrenal glands and kidneys (Tisserand & Balacs 1995). The rate of elimination of a drug from the body is proportional to the concentration of that drug in the bloodstream. It is a complicated equation because the drug (or essential oil) begins to be eliminated while it is still being absorbed (Balazs 2002) In most instances, the biologic half-life ($t_{1/2}$), rather than the elimination rate, is documented. The half-life is the time taken for the drug concentration in the blood to decrease by one half. It depends on both the volume of distribution of the drug and the rate at which that drug is eliminated from the body (known as clearance) (Gwilt 1994).

Drugs and essential oils are excreted via the kidneys, lungs, skin, and feces. In addition, many nursing mothers also excrete drugs, and therefore components of essential oils, in their breast milk (Berndt & Stitzel 1994). Theoretically, essential oils could interact with orthodox drugs in several ways: by combining with a cellular receptor (and thereby competing with the drug), by combining with plasma protein, or by combining with and somehow altering the chemistry of the drug to produce a different compound with different effects (Tisserand & Balacs 1995).

Cellular Receptors

Most drugs combine with a molecular structure called a receptor, which is found on the surface of cells. This produces a molecular change in the receptor and leads to a chain of events called a response. The same situation occurs with naturally formed neurotransmitters and hormones secreted by the body itself. Some drugs produce the same effects as naturally occurring substances because they combine with the same receptors at a cellular level. An example of this is morphine mimicking the effects of endorphins (Fleming 1994).

It is known that receptors only react with a limited number of substances that have a similar molecular structure. Therefore an essential oil with a molecular structure similar to that of a drug known to bind to a particular receptor may also combine with that receptor. An example of this is anethole and its polymers, dianethole and photoanethole, which bear a striking resemblance to the catecholamine dopamines adrenaline and noradrenaline (Albert-Puleo 1980). Also worthy of mention are the nonsteroidal compounds with estrogenic activity found in plants, which mimic the A-ring of steroids (Murad & Kuret 1990). However, just because a molecule has a similar structure does not mean it will mimic a neurotransmitter (Balazs 2002).

Combining at the Plasma Level

Most drugs found in the vascular compartment bind with one of the macromolecules in the plasma. Compartmental modeling is used as a theoretical vehicle for assessing the distribution of drugs (Blaschke & Bjornsson 1995). This binding is reversible because only an unbound drug can diffuse through the capillary wall, produce systemic effects, be metabolized, and then be excreted. As the macromolecule circulates within the bloodstream, so the vascular system works as a human drug distributor.

There is no reason to suppose an essential oil could not also bind with plasma proteins. It could bind with one of the most important plasma proteins, albumin, because most albumin-bound drugs are only slightly soluble in water. Drug binding at this level is nonspecific, and displacements frequently occur when a newer drug with a higher affinity comes along. This means the previous drug is suddenly free to be distributed to another part of the body. In some diseases, such as uremia, plasma-protein binding is reduced.

Changing the Action or Potency of a Drug

Certain components found in essential oils aid the penetration of drugs through the skin of animals (Williams & Barry 1989). Therefore it is possible that the topical application of an essential oil could increase the level of drug being received by a patient using patch therapy (e.g., hormone replacement therapy) if the oil is applied at the site of drug absorption. However, no documented information has confirmed this yet.

Freitas et al (1993) found that b-myrcene affected the metabolism of barbiturates in rats. The rats were given b-myrcene orally 1 hour before an intraperitoneal injection of pentobarbital. This enhanced the sleeping time and was attributed to the pentobarbital-biotransforming enzymes found in b-myrcene. However, when b-myrcene was given 1 day before the barbiturate injection, the sleeping time was reduced by 50%. b-myrcene is found in lemongrass (Sheppard-Hangar 1995).

Wintergreen and sweet birch are essential oils not commonly used in aromatherapy, mainly because they contain high levels of methyl salicylate (closely related to acetylsalicylic acid or aspirin). Some safety data manuals call them hazardous (Tisserand & Balacs 1995; Anonymous 1993). However, they are found in many proprietary creams (such as Deep Heat) for sprains and strains, as well as in chewing gum and candy (Guba 2000). Wintergreen and sweet birch essential oils are easy to purchase. Guba (2000) suggests that 10 ml of a 2.4% mix of wintergreen in carrier oil would give approximately 250 mg methyl salicylate, equivalent to one tablet of aspirin. Methyl salicilate is absorbed through the skin and can affect warfarin anticoagulation therapy (Littleton 1990; Yip et al 1990). Guba

(2000) suggests that because only 50% of methyl salicilate would be absorbed, the amount produced from wintergreen oil in this experiment would be no more toxic than rubbing half an aspirin on the skin. However, aspirin is known to affect the blood-clotting mechanism and prostaglandin production. The combination of regular amounts of an aspirinlike substance (wintergreen) and warfarin could lead to hemorrhage. Collins et al (1984) showed that blood salicylate reached maximum level 20 minutes after Deep Heat cream was applied to the skin. Guba (2000) recommends not using wintergreen for full body treatments or when the patient is taking warfarin or some other anticoagulant therapy. However, several proprietary brands of creams for arthritis contain similar acetylsalicylic acid-like components and do not offer warnings. Many volatile chemicals are absorbed though the skin (Riviere et al 1997). There seems to be a question as to whether essential oils reach the bloodstream in sufficient quantities after a topical aromatherapy treatment to have a pharmacologic effect (Balazs 2002).

Essential oils containing b-asarone or d-pulegone may increase the toxic effects of a drug because they both induce the detoxifying enzyme cytochrome P450. (These substances are found in essential oils that are rarely used because they are thought to be toxic themselves.) Drugs that induce this enzyme include progestogens (found in the contraceptive pill), diphenhydramine (an antihistamine), pethidine, nitrazepam, phenobarbitone, and phenytoin, the last four being frequently used hospital drugs (Tisserand & Balacs 1995). Fortunately, very few essential oils contain b-asarone or d-pulegone, and few that do are in regular use. They include wintergreen, cultivated carrot seed, calamus (which contains b-asarone), and pennyroyal (which contains d-pulegone). Madhava-Madyastha and Chadha (1986) found that 1,8-cineole, administered by inhalation, induced the liver microsomal cytochrome P450 to a significant extent in rats. However, Tisserand and Balacs (1995) state the amounts used in aromatherapy is insufficient to induce changes in cytochrome P450 activity. Chiou et al (1997) found that beta-uedesmol, a sesquiterpene found in West Indian sandalwood, alleviated electric shock-induced seizures in rat tissue and may enhance the effect of epilepsy drugs such as phenytoin.

A study by Perez Raya et al (1990) has shown that two different species of mint enhance the effect of pentobarbitone in rats. Both *Mentha rotundifolia* and *Mentha longifolia* significantly enhanced sodium-pentobarbital induced sleep. Lavender was also shown to enhance sodium-pentobarbital-induced sleep in rats, although the effect ceased if treatment lasted longer than 5 days (Delaveau et al 1989). Guillemain et al (1989) also demonstrated the ability of lavender *(Lavandula angustifolia)* to enhance neurodepressant effects. However, these findings are a long way from proving a similar action on enzymes in humans.

Almirall et al (1996) found that 1,8-cineole, d-limonene, and pinene permeated the skin and affected topical application of conventional drugs such as haloperidol and chlorpromazine. Whereas 1,8-cineole and d-limonene enhanced the transdermal permeability of haloperidol, d-limonene reduced the transdermal permeability of chlorpromazine. The oxide 1,8-cineole (also called eucalyptol) is found in rosemary, cardamon, spike lavender, sage, and eucalyptus (Bowles 2000), and d-limonene is found in many citrus-peel oils.

Jori et al (1969) studied the effects of several components of essential oils on the metabolism of drugs in rats. The components, which were delivered by aerosol or subcutaneously, were eucalyptol (1,8-cineole), guaiacol, menthol, and essential oil of *Pinus pumilio* (which contained a-pinene, phellandrene, dipentene, sylvestrene, and bornyl acetate). Eucalyptol was shown to increase the activity of the microsomal enzymatic reaction and altered the metabolism of drugs. The disappearance rate from brain and plasma of amphetamine and pentobarbital was increased after eucalyptol administration, but eucalyptol had no influence on phenylbutazone. An increased plasma disappearance was also shown to occur in humans after 10 days' treatment with eucalyptol aerosol.

Hohenwaller and Kima (1971) found that eucalyptol, either given subcutaneously or by aerosol, raised in vivo phenobarbital metabolism. The change of enzyme activity with time resembled the change of drug concentration in blood serum. The mechanism of eucalyptol appeared to be quite different from the mechanism of phenobarbital in three ways. First, unlike the rapid decrease of phenobarbital, eucalyptol disappeared gradually. Second, enzyme activity continued after the end of treatment with eucalyptol. Third, a single treatment of eucalyptol caused reduction in enzyme activity, but several doses of phenobarbital were required. Hohenwaller and Kima (1971) concluded "many other mechanisms beside enzyme synthesis must be involved in producing the striking differences on the action of the two drugs." Eucalyptol is used extensively in the pharmaceutical preparations for external application and as a nasal spray. However, Tisserand and Balacs (1995) state that because essential oils are used in such small amounts compared with orthodox drugs, even if they are given orally, they are unlikely to affect the therapeutic action of most orthodox pharmacology.

Certain essential oils may react with other medications. In some instances essential oils may enhance the effects of orthodox drugs, whereas in other cases they may interfere at a cellular level, reducing the effectiveness of medication. Ylang ylang *(Cananga odorata)* enhances the dermal absorption of 5-Fluorouracil sevenfold (Williams & Barry 1989). Blue gum eucalyptus *(Eucalyptus globulus)* enhances the activity of streptomycin, isoniazid, and sulfetrone in *Mycobacterium tuberculosis* (Kufferath & Mundualgo 1954; Guillemain et al 1989). Eucalyptol (1,8-cineole) found in gully gum *(Eucalyptus smithii)*, and blue gum eucalyptus *(E. globulus* and *E. fruticetorum)* produced a significant decrease in pentobarbital effects and dose-related effects on the liver-enzyme activity of rats (Jori et al 1969). The reduction in sedative effect occurred even when the eucalyptus had been administered 36 hours previously.

Roman chamomile *(Chamaemelum nobile)* was found to be incompatible with the administration of products containing Peruvian bark, tannin, or silver salts (Chiej 1984). These are sometimes present in old-fashioned preparations used for pressure-area care.

Acetaminophen (paracetamol) is a common analgesic that reduces the level of glutathione in the liver. Glutathione is responsible for absorbing free radicals, and when the level of glutathione falls, reactive molecules such as free radicals can attack the liver cells with potentially fatal consequences. It is extremely unlikely that the small amounts of essential oils used in aromatherapy could adversely affect glutathione production. However, in a patient using the maximum recommended dosage of Tylenol, it might be advisable to avoid essential oils containing transanethole, estragole, and eugenol (Tisserand & Balacs 1995). This means avoiding the following essential oils: fennel *(Foeniculum vulgare),* aniseed *(Pimpinella anisum),* basil *(Ocimum basilicum),* and clove *(Syzygium aromaticum).*

Terpineol is thought to enhance prednisolone absorption through the skin (Williams & Barry 1989). Terpineol is found in many essential oils, including niaouli, ravansara, and tea tree. Godwin and Michniak (1999) found that terpinen-4-ol and a-terpineol enhanced the dermal penetration of hydrocortisone four to five times in mice. Both of these chemical components are found in tea tree oil. Limonene is thought to increase indomethacin absorption through the skin. Indomethacin is a drug commonly used in arthritis. Limonene is a monoterpene that occurs in many essential oils from citrus peels. Menthol lowers the melting point of testosterone (which is solid at room temperature) and increases the permeation of testosterone through the skin eightfold (Kaplun-Frischoff & Touitou 1997). Bowles (2000) suggests that there could be a remote possibility of myristicin (found in nutmeg) compounding the effect of serotonin-altering drugs.

Cedarwood *(Cedrus atlantica)* reduces the effect of barbiturate-induced sleep (Wade et al 1968). This study also showed that cedarwood could reduce the amount of dicoumarol in the blood. Dicoumarol is an anticoagulant that can be obtained from sweet clover (Budavari 1996). Eugenol has been shown to have antiplatelet activity (Janssens et al 1990), and should be avoided in patients receiving anticoagulant therapy. Eugenol occurs in clove leaf and bud, pimento berry and leaf, and cinnamon leaf. Cinnamon leaf is thought to depress liver glutathione levels in rats and may interfere with the body's metabolization of acetamionphen.

Finally, some patients with particular enzyme deficits or specific conditions may be affected by certain essential oils. Male children of Chinese, West African, Mediterranean, and Middle Eastern origin are susceptible to a deficiency of glucose-6-phosphate dehydrogenase. This enzyme is responsible for liver detoxification of menthol. When the enzyme is missing, toxic build-up of menthol can occur (Owole & Ramson-Kuto 1980). Large amounts of peppermint should be avoided in these children.

Rosemary has been shown to interfere with calcium influx into the myocardial cells (Tisserand & Balacs 1995) and should be not be used orally in cardiac patients. Patients with glaucoma should avoid taking oral citral-rich essential oils (Leach & Lloyd 1956). Tisserand and Balacs (1995) suggest that hormone replacement therapy (HRT) is not adversely affected by aromatherapy because the hormonal effect of the essential oil is considerably weaker than the effect of the HRT.

ESSENTIAL OILS AND HOMEOPATHY

Although Hippocrates may have been the first to say "like cures like," this tenet is associated with homeopathic medicine, which dates back to 1810 and Samuel Hahnemann, a German physician. Hahnemann discovered that cinchona bark taken by a healthy person produced the symptoms of malaria. At that time, cinchona bark was administered as a herbal remedy to cure malaria. (Much later cinchona bark was found to contain quinine, a component that became a classic drug to treat malaria.) Hahnemann thought giving a minute dose of the substance that may have caused the disease would stimulate the body to fight that disease.

He tested this hypothesis on himself and his family, compiling a huge encyclopedia of knowledge that now forms the foundation of homeopathic literature. The first homeopathic hospital opened its doors in 1850. In addition to "like cures like," homeopaths believe the more diluted the dose, the more potent it may be. Often their medicines are so diluted that there are no molecules of medicine left in them. This has caused much derision among members of the medical profession, who feel that leaving the curing of the patient to the "learned memory of water" is something of a joke. However, rigorous scientific studies are now showing that homeopathy is indeed a valid and useful form of medicine (Kleijinen et al 1991).

There is some controversy among homeopaths concerning the use of essential oils for patients receiving homeopathy. The traditional view has always been that essential oils and homeopathic remedies do not mix. Many aromatherapy courses teach that the two should not be combined. They are very different therapies at opposite ends of the spectrum—one very concentrated and one very dilute. Peppermint, eucalyptus, thyme, and essential oils with strong aromas are some of those best avoided by patients using homeopathy.

Stevensen (1995), who worked for many years using both homeopathy and essential oils on a daily basis, wrote "I would find it difficult to envisage a clash of effects between homeopathy and aromatherapy." However, the safest option is to restrict the choice of essential oil to florals such as rose, lavender, geranium, neroli, and the softer herbs.

SPECIFIC CONTRAINDICATIONS

Some essential oils are contraindicated in certain aromatherapy situations, or contraindicated altogether, although they may be used as food flavorings or in perfumery. The amount of essential oil used in flavoring is often very tiny. For example, mustard, a well-known flavoring, is contraindicated in aromatherapy because it is extremely toxic. Tisserand and Balacs (1995) describe the dose used by the food industry as one-hundredth of a drop of mustard to 50 g of pickle. It would be impossible to measure one-hundredth of a drop in aromatherapy.

However, if just one drop was used (1%), the resulting dilution would be 1000 times greater than that in pickles!

There are several safety data manuals available that go into detail regarding why some essential oils are contraindicated. *Essential Oil Safety* (Tisserand & Balacs 1995) is particularly recommended. If hospitals are to become involved in the use of essential oils, they should have a safety data manual. Hazardous oils are still on sale in many health-food shops, and sometimes in bottles without integrated droppers.

Some essential oils are generally contraindicated for all therapeutic uses. These include boldo leaf, calamus, cassia, bitter fennel, mugwort, mustard, rue, sassafras, tansy, wintergreen, and wormwood. These oils all contain toxic constituents. The essential oils contraindicated for undiluted topical application include oregano, clove bud and leaf, cinnamon bark, camphor, and red thyme. Essential oils that should be used with caution in patients with hypertension include rosemary, spike lavender, hyssop, juniper, thyme, and clove, although there is no published report of blood pressure being substantially raised by essential oils. Contraindicated in patients with epilepsy are hyssop, fennel, peppermint, and rosemary, although there is no published report of any of these triggering a seizure. However, Guba (2000) writes that large doses of ketones, in particular camphor, pinocamphone, pulegone, and thujone have been found to cause seizures (NDPSC 1998).

Contraindications in Oncology

Some malignant growths depend on estrogen, so perhaps the use of essential oils that are mildly estrogenlike should be avoided. However, soy products, which also contain phytoestrogens, have cancer-fighting compounds (Weil 1998), so estrogen stimulating or estrogenlike essential oils may be good for estrogen-dependent tumors. Barrett (1997) gives an interesting discussion of the pros and cons of using phytoestrogens. Franchomme & Penoel (1991) list the specific chemical components associated with estrogen stimulation or estrogenlike properties as sclareol and viridiflorol (sesquiterpenic alcohols), anethole (a phenyl methyl ether), and "certain" ketones not specified. Citral was found to have an estrogenic action by Geldof et al (1992). Animal studies suggest the topical use of citrus-peel oils such as bergamot should be avoided in patients who have a history or symptoms of melanoma (Elegbede et al 1986).

Contraindications in Pregnancy

The use of essential oils in pregnancy is a contentious subject, especially during the vital first 3-month period. Some aromatherapists will not treat expectant mothers. Because lipophilic substances can diffuse between two circulations, it is likely that essential oils cross the placenta (Burfield 2001). Balacs suggests the best advice is to "urge caution when giving oils to pregnant women and to avoid pennyroyal at all costs." However, to put this in context, remember that perfume does not carry a warning not to be used in pregnancy. It is extremely unlikely that a nightly bath containing a few drops of essential oil will cause any problems for the unborn child.

Many midwives are happy to use essential oils during labor to promote contractions and for their analgesic properties. Mason (1996) suggests avoiding essential oils during the first 24 weeks of pregnancy. Tiran suggests avoiding them during the first trimester only (1996). Several hospital labor units using essential oils during labor and delivery report that aromatherapy is useful, safe, and pleasant. More details on obstetrics can be found in Chapter 21.

SAFETY AND STORAGE OF ESSENTIAL OILS

Safety

Aromatherapy requires knowledge, and yes, in the wrong hands, essential oils can be hazardous. Just like Tylenol and aspirin, which can be bought over the counter almost anywhere, essential oils should always be kept away from children. See Table 4-2 for potentially lethal dosages in children.

If a child appears to have drunk several spoonfuls of essential oil, contact the nearest poison unit (often listed in the front of a telephone directory). Keep the bottle for identification and encourage the child to drink whole milk. Do not try to induce vomiting. If essential oils (diluted or not) get into the eyes it is important to irrigate the eyes as rapidly as possible with whole milk or carrier oil followed by water and then to seek medical help. If there is a skin reaction to an essential oil, dilute the essential oil with carrier oil, then wash the area with a nonperfumed soap. The majority of the components found in essential oils are nonpolar; therefore essential oils do not mix well or dissolve in water.

Storage

Essential oils are powerful, and it is important that they be stored away from children, the confused, or those unaware of what essential oils are. It takes just 4 ml (less than a teaspoonful) of ingested blue gum eucalyptus to produce severe effects. Gurr & Scroggie (1965) reported on a case that necessitated emergency peritoneal dialysis, hemodialysis, and a mannitol infusion.

Essential oils kept in a hospital should be stored in a locked container. If stored in a cool, dry, dark place, undiluted essential oils can stay fresh for up to 6 years. They should be kept in colored (blue or amber) glass bottles to protect them from ultraviolet light, with the bottles sealed. Bottles should have an integral dropper contained in the lid to prevent spillage. All opened bottles should be stored away from heat and sunlight (ideally in a refrigerator, similar to the storage of heparin). All bottles should carry a firmly attached label, stating the botanical name, the supplier's name, and the batch number. Most reputable companies also include a label warning that the oils should be kept away from the eyes, out of reach of children, and not be taken by mouth. Some also have a note printed on them stating they are of medicinal strength. It is helpful to keep a record of when each es-

Table 4-2 ❧ *Potentially Lethal Oral Doses of Essential Oil for a Child.*

Common Name	Botanical Name	Oral Lethal Dose for a Child
Basil	*Ocimum basilicum* (estragole above 55%)	8 ml
Aniseed	*Pimpinella anisum*	25 ml
Clove	*Syzygium aromaticum*	19 ml
Eucalyptus	*Eucalyptus globulus*	5 ml
Hyssop	*Hyssopus officinalis*	19 ml
German spearmint	*Mentha longifolia*	6.5 ml
Egyptian round leaf	*Mentha rotundifolia*	10 ml
Oregano	*Oreganum vulgare*	21 ml
Parsley seed oil	*Petroselinum sativum*	21 ml
Pennyroyal	*Mentha pulegium*	3 ml
Sage	*Salvia officinalis*	26 ml
Savory, Summer	*Satureja hortensis*	19 ml
Tansy	No botanical name given	5 ml
Tarragon	No botanical name given	26 ml
Thuja	*Thuja occidentalis*	10 ml
Wintergreen	*Methyl salicylate*	5 ml

Adapted from Watt M. 1991. Essex, UK: Witham. This book discusses adverse reactions and toxicity in greater detail. Not all the botanical names are given.

sential oil was purchased, the supplier's name, and the price. A separate list should be kept with the patient's name, the name of the physician, the dates the patient received aromatherapy, and any therapeutic (or adverse) results. Recording this information makes a portfolio on the use of essential oils easily available.

Essential oils are highly flammable, so they must be stored away from open flame such as candles, fire, matches, cigarettes, and gas cookers. Sprinkling them on top of light bulbs is not a good idea!

Although essential oils have been used for thousands of years, there have been few recorded cases of sensitivity, allergy, or fatality. Lovell (1993) suggests that the family *Lamiacea*, which contains many aromatic plants used in perfumery, cooking, and medicine, could possibly produce allergic contact dermatitis. He cites Canlan, who recorded six positive reactions to lavender oil patch tests in 1147 patients. The incidence of adverse reactions to essential oils is considerably lower than the incidence of adverse reactions to synthetic drugs, and the reactions are generally less severe. However, this could be because essential oils are used much less often than orthodox drugs. In a Japanese study carried out between 1990 and 1998, a 2-day, closed patch test using 2% essential oil of lavender on people who had suspected cosmetic contact dermatitis found a sudden increase in reactions for the year 1997 (Sugiura et al 2000). Researchers suggested this increase could be due to the trend of placing lavender flowers in pillows and drawers. Essential oils are wonderful things, but over-use may lead to sensitivity—even with the ubiquitous lavender.

REFERENCES

Albert-Puleo M. 1980. Fennel and anise as estrogenic agents. Journal of Ethnopharmacology. 2(4) 337-344.

Almirall M, Montana J, Escribano E et al. 1996. Effect of d-limonene, alpha-pinene and cineole on in vitro transdermal human skin penetration of chlorpromazine and haloperidol. Arzneimittelforschung. 46(7) 676-680.

Balacs T. 1992. Safety in pregnancy. International Journal of Aromatherapy. 4(1) 12-15.

Barrett E. 1997. Environmental health: Phytoestrogens. Focus. 104(5). Retrieved September 2002 from http://ehpnet1.niehs.nih.gov/docs/1996/104(5)focus.html.

Bartlett J. 1977. Bartlett's Familiar Quotations, 14th ed. London: Macmillan Press, 208.

Berndt W, Stitzel R. 1994. Excretion of drugs. In Craig C, Stitzel R (eds.), Modern Pharmacology. Boston: Little, Brown & Co., 47-53.

Bilsland D, Strong A. 1990. Allergic contact dermatitis from the essential oil of French marigold (*Tagetes patula*) in an aromatherapist. Contact Dermatitis. 23(1) 55-56.

Blaschke T, Bjornsson T. 1995. Pharmacokinetics and pharmacoepidemiology. Scientific American. 8:1-14.

Bowles J. 2000. The Basic Chemistry of Aromatherapeutic Essential Oils. Sydney, Australia: Pirie Printers.

Brandao F. 1986. Occupational allergy to lavender oil. Contact Dermatitis. 15(4) 249-250.

Budavari S (ed.). 1996. Merck index, 12th ed. Whitehouse Station, NJ: Merck & Co. Inc.

Burfield T. 2001. Safety of essential oils. International Journal of Aromatherapy. 10(1/2) 16-30.

Calnan C. 1976. Cinnamon dermatitis from an ointment. Contact Dermatitis. 2(3) 167-170.

Chiej R. 1984. The Macdonald Encyclopedia of Medicinal Plants. London: Macdonald.

Chiou L, Ling J, Chang C. 1997. Chinese herb constituent beta-eudesmol alleviated the electroshock seizures in mice and electrographic seizures in rat hippocampal slices. Neuroscience Letters. 231(3) 171-174.

Collins A, Notarianni L, Ring E et al. 1984. Some observations on the pharmacology of 'deep-heat,' a topical rubifacient. Annals of Rheumatic Diseases. 43(3) 411-415.

De Groot A, Weyland J. 1992. Systemic contact dermatitis from tea tree oil. Contact Dermatitis. 27(4) 279-280.

De Groot A, Frosch P. 1997. Adverse reactions to fragrances. Contact Dermatitis. 36(2) 57-86.

Delaveau P, Guillemain J, Marcisse, G et al. 1989. Neuro-depressive properties of essential oil of lavender (French). Comptes Rendus des Séances de la Societié de Biologie et de ses Filiales. 183(4) 342-348.

Elegbede J, Maltzman T, Verma A et al. 1986. Mouse skin tumor promoting activity of orange peel oil and d-limonene: A re-evaluation. Carcinogenesis. 7(12) 2047-2049.

Fleming W. 1994. Mechanisms of drug action. In Craig C, Stitzel R (eds.), Modern Pharmacology. Boston: Little, Brown & Co., 9-18.

Freitas J, Presgrave O et al. 1993. Effect of b-myrcene on pentobarbital sleeping time. Brazilian Journal of Medical and Biological Research. 26(5) 519-523.

Geldof A, Engel C, Rao B. 1992. Estrogenic action of commonly used fragrant agent citral induces prostatic hyperplasia. Urology Research. 20(2) 139-144.

Godwin D, Michniak B. 1999. Influence of drug lipophilicity on terpenes as transdermal penetration enhancers. Drug Development & Industrial Pharmacy. 25(8) 905-915.

Grant T. 1994. Metabolism of drugs. In Craig C, Stitzel R (eds.), Modern Pharmacology. Boston: Little, Brown & Co., 33-46.

Guba R. 2000. Toxicity myths: The actual risks of essential oil use. International Journal of Aromatherapy. 10(1/2) 37-49.

Guillemain J, Rousseau R, Delaveau P. 1989. Neurodepressive effects of the essential oil of *Lavandula angustifolia.* Annales Pharmaceutiques Francais. 47(6) 337-342.

Gurr F, Scroggie J. 1965. Eucalyptus oil poisoning treated by dialysis and mannitol infusion, with an appendix on the analysis of biological fluids for alcohol and eucalyptol. Australasia Annals of Medicine. 14(3) 238-249.

Gwilt R. 1994. Pharmacokinetics. In Craig C, Stitzel R (eds.), Modern Pharmacology. Boston: Little, Brown & Co., 55-64.

Hansten P, Horn J. 1989. Drug Interactions: Clinical Significance of Drug–Drug Interactions, 6th ed. New York: Lea & Febiger.

Hohenwaller W, Kima J. 1971. In vivo activation of glucuronyl transferase in rat liver by euacalyptol. Biochemical Pharmacology. 20(12) 3463-3472.

International School of Aromatherapy. 1993. A Safety Guide for the Use of Essential Oils. London: Nature by Nature Oils.

Janssens J, Laekeman G, Pleters L et al. 1990. Nutmeg oil: Identification and quantification of its most active constituents as inhibitors of platelet aggregations. Journal of Ethnopharmacology. 29(2) 179-188.

Jori A, Bianchetti A, Prestinit P. 1969. Effect of essential oils on drug metabolism. Biochemical Pharmacology. 18(9) 12081-12085.

Kaplun-Frischoff Y, Touitou E. 1997. Testosterone skin permeation enhancement by menthol through formation of eutectic with drug and interaction with skin lipids. Journal of Pharmaceutical Science. 86(12) 1394-1399.

Kleijnen J, Knipschild P, ter Riet G. 1991. Clinical trials of homeopathy. British Medical Journal. 301(6772) 316-332.

Kligman A. 1996. The identification of contact allergens by human assay. Journal of Investigative Dermatology. 47(5) 393-409.

Kufferath F, Mundualgo G. 1954. The activity of some preparations containing essential oils in TB. Fitoterapia. 25:483-485.

Larsen W. 2000. How to test for fragrance allergy. Cutis. 65(1) 39-41.

Larsen W, Nakayama H, Lindberg M et al. 1996. Fragrance contact dermatitis: a worldwide multicenter investigation (part 1). American Journal of Contact Dermatitis. 7:77-83.

Leach E, Lloyd J. 1956. Experimental ocular hypertension in animals. Transactions of the Ophthalmological Societies of the UK. 76:453-460.

Lesesne C. 1992. The postoperative use of wound adhesives. Gum mastic versus benzoin, USP. Journal of Dermatologic Surgery and Oncology. 18(11) 990-991.

Littleton F. 1990. Warfarin and topical salicylates (letter). Journal of the American Medical Association. 263(21) 2888.

Lovell C. 1993. Plants and the Skin. Oxford, UK: Blackwell Scientific Publications.

Madhava-Madyastha K, Chadha A. 1986. Metabolism of 1,8 cineole in rats: Its effect on liver and lung microsomal cytochrome P-450 systems. Bulletin of Environmental Contaminants and Toxicology. 37:759-766.

Marks J, Belsito D, DeLeo V et al. 1998. North American Contact Dermatitis Group patch test results for the detection of delayed-type hypersensitivity to topical allergens. Journal of the American Academy of Dermatology. 38(6 Pt 1) 911-918.

Mason M. 1996. Aromatherapy and midwifery. Aromatherapy. Quarterly spring issue. 32-34.

Meyer J. 1970. Accidents due to tanning cosmetics with a base of bergamot oil. Bulletin de la Societé Francaise de Dermatologie et de Syphiligraphie. 77(6) 881-884.

Murad F, Kuret J. 1990. Estrogens and progestins. In Goodman and Gilman's The Pharmacological Basis of Therapeutics, 8th ed. New York: McGraw-Hill, 1384-1386.

Naganuma M, Hirose S, Nakayama K, et al. 1985. A study of the phototoxicity of lemon oil. Archives of Dermatological Research. 278(1) 311-316.

National Drugs and Poisons Schedule Committee (NDPSC) Working Party on Essential Oils. 1998. Essential Oil Monographs. Canberra: Australian Therapeutic Goods Administration.

Olleveant N, Humphris G, Roe B. 1999. How big is a drop? A volumetric assay of essential oils. Journal of Clinical Nursing. 8(3) 299-304.

Owole S, Ramson-Kuto O. 1980. The risk of jaundice in glucose-6-phosphate dehydrogenase deficient babies exposed to menthol. Acta Paediatrica Scandinavica. 69(3) 341-345.

Parys B. 1983. Chemical burns resulting from contact with peppermint oil: a case report. Burns Including Thermal Injury (Bristol). 9(5) 374-375.

Perez Raya M, Utrilla M, Navarro M et al. 1990. CNS activity of *Mentha rotundifolia* and *Mentha longifolia* essential oil in mice and rats. Phytotherapy Research. 4(6) 232-234.

Price S, Price L. 1999. Aromatherapy for Health Professionals, 2nd ed. London: Churchill Livingstone.

Rademaker M, Kirby J. 1987. Contact dermatitis to a skin adhesive. Contact Dermatitis. 16(5) 297-298.

Riviere J, Brooks J, Qiao G et al. 1997. Percutaneous absorption of volatile chemicals. Airforce Office of Scientific Research G49620-95-1-0017. National Technical Information Service Report American Disability Act 1-23.

Roethe A, Heine A, Rebohie E. 1973. Oils from juniper berries as an occupational allergen for the skin and the respiratory tract. Berufs-Dermatosen. 21(1) 11-16.

Schaller M, Korting H. 1995. Allergic airborne contact dermatitis from essential oils used in aromatherapy. Clinical and Expermental Dermatology. 20(2) 143-145.

Scheinman P. 1997. Is it really fragrance free? American Journal of Contact Dermatitis. 8(4) 239-242.

Sheppard-Hangar S. 1995. The Aromatherapy Practitioner's Reference Manual, Vol. II. Tampa, FL: Atlantic Institute of Aromatherapy.

Sieben S, Hertl M, Masaoudi T, et al. 2001. Characterization of T cell responses to fragrances. International Journal of Aromatherapy. 11(3) 157-166.

Sugiura M, Hayakawa R, Kato Y et al. 2000. Results of patch testing with lavender oil in Japan. Contact Dermatitis. 43(3) 157-160.

Tiran D. 1996. Aromatherapy in midwifery: Benefits and risks. Complementary Therapies in Nursing and Midwifery. 2(4) 88-93.

Tisserand R, Balacs T. 1995. Essential Oil Safety. London: Churchill Livingstone.

Van Ketel W. 1982. Allergy to *Matricaria chamomilla*. Contact Dermatitis. 8(2) 143.

Van Ketel W. 1987. Allergy to *Matricaria chamomilla*. Contact Dermatitis. 16(1) 50-51.

Vessell ES, Lang CM, White GT et al. 1976. Environmental and genetic factors affecting response of laboratory animals to drugs. Federation Proc. 35:1125-1132.

Watt M. 1991. Plant Aromatics. Essex, UK: Witham.

Weil A. 1998. Complementary care for cancer. Dr. Andrew Weil's Self-Healing. Jan. 1, 6-7.

Williams A, Barry B. 1989. Essential oils as novel human skin penetration enhancers. Journal of Pharmaceutics. 57:R7-R9.

Yip A, Chow W, Tai Y. 1990. Adverse effect of methyl salicylate ointment on warfarin anticoagulation: an unrecognized potential hazard. Postgraduate Medical Journal. 66(775) 367-369.

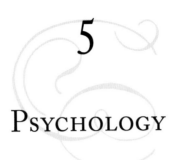

5

PSYCHOLOGY

"Why do women sniff bread?" I asked. It was something I often noticed Ma doing. "To see if it is fresh I suspect," Uncle Seth said. "I have never sniffed bread in my life, which is the difference between me and a woman. . . . And when a woman comes to decide who to marry it comes down to the same test," he added.

"You mean they sniff men?" I asked. I could not imagine what it would feel like to have a woman sniff me.

"Yes, to determine if the fellow's fresh," Uncle Seth said. "I guess I don't smell fresh, which is why I'm a bachelor still."

Larry McMurtry
Boone's Lick

Dodd (1991) described stimulation of olfactory responses by odorants as "a branch of molecular pharmacology that was similar to mood changes brought about by some psychotropic drugs." Responses to pleasant odors are conducted unconsciously, although both olfactory nerve connections and measured physiologic changes indicate that the response is of an emotional and hormonal nature.

Jellinek (1999) describes four different mechanisms through which essential oil odors affect psychologic states. He calls these mechanisms quasipharmacologic, semantic, hedonic, and placebo. Quasipharmacologic refers to the small amounts of essential oil components found in the bloodstream following inhalation. Semantic refers to the odor within the context of life experience. Hedonic refers to feelings of pleasure or displeasure on inhaling an essential oil. Placebo refers to the expectations of the person inhaling the essential oil, which color his or her response.

PHEROMONES

Smell is very important in life, beginning with newborn babies' identification of their mothers (Macfarlane 1975) and continuing into old age. Even subliminal smell is important. Partners, lovers, and friends are chosen through subliminal smells called pheromones (Watson 2000). Pheromones are airborne chemicals involuntarily expelled into the air that affect the physiology or behavior of other members of the same species. Pheromones were discovered in the 1930s by Adolph Butenandt, a German biochemist who won the Nobel Prize in 1939 for his work on human hormones. He was forbidden to accept the award by Hitler, and he changed his research focus to how female moths attract males at great distance. It took Butenandt the next 20 years to identify the first pheromone, bobykol, "a substance so powerful that if any one female moth were to release all her store in a single spray, there would be enough to bring a trillion males to her side" (Dossey 2001). Pheromones are linked to the vomeronasal organ: two tiny pits just inside the nostrils (Watson 2000).

Although a person may not be aware of another person's pheromones, they are what really attracts him or her to that person. Couples going through marriage breakdown often say their partner "no longer smells the same" (Needham 1999). This is much truer than they realize because the chemical attraction between them has changed from attracting mode to repelling mode, just as their emotions have changed. Pheromones work in a subliminal way, meaning humans are unaware of them, although they may still sense "something" is different.

Everyone's body odor is unique—a "smellprint." An electronic device known as the Bloodhound, an artificial sniffing dog, was built at Cambridge University. This device could identify a person's smellprint, and by recording a particular person's unique body odor, the machine could recognize that smellprint anywhere in the world.

PSYCHOAROMATHERAPY

It is also possible, using psychoaromatherapy (environmental fragrancing), to manipulate mood or change perception through the use of subliminal smell. A certain amount of research has been conducted on this, and the results show people can be encouraged or manipulated using this method of aromatherapy (Kirk-Smith 1993). For example, customers in a store can be encouraged to purchase an item, rather than another identical item, by impregnating it with a pleasant subliminal smell. Companies can "persuade" customers to pay bills on time by impregnating invoices with subliminal, offensive odors. The concept is disturbing, and the possible repercussions arguably unethical.

Psychoaromatherapy is not just about subliminal smell. The perfume industry is very concerned with how our choice of scent affects us (Mensing & Beck 1988). Millions of British pounds and American dollars are spent each year on olfaction research (Dossey 2001).

Aromas have measurable effects on how we feel. Torii et al (1988) report on the psychological stimulating effect of jasmine. Manly (1993) found the effect of lemon, lemongrass, peppermint, and basil to be psychologically stimulating, and the effects of bergamot, chamomile, and sandalwood to be relaxing. Other aromas found to be relaxing were rose and lavender (Kikuchi et al 1991). Peppermint and lavender improved the efficiency of proofreaders (Kliauga et al 1995). Sweet orange essential oil was effective in children for both induction of anesthesia and recovery time following surgery (Mehta et al 1998).

It is not necessary to be awake for an aroma to affect a person physiologically. Whereas Sugano (1992) found jasmine stimulating to subjects who were awake, Badia et al (1990) found the effect of jasmine was still stimulating when subjects were asleep. Badia et al (1990) found that peppermint was also simulating. Heliotropin relaxed some subjects and disrupted sleep in others. The aroma appeared to cause changes in subjects' electroencephalogram (EEG) results and blood pressure, but did not affect respiration.

Yamaguchi (1990) found that aromas could affect heart rate. Van Toller et al (1992) mapped the brain while subjects wearing a special 28-lead "hat" inhaled aromas. Schulz et al (1998) used EEG activity to screen acute sedative effects of several essential oils compared against diazepam, and the use of EEGs to monitor the effects of aromas is becoming more commonplace. Lorig et al (1990) also measured EEG activity during olfaction. Masago et al (2000), using lavender, chamomile, and sandalwood, found that alpha 1 activity significantly decreased during odor conditions in which the subjects felt comfortable, and showed no significant change under odor conditions in which the subjects felt uncomfortable. Alpha 1 is the 8.5-10.5 Hz frequency band of an EEG signal.

Smell is also a language, a method of communication. We involuntarily communicate through subliminal smell—our pheromones. We talk about "smelling danger," say that someone or something "smelled wrong," or refer to "sniffing it out." The French have a saying, *Je ne peux pas le sentir,* which means "I don't trust him"; the literal translation is "I can't smell him." Unconsciously we choose our friends and partners by smell. Research has shown that subliminal smell placed on a waiting-room chair attracted a statistically significant proportion of patients entering that waiting room (Kirk-Smith & Booth 1987).

Learned memory is a reaction to a smell that has been learned through experience, for example, trauma linked to an aroma. When that odor is smelled again, fear, or the emotion originally experienced, is triggered. An example of this phenomenon of learned memory is the use of lavender in older adults. For many elderly people in Europe, lavender is associated with linen chests, and for some the odor is closely linked with care of the dying. Lavender has undergone a tremendous revival thanks to aromatherapy, and although it appears to be universally enjoyed by those younger than 60 years of age, this learned memory association between lavender and death could be why those Europeans in their 70s or older are sometimes not quite so enthusiastic.

Kirk-Smith (1993) tells the story of a 55-year-old man who, as a child, was terrified of a teacher who wore a particular perfume. In later life, that same perfume still evoked a sense of anxiety. Learned memory of smell is hard to undo. The functioning of the human body is greatly affected by the mind. In recent years, medicine has begun to accept the mind/body connection. Our immune system has receptors for endorphins and is strongly affected by our sense of well being. Bereavement, anxiety, and stress (Quinn & Strelkauskas 1993) affect this continual conversation between brain and immune system. By combining two external communicators, smell and touch, our patients' abilities to communicate internally are greatly enhanced.

Smell is closely linked to taste (although smell is considerably more sensitive), which is why when we have a cold, food does not smell appetizing. We eat to live: food has a molecular structure, which our bodies break down into atoms; this has both physiologic and psychologic effects. We also eat because food tastes good. Smells can give us similar pleasure, and they too affect us physiologically and psychologically. Aromas have also been shown to enhance the output of the workforce, raise feelings of job satisfaction, and reduce sick-leave absences (Chadwick & Mann 1983). Specific aromas have specific effects. Melissa has been used for grief, lemongrass to mask offensive smells, marjoram and lavender to aid insomnia in the elderly, and geranium and mandarin to enhance memory recall in patients with Alzheimer's disease.

Saeki and Shiohara (2001) investigated the physiologic response to inhaled lavender, rosemary, and citronella on nine healthy women aged 21 to 23 who were recruited from Nagano College of Nursing in Japan. The study measured the responses to R-wave intervals on an electrocardiogram, blood flow in the fingertips, galvanic skin conduction (GSC), and blood pressure. Tests were performed in an air-conditioned room at 22° to 25° C. The study began by measuring baselines. Then 6 drops of one of the three aromas were heated in 10 ml of hot water in an aroma pot. The subject entered the room and inhaled the essential oil for 10 minutes. A break of 90 minutes was allowed between each aroma to allow for aroma dispersal.

The results showed lavender decreased systolic blood pressure within 10 minutes, decreased GSC within 2 minutes, and increased blood flow within 6 minutes. The R-R interval did not change. Rosemary increased the systolic blood pressure and decreased the blood flow immediately, but these responses returned to normal within minutes. There were also changes in the ECG, and the two frequency components of heart rate variation, (which, simply put, means the ratio between respiration and heart beat) increased significantly and immediately. This appears to confirm that rosemary has stimulant effects, although they appear to be transitory. Citronella did not change blood flow or blood pressure, but it did increase the R-R interval after 10 minutes, although GSC decreased immediately. Each participant's like or dislike of the aroma could explain these conflicting results.

MIND/BODY CONNECTIONS

Sugawara et al (1999) found that a perception of fragrance is related to the type of work a person does. In this study the difference between mental and physical work altered perceptions of scent. Scores were recorded for seven essential oils before and after specific types of work. Cypress had a more favorable impression after physical work than before. (This is interesting because cypress has a deodorant effect!) Orange had a less favorable reaction after physical work. Degel & Koster (1999) found that ambient odor could have a negative or positive effect on a variety of tests. The researchers gave 108 subjects a variety of tests in a room weakly scented with jasmine or lavender or in an odorless room. The tests included viewing slides of different surroundings (including the room in which they were located). Subjects were asked to rate how well specific odors matched the slides. Jasmine appeared to have a negative and lavender a positive effect on test performance.

Jelinek and Novakova (2001) give a moving account of how aromatherapy had a positive effect on a 14-year-old boy in prison in Bohemia. The teenager was aggressive and had behavior problems. What was most interesting was how each aroma triggered his memory and how that memory allowed the boy to communicate his feelings. For example ylang ylang evoked the smell of his father's Sunday-morning shave and the good things they did together, but after smelling peppermint the boy said "I don't know any more."

Aromas affect even the unborn child. A French study (Schaal et al 2000) examined whether prenatal exposure to aroma could influence selective response. In this randomized study the test group of mothers consumed anise-flavored candy containing up to an estimated intake of 121 mg of anethole. When the newborn babies were exposed to a swab with anethole, videos recorded facial and head responses in favor of the smell. The babies of the control mothers (who did not eat any anethole candy) demonstrated an aversive or neutral response. The other babies turned toward the anethole swab.

Smell can help people cope with a traumatic experience, and may be of use in treating panic attacks. Redd and Manne (1995) investigated the effect of using aroma to reduce distress during magnetic resonance imaging. A small tube was inserted in the nostrils of 57 participants who received either heliotropin (a vanilla-like scent) or plain air. Patients who received the heliotropin reported 64% less anxiety than the control group who had plain air, even though the respiration and heart rate of the experimental group showed no change.

Not all aromatherapy studies have been successful in reducing perception of anxiety. Wiebe (2000) found that vetiver (a common ingredient in men's cologne and aftershave), bergamot, and geranium did not reduce the stress of women about to have an abortion. The essential oils were smelled for 10 minutes. The control group smelled a hair conditioner containing synthetic scent.

Certain aromas may help reduce stress before and during examinations. Fillian (2000) studied the effect of a mixture of lavender *(Lavandula angustifolia)* and rosemary *(Rosmarinus officinalis)* on 13 adult volunteers of an advanced physiology class at a graduate college All students were patch tested before the study began. During the study, subjects were asked to apply 5 drops of 2% solution to their wrists, rub their wrists together and inhale deeply for 5 minutes before the examination. This could be repeated as necessary during the examination. The average mean score of the tests taken previously by the subjects was 85.4%. The average score of the tests when aromatherapy was used was 89.7%. Although the students could have become more familiar with the testing procedure (this was their fifth test out of six), and the test itself could have been simpler, the students all reported a feeling of calmness and clear thought.

Lavender and rosemary were the subjects of a randomized, controlled study reported in Reuters Health (an on-line health bulletin service) on March 28, 2002. Either lavender or rosemary was given to 144 young adults; they were then given tests of their working memory and reaction times. Mood tests were completed before and after the memory exercises. Study participants in the lavender group reported feeling less alert in the lavender-scented cubicles, participants in the rosemary group reported feeling more content after they completed the memory tests than they did before. The study findings were presented at the British Psychological Society's annual meeting in Blackpool, UK.

Age, sex, and exposure to noxious agents all affect our sense of smell. As we become older our sense of smell deteriorates. Women are thought to have a greater sense of smell than men. This is particularly interesting as most 'noses' or professional perfumers are men. Results from a National Geographic Smell Survey (712,000 respondents) indicate that certain medicinal and environmental agents adversely affect the sense of smell. Workers in a factory reported poorer sense of smell after the suggestion that exposure to the factory workplace had impaired their sense of odor (Corwin et al 1995). Russell et al (1993) interpreted the Smell Survey to show that there were marked changes in odor categorization across the life span. After the age of 60, there was marked displacement for some odors—some odors were more difficult to smell or identify.

Essential oils make up very complicated aromas that are difficult to emulate. Rose oil is one of the most complicated and has baffled synthetic chemists for some time. Scientists suspect that the sweet component of rose odor is made by the breakdown of carotenoids, a compound found in the petals that gives red roses their color. *Science News* describes how Japanese researchers have identified an enzyme that turns carotenoids into the chemical precursor to beta-damascenone, but have been unable to replicate it. (April 15, 2000).

Espenshade (1999) discussed a select mute child in the second grade who had not responded in class to any questions since kindergarten. He had arrived at the school 2 years previously. The child was from Sardinian parents but was born in the United States. He behaved normally at home. Espenshade, a teacher, worked with the family and suggested six essential oils for the boy to choose from. The boy chose three: frankincense, bergamot, and Scotch pine. Each morning when he arrived at school he came to Espenshade and selected one of the scents. Several drops were placed on a tissue he kept in his pocket. There was a gradual but definite change. A few weeks into the study, the boy spoke for the first time in class. One particular essential oil, Scotch pine, seemed to help him. When his father learned his son had spoken in class for the first time, he asked which scent had worked. On hearing that it was Scotch pine, his comment was, "That is just how Sardinia smells!" The boy had never visited Sardinia. Table 5-1 indicates some essential oils and the research carried out on them regarding their psychologic effects.

DEPRESSION

Depression is one of the most widespread mental-health problems in the world (Yarnell & Abascal 2001). It is estimated that more than 20 million Americans suffer from depression, but only one in three seeks professional help (Papoloso & Papoloso 1997). Although the majority of patients are treated with medication or psychotherapy, some medications can be unacceptable because of side effects, potential drug interactions, or potentially dangerous overdose (Davidson et al 1997). Psychotherapy can be rejected as an alternative to drugs because of time, effort, and cost. Many patients in the United States are turning to complementary

Table 5-1 ❧ *Selected Studies on the Psychologic Effect of Essential Oils.*

Basil	Manly 1993
Bergamot	Manly 1993
Chamomile	Manly 1993
Eucalyptus	Berg 1987
Citronella	Saeki & Shiohara 2001
Jasmine	Sugano 1992, Torii et al 1988
Lavender	Kikuchi et al 1991, Kliauga et al 1995, Yamaguchi et al 1995
Lemon	Sakakibara et al 1995
Lemongrass	Manly 1993
Orange	Baron & Thomley 1994, Mehta et al 1998
Rose	Kikuchi et al 1991
Peppermint	Kliauga et al 1995, Warm et al 1992
Rosemary	Kubota et al 1992
Sandalwood	Steiner 1994

medicine and are either self-medicating or are being treated by therapists outside conventional medicine.

Depression can go unnoticed and sometimes be misdiagnosed as exhaustion (Castro 1997). Depression is not always caused by emotional stress. Alcohol, substance abuse, prolonged lack of sleep, environmental pollutants, and conventional medicines such as antibiotics or the contraceptive pill can be contributors. Seasonal affective disorder (SAD) thought to be caused by lack of sunlight which manifests in depression is particularly relevant to those living in Alaska, or other places in the far north. Postpartum depression was thought by many to have influenced the mood and behavior of Andrea Yates, who drowned her five children (Slater 2001).

Few patients are able to articulate their feelings of depression to a physician, and may say they feel generally unwell. A diagnosis of clinical depression is made when five or more of the following symptoms have been present every day, or nearly every day, for 2 weeks or more (Diagnostic and Statistical Manual of the American Psychiatric Association–IV [DSM-IV] 1994):

- Feelings of sadness, gloom, emptiness
- General lack of interest (apathy)
- Significant weight loss or gain or increase in appetite
- Insomnia or hypersomnia
- Physical restlessness or lack of physical motivation
- Exhaustion, not helped by sleep
- Feelings of worthlessness or excessive or inappropriate guilt
- Difficulty making decisions, thinking, remembering, and concentrating
- Recurrent thoughts of death or suicide without specific plan

Since March of 1998, psychologists in New Mexico have had prescriptive powers and this is set to be repeated in several other states across the USA. Therefore it is pertinent to mention the most commonly prescribed anti-depressant drug in the USA, which is imipramine, a tricyclic antidepressant. Unlike essential oils, there are considerable side effects to imipramine that include lethargy, disorientation, dry mouth, weight gain, impaired concentration, and memory disorientation (Lieberman 1998). These symptoms alone could lead to depression.

Although most people agree that a foul-smelling odor does not enhance their mood but a pleasant one might, there has been little scientific research to substantiate this. Yarnell and Abscal (2001) suggest essential oils should not be overlooked in the treatment of depression because "inhaled volatile oils pass through the olfactory nerve directly to the cerebrum." Whereas antidepressants work by making the neurotransmitter serotonin linger in the gaps between brain cells, essential oils may work as serotonin agonists, which can push the serotonin system into overdrive. This makes the brain more sensitive, rather like turning up the volume on a radio: Suddenly you can hear very weak stations.

Erlichmann and Bastone (1992) found that odors could produce psychologic effects similar to mood states. Subjects were presented with pleasant and unpleasant odors while engaging in mood-sensitive tasks. The pleasant odors tested were almond and coconut, representing food, and muguet and water lily, representing flowers. The unpleasant odors were pyridine and butyric acid, representing chemicals, and limburger cheese and cigar butt, representing natural substances. Synnott (1995) discusses the meaning of smell and relates that 50% of people who use public transportation in the United States object first and foremost to wearers of heavy perfume. Crying babies came after that!

Knasko (1992) tested the effect of ambient odor of lemon, lavender, and dimethyl sulfide (DSM) on the creativity, mood, and perceived health of 30 subjects (15 women and 15 men). The test room was scented by placing five perfume blotters, each containing four drops of the essential oil or four drops of DSM, in the ceiling ducts of the room, as well as under the table and chair of the subject. On control days, blank perfume blotters were used. During testing the room's vents were closed to keep the aroma in the room. Between subjects the vents were opened and the fans run for at least 1 hour to clear the room. Before the study, 12 people rated the intensity of all 3 aromas as weak-moderate.

Subjects in the DSM group appeared to be in a less-pleasant mood after exposure to the scent. Subjects in the lemon group appeared to feel healthier. There was no demonstrated difference in creativity, but relationships emerged between the personality of the person and the effect of the odor. The lack of impact on creativity may have been related to the weakness of the odor. Ludvigson and Rottman (1989) found an effect from lavender and cloves on cognition, memory, affect, and mood, but the aroma had been classified as "strong." Warm et al (1990) also reported a positive effect from fragrances, but they used a facemask to deliver an intermittent scent.

Knasko (1995) found that areas diffused with a pleasant smell produced a more positive mood in the public. One of her studies involved an exhibit at an anthropological museum displaying North American crafts and clothing. Three odors—bubble gum, incense, and leather—were tested during a 3-week period, following a first week with no odor. A surveillance camera recorded the length of time an individual lingered by the exhibit and exit interviews were conducted. The visitors reported the most positive mood effect during the bubble gum week. However, visitors in the incense week felt they had learned more from the exhibit.

Itai et al (2000) found that hiba oil reduced depression and anxiety in 14 patients receiving hemodialysis in a controlled study. Hiba oil is obtained from *Thujopsis dolabrata*, a Japanese tree (Guenther 1976). Hamilton rating scales for depression (HAMD) and anxiety (HAMA) were used. Lavender reduced anxiety but not depression.

Studies have shown the depression levels of elderly people living in assisted-care facilities were reduced with the aromas of fruit and flowers (Schillmann & Siebert 1991). Citrus was found to relieve depression (and improve immune function) by Komori et al (1995). A number of essential oils, including lavender, jasmine, rosemary, rose, and chamomile are used for treating depression. They are primarily given as inhalants, but Valnet (1980) also suggests taking thyme and lavender orally using between 2 to 5 drops two or three times a day.

Research indicates that there is a link between depression and increased deep-limbic activity when the amygdala becomes overactive (Drevets et al 1992). Herz (2000) found most people choose to lose their sense of smell rather than any other sense or a part of their anatomy. However, people who did lose their sense of smell though illness or accident reported a loss of emotional richness in their lives and tended toward depression. The link between smell and emotion is very strong. Following bereavement, a photo may elicit sad memories, but the smell of a loved one's clothes is more likely to produce tears.

Depression, anger, and fear are closely related. The amygdala is the key to our sense of fear and is thought to play a pivotal role in survival behavior. Somatosensory stimuli have direct input into the amygdala and do not go through the thalamus to reach the cortex. This process is unique and is thought to occur because the olfactory cortex has only four cellular layers. Every other part of the frontal, parietal, occipital, and temporal lobes of the brain has six layers. To facilitate an instant response to stimuli, the amygdala is thought to control the autonomic nervous system. The main outputs of the amygdala are to the hypothalamus and brainstem autonomic centers. These include the vagal nuclei and the sympathetic neurons (www.limbic.html).

DREAMS

Dossey (1999) describes the divide between how dreams are perceived by Western culture and by traditional cultures. Whereas orthodox medicine perceives activity of the mind as a local event happening solely within the brain, the approach of many other health care systems is that dreams have the ability to make people ill or restore them to health (Severson 1979). Therefore anything that impacts dreams and their link to our subconscious is not to be taken lightly.

Badia et al (1995) investigated the impact of odor on the sleep and dreams of 20 undergraduate students (6 male and 14 female) using a 5-band EEG (delta, theta, alpha, beta 1, and beta 2). Previous research had shown that stimuli presented during sleep could be detected and that the right side of the brain, specifically the frontal region, was more active during rapid eye movement (REM) sleep. REM is the period of sleep when dreams occur. (Humans may not be the only creatures who dream; dolphins also experience REM sleep.) Test subjects slept in a room with either filtered air or one of two odors: androsterone or peppermint. Contrary to expectations, there was no significant difference found in most subjects' EEG bands. However, there was significantly more power in the theta band of subjects in the room with androsterone, suggesting androsterone was disruptive to sleep, regardless of whether the subject could smell it. However, there was little incorporation of either aroma into the participants' dreams.

Trotter et al (1994) introduced 16 olfactory stimuli of different kinds (ranging from roses and coffee to dog feces and hand lotion) for 1 minute after subjects had displayed REM sleep for a minimum of 5 minutes. There were 5 subjects, and they were examined during 15 nights with 48 tests during this time.

The scents were incorporated into the subjects' dreams 22% of the time. One subject described a dream of walking by some gardenias that smelled like lemons.

Hoffman (1999) investigated the effect of frankincense on dreaming. Seven subjects, who were all women and had been recording their dreams for many years, took part in the study. During the first week the scientists took base-line measurements: number of dreams, vividness, color intensity, length, clarity, and quality. Each measurement was graded between 0 and 10 (0 the lowest, 10 the greatest). For the next 2 weeks, the women put 2 drops of frankincense on a cotton ball and placed the cotton ball underneath their pillowcases each night. Three participants had a significant positive change in their dream recall. Another stated she had solved a problem that, in her waking state, she had been working on for some time. Two others believed that their dream recall was enhanced slightly. The remaining two at first believed that frankincense had decreased their ability to recall dreams, but during the second week the quality of their dreams was enhanced.

Fabrici (1998) carried out a similar study using the same methodology but used angelica *(Angelica archangelica)*. Her four subjects were all women and were seasoned dreamers used to recording their dreams. Each of the four women found that angelica either stopped her dreams or interfered with them in such a way that she did not want to continue with the study. This is a fascinating area of research and one that has hardly been touched. As we become more aware of the subtle messages dreams can give us, anything that can encourage the messenger is potentially very valuable.

REFERENCES

Badia P, Wesensten N, Lammers W et al. 1990. Responsiveness to olfactory stimuli presented in sleep. Physiology and Behavior. 48(1) 87-90.

Badia P, Boecker M, Wright K. 1995. Some effects of fragrances on sleep. In Gilbert A (ed.), Compendium of Olfactory Research 1982-1994. New York: Olfactory Research Fund Ltd, 31-39.

Baron R, Thomley J. 1994. A whiff of reality. Environment and Behavior. 26(6) 766-784.

Berg K. 1987. The effect of smell on cognitive processes. DRAGOCO Report. 39, 128-129.

Castro M. 1997.The treatment of depression with homeopathy. Alternative & Complementary Therapies. 1(4) 300-305.

Chadwick J, Mann W (eds.). 1983. Hippocratic Writings. Harmondsworth, UK: Penguin Books, 24.

Corwin J, Loury M, Gilbert A. 1995. Workplace, age, and sex as mediators of olfactory function: Data from the National Geographic Smell Survey. The Journals of Gerontology. Series B, Psychological Sciences and Social Sciences. 50(4) 179-186.

Davidson J, Morrison R, Shore J et al. 1997. Homeopathic treatment of depression and anxiety. Alternative Therapies in Health and Medicine. 3(1) 46-49.

Degel J, Koster E. 1999. Odors: Implicit memory and performance effects. Chemical Senses. 24(3) 317-325.

Diagnostic and Statistical Manual of the American Psychiatric Association–IV [DSM-IV]): 1994.

Dodd G. 1991. The molecular dimension of perfumery. In Van Toller S, Dodd G (eds.), Perfumery: The Psychology and Biology of Fragrance. London: Chapman and Hall, 19-46.

Dossey L. 1999. Dreams and healing: Reclaiming a lost tradition. Alternative Therapies in Health and Medicine. 6(6) 12-17, 111-117.

Dossey L. 2001. Surfing the odornet: Exploring the role of smell in life and healing. Alternative Therapies in Health and Medicine. 7(2) 12-16, 100-107.

Drevets W, Videen T, Price J et al. 1992. A functional anatomical study of unipolar depression. Journal of Neuroscience. 12(9) 3628-3641.

Erlichmann H, Bastone L. 1992. The use of odor in the study of emotion. In Van Toller S, Dodd G (eds.), Fragrance: The Psychology and Biology of Perfume. London: Elsevier Applied Science, 143-159.

Espenshade T. 1999. The effects of aromatherapy on a select mute. Unpublished dissertation, Hunter, New York, RJ Buckle Associates.

Fabrici M. 1998. What is the effect of angelica on dreams? Unpublished dissertation, Hunter, New York, RJ Buckle Associates.

Fillian C. 2000. Does aromatherapy have any impact on human performance Unpublished dissertation, Hunter, New York, RJ Buckle Associates.

Guenther E. 1976. The Essential Oils, Vol. IV. Malabar, FL: Krieger, 323-325.

Herz R. 2000. Scents of time. The Sciences. 40(4) 34-39. Retrieved October 12, 2002 from http://infotrac.galegroup.com.

Hoffman C. 1999. Does aromatherapy enhance dream recall? Unpublished dissertation, Hunter, New York, RJ Buckle Associates.

Itai T, Amayasu H, Kuribayashi M et al. 2000. Psychological effects of aromatherapy on chronic hemodialysis patients. Psychiatry and Clinical Neurosciences. 54(4) 393-397.

Jelinek A, Novakova B. 2001. The psychotherapeutic use of essential oils. International Journal of Aromatherapy. 11(1) 100-102.

Jellinek A, 1999. Odors and mental states. International Journal of Aromatherapy. 9(3) 115-120.

Kirk-Smith M, Booth D. 1983. Unconscious odor conditioning in human subjects. Biological Psychology. 17: 221-231.

Kirk-Smith M. 1993. Human olfactory communication. In Aroma 93 Conference Proceedings. Brighton, UK: Aromatherapy Publications, 83-103.

Kliauga M, Huberts K, Cenci T. 1995. Consumer panel study of fragrance and proofreading efficiency. In Gilbert A (ed.), Explorations in Aroma-chology: Compendium of Aroma-chology Research 1982-1994. New York: Olfactory Research Fund Ltd., 131-135.

Knasko S. 1992. Ambient odor's effect on creativity, mood, and perceived health. Chemical Senses. 17(1) 27-35.

Knasko S. 1995. Congruent and incongruent odors: Their effect on human approach behavior. In Gilbert A (ed.), Compendium of Olfactory Research 1982-1994. New York: Olfactory Research Fund Ltd., 117-128.

Komori T, Fujiwara R, Tanida M et al. 1995. Effects of citrus fragrance on immune function and depressive states. Neuroimmunomodulation 2(3) 174-180.

Kubota M, Ikemoto T, Komaki R et al. 1992. Odor and emotion—Effects of essential oils on contingent negative variation. In Buchbauer G, Woidich H (eds.), Proceedings:

12th International Congress of Flavors, Fragrances and Essential Oils. Vienna: Austrian Association of Flavor & Fragrance, 456-461.

Lieberman S. 1998. Treating depression with St John's Wort. Alternative & Complementary Therapies. 4(3) 163-168.

Lorig T, Schwartz G. 1988. Brain and Odor: Alteration of human EEG by odor administration. Psychobiology. 16(3) 281-284.

Ludvigson H, Rottman T. 1989. Effects of lavender and cloves on cognition, memory, affect and mood. Chemical Senses. 14(4) 525-536.

Macfarlane A. 1975. Olfaction in the development of social preferences in the human neonate. In Parent-Infant Interaction (Ciba Foundation Symposium No. 33). Amsterdam: Elsevier, 103-107.

McMurtry L. 2000. Boone's Lick. New York: Simon & Schuster, 87-88.

Manley C. 1993. Psychophysiological effects of odor. Critical Review of Food Science Nutrition. 33(1) 57-62.

Masago R, Matsuda T, Kikuchi Y et al. 2000. Effects of inhalation of essential oils on EEG activity and sensory evaluation. Journal of Physiological Anthropology & Applied Human Science. 19(1) 35-42.

Mehta S, Stone D, Whitehead H. 1998. Use of essential oils to promote induction of anesthesia in children. Anaesthesia. 53(7) 720-721.

Mensing J, Beck C. 1988. The Psychology of fragrance selection. In Perfumery: the psychology and biology of fragrance. Edited by Van Toller S and Dodd G. Chapman & Hall, London.

Needham S. 1999. Personal communication.

Papoloso D, Papoloso J. 1997. Overcoming Depression, 3rd ed. New York: Harper Perennial.

Quinn J, Strelkauskas A. 1993. Psychoimmunologic effects of therapeutic touch on practitioners and recently bereaved recipients: A pilot study. Advances in Nursing Science. 15(4) 13-26.

Redd W, Manne S. 1995. Using aroma to reduce distress during magnetic resonance imaging. In Gilbert A (ed.), Compendium of Olfactory Research 1982-1994. New York: Olfactory Research Fund Ltd., 47-52.

Russell M, Cummings B, Profitt B, et al. 1993. Life span changes in the verbal categorization of odors. Journal of Gerontology. 48(2) 49-53.

Saeki Y, Shiohara M. 2001. Physiological effects of inhaling fragrances. International Journal of Aromatherapy. 11(3) 118-125.

Sakakibara K, Iguchi H, Satoh S et al. 1995. Psychological and physiological effects of odors on mental workload. Chemical Senses. 20(3) 382.

Schaal B, Marlier L, Soussignan R. 2000. Human foetuses learn odours from their pregnant mother's diet. Chemical Senses. 25(6) 729-737.

Schillmann S, Siebert J. 1991. New frontiers in fragrance use. Cosmetics & Toiletries. 106(6) 39-45.

Schulz H, Jobert M, Hubner W. 1998. The quantitative EEG as a screening instrument to identify sedative effects of single doses of plant extracts in comparison with diazepam. Phytomedicine. 5(6) 449-458.

Severson R. 1979. The alchemy of dreamwork: Reflections on Freud and the alchemical tradition. Dragonflies. Spring, 109.

Slater L. 2001. Beginning and end. New York Times Magazine. July 8, 11.

Sugano H. 1992. Psychophysiological studies of fragrances. In Van Toller S, Dodd G (eds.), Fragrance: The Psychology and Biology of Perfume. London: Elsevier Applied Science, 221-226.

Sugawara Y, Hino Y, Kawasaki M et al. 1999. Alteration of perceived fragrance of essential oils in relation to type of work: A simple screening test for efficacy of aroma. Chemical Senses. 24(4) 415-421.

Steiner W. 1994. The effects of odors on human experience and behavior. In Jellinek P (ed.), The Psychological Basis of Perfumery. London: Blackie Academic & Professional, 200-217.

Synnott A. 1995. Roses, coffee and lovers: The meaning of smell. In Gilbert A (ed.), Compendium of Olfactory Research 1982-1994. New York: Olfactory Research Fund Ltd., 117-128.

Tanida M, Kikuchi A, Uenoyama S et al. 1992. Effect of odor on cardiac response patterns during a fore period in reaction time task. J Soc Cosmet Chem Jap. 26(2) 113-119.

Torii S, Fukuda H, Kanemoto H et al. 1988. Contingent negative variation and the psychological effects of odor In Van Toller S, Dodd G (eds.), Perfumery: The Psychology and Biology of Fragrance. London: Chapman and Hall, 107-120.

Trotter K, Dallas K, Verdone P. 1994. Olfactory stimuli and their effects on REM dreams. In Dossey L. 2001. Surfing the odornet: Exploring the role of smell in life and healing. Alternative Therapies in Health and Medicine. 7(2) 12-16, 100-108.

Valnet J. 1990. The Practice of Aromatherapy. Saffron Walden, UK: CW Daniels.

Van Toller S, Hotson S, Kendal-Reed M. 1992. The brain and the sense of smell. In Van Toller S, Dodd G (eds.), Fragrance: The Psychology and Biology of Perfume. London: Elsevier Applied Science, 195-217.

Warm J, Dember W, Parasuraman R. 1990. Effects of fragrances on vigilance performance and stress. Perfumer & Flavorist. 15(15) 17-18.

Warm J, Dember W, Parasuraman R. 1992. Effects of olfactory stimulation on performance and stress of a visual sustained attention task. Journal of the Society of Cosmetic Chemists. 42 199-210.

Watson L. 2000. Jacobson's Organ. New York: WW Norton & Co.

Wiebe E. 2000. A randomized trial of aromatherapy to reduce anxiety before abortion. Effective Clinical Practice. 3(4) 166-169.

Yamaguchi A, Koga Y, Fujimura A et al. 1995. The psychological study on the effect of odor absorbed in cloth. Chemical Senses. 20(3) 381.

Yamaguchi H. 1990. Effect of odor on heart rate. In Indo M (ed.), The Psychophysiological Effect of Odor. Tokyo: Koryo, 168.

Yarnell K, Abascal K. 2001. Botanical treatments for depression. Alternative & Complementary Therapies. 7(2) 82-87.

6

EVIDENCE-BASED
AROMATHERAPY IN
NURSING PRACTICE

Nurses are the real backbone behind the care delivered within our walls and the key to patient and physician satisfaction.

Brian Keeley, CEO of Baptist Health Systems
(in Bender J 2001)

NURSES COULD be described as an endangered species because an Internet search for "nursing shortages" produces more than 58,000 sites. Although nurses are the largest group of health care workers in the United States—some 2.3 million—the number of people entering the profession has dropped drastically since managed care came into being (Box 6-1). The American Medical Association estimates there will be a shortage of 114,000 registered nurses by 2015 (Jacob 2001). One could argue that managed care has managed the care *out* of nursing because care itself is not reimbursable.

Disillusioned with their choice of career, many nurses are leaving the clinical environment and setting up practice on their own. The situation is so devastating that the nursing shortage dominates much of the discussion surrounding health care concerns.

Of the 2.3 million registered nurses (RNs) in the United States, 1.8 million work in hospitals (Nevidjon & Erickson 2001). There is a direct correlation between RN's providing patient care and better patient outcome (DeMetro 2001). Despite this rather obvious fact, managed care continues to reduce the number of RNs and reduce the length of a patient's stay in the hospital so the nurses' workloads become more intense and demanding. Nurses often have to work 12-hour shifts, and overtime is frequently mandatory. Burnout is commonplace (Crow 2001). Nurses' morale was at an all-time low in 1999 (McNeese-Smith 1999) and remains so.

Box 6-1	Nursing Shortfalls

Percentage of nurses aged 50-64: 20%
Percentage of nurses aged 30-45: 65%
Percentage of nurses aged 30 or younger: 10%
Decline in entry-level nursing enrollment each of the past 4 years: 5-7%
Estimated increase in nursing positions by 2008: 23%
Percentage of New York hospitals that reported a shortage of nurses in April 2000: 82%
Average vacancy rate for hospital nursing jobs in first quarter of 2000: 14.7%
Average time it takes to fill an RN vacancy: 3 months
Average nurse's salary (unchanged since 1992): $46,782
Salary offered by Kaiser (one of the largest health systems) for clinic nurses in 2001: $15.84 per hour

Sources: AMA Council on Medical Service Report "Growing Nursing Shortage in the USA. South Florida Business Journal (http://southflorida.bcentral.com); California Nurses Association.

Despite this, nurses are trusted by a society who ranks them above physicians and other health care workers (Nevidjon & Erickson 2001). Although they are frequently referred to as angels (Short 2001), nurses remain financially undervalued. The average nurse's salary of $46,782 in 2001 had not changed in almost 10 years. However, the reason nurses no longer want to enter the profession is not just money. It is inflexible, long working hours. It is looking after an increasing number of patients so quality of care becomes compromised, and the nurse leaves the shift feeling frustrated and angry. It is forced overtime and a poor retirement plan. Today's workforce has many other career choices, and they are making it plain nursing is no longer attractive.

Many believe the growth of complementary therapies among nurses is the result of their frustration with the limited care they can provide (Thompson 2001). Others believe nurses are simply responding to the market and giving patients what they want. Certainly complementary therapies give nurses a means of demonstrating they care at a deep level. Many nurses combine aroma and touch, and this mixture is proving the most popular of all complementary therapies with patients (Reid 2001).

For many years nursing has been called a profession, but it may be more accurate to describe it as an "emerging profession with a concept of mission which is open to change"(Leddy & Pepper 1993). This ability to change makes nursing an art as well as a science. There have been many changes since Florence Nightingale's day. The nurse's role has become increasingly technological, with more and more medical breakthroughs. Surgical procedures became more intricate, and a field of critical-care nursing developed. Babies survived at 22 weeks gestation, and neonatal nursing was born. Spare-part surgery became so normal that donor cards vie for space with our credit cards.

However, even with all the changes, there is an enduring conceptual framework that underlies nursing. Two other words share the same Latin derivation as the word *nurse*. They are *nourish* and *nurture*. Nurses have nourished and nurtured their patients to the best of their abilities no matter what the drug regime, surgical operation, or hospital constraints. Nursing the world over shares a common aim: to facilitate a speedy return to health (or a peaceful and dignified death) through nurturing the body and nourishing the soul.

How do nurses know how to nurse? The answer is a mixture. Much of what nurses do is based upon experience. However, some of what they do is learned in the classroom, and some is based on research. If one accepts (as many do) that nursing is a calling —a vocation—there is a prevailing belief that much of what a nurse does is "learned" intuition. How many nurses just "know" a patient will not make it through the night? How many nurses just "know" they must go into that room before a patient crashes or "know" a child's temperature has just returned to normal? These are similar to the instincts of a mother for her child. It is the nurturing instinct in nursing that gives it the dignity of a noble profession.

Leddy and Pepper (1993) think nurses' "body of knowledge" is derived from the experience of thousands of nurses who have gone before and from their own intuition. However, in recent years, nursing theorists have developed frameworks to explain the experience of nursing and put it in a theoretical context. Nursing diagnosis is a method of defining what nurses do and the rationale behind those actions.

There will always be resistance to change, and there will be those who ask where the body of knowledge was when Florence Nightingale put lavender oil on the brows of her soldier patients. Where was her nursing diagnosis and her nursing plan? There will be others who agree with Dossey (1993) who says "a body of knowledge that does not fit with prevailing ideas can be ignored as if it does not exist, no matter how scientifically valid it may be."

In today's world, nurses are being asked to define their role, so the appearance of nurse academicians is apposite as they struggle to give some kind of status to nursing. A change in status usually brings with it a change in language. This language needs to be understood by nurses, and by others outside the field of nursing, so everyone can be clear as to what nurses do, why they do it, and what they hope to achieve by doing what they do.

Some might argue this is all reductionist and mechanistic. How can the theory of nursing diagnosis have validity when every patient is different? The answer is nurses are fighting for their survival and need to show a clear protocol of what they do. This can only help the development and future of nursing, which lies in the ability to integrate holism, nursing theory, and nursing diagnosis symbiotically. Nurses need to use the science of language to reveal the true art of nursing.

Behind the scientific framework of nursing is increased discussion of the role of holism in nursing: the art or skill of the nurse to care for the whole patient, rather than just for the symptoms the patient is presenting. No complementary therapy on its own can make a nurse holistic because holism is something that grows from within.

Aromatherapy involves smell and touch, which are basic needs. They are also both learned memories of (hopefully) pleasurable and comforting experiences for nurse *and* patient: basic needs. Clinical aromatherapy uses essential oils to target specific outcomes that are measurable, so it gives nurses a documentable way to nurture their patients in a truly holistic manner. Nurses can argue their case for using essential oils with nursing theory and nursing diagnosis.

Clinical aromatherapy empowers nurses as it allows them to use the art as well as the science of nursing. In a nutshell, aromatherapy puts some "good scents" back into nursing and, in the process, allows nurses to feel good about what they do. Nursing is evolving, and it is wonderful to see nurses using complementary therapies as they were intended: to complement nursing.

NURSING DIAGNOSIS*

Bulechek and McCloskey (1985) state nursing interventions are "any direct care treatment that a nurse performs on behalf of a client." Using this definition, all treatments initiated by a nurse are related to nursing diagnosis. So if aromatherapy is part of nursing, then aromatherapy would be an appropriate response to a nursing diagnosis. Many nurses believe nursing diagnosis allows them to assess their patients and write care plans more easily.

The development of nursing diagnosis gives focus to the specifications of nursing needs by creating an exact language to analyze how the nurse can reach the correct decision. Although resented by some who feel this language is just what nursing does *not* need, nursing diagnosis is probably exactly what nursing needs: a practical tool to clarify the nature, origin, and manifestations of nursing needs. Nursing diagnosis can also give validity to a complementary therapy (like aromatherapy) within the concept of a care plan. Gordon (1982; 1990) suggests "a nursing diagnosis is a health problem a nurse can treat but does not mean that non-nursing consultants cannot be used. The critical element is whether nurse-prescribed interventions can achieve the outcome established with the client."

The term *nursing diagnosis* was first introduced in 1953 by Fry, who was attempting to set a standardized language for nursing care plans. However, nurses disliked the idea of the word *diagnosis*, as it was too medical. They believed nursing had a tradition of avoiding making statements about patients. Twenty years went by before the first meeting of the National Group for the Classification of Nursing Diagnosis was held. Eventually, in 1990, the North American

---

*For this section of the book, I relied heavily on the standard textbook *Nursing Diagnosis: Applications to Clinical Practice* (Carpenito 1993). Sometimes similar examples have been used, followed by parallel analysis to show how aromatherapy can be part of nursing diagnosis.

Nursing Diagnosis Association approved the following definition of nursing diagnosis: "Nursing diagnosis is a clinical judgment about individual, family, or community responses to actual or potential health problems/life processes. Nursing diagnosis provides the basis for selection of nursing interventions to achieve outcomes for which the nurse is accountable" (Carpenito 1993).

It is the independent function of a professional nurse to make a nursing diagnosis and decide upon a course of action to be followed for the solution of the problem (Abdellah & Levine 1965). The practice of nursing often interfaces with the practice of other health professionals; physicians and nurses collaborate in common areas. This can necessitate a nurse having to choose between a nursing or medical diagnosis. Sometimes a nurse can only attend to a medical diagnosis because of time constraint. Sometimes the nurse may decide the medical diagnosis is more important than her own nursing diagnosis.

Looking at the areas of nursing diagnosis, it is obvious they carry very generalized headings under which more specific headings are given. There are many headings that could lend themselves to the use of aromatherapy. These could include the following:

Altered comfort
Anxiety
Constipation
Fatigue
Fear
Grieving
Impaired communication
Infection
Pain
Powerlessness
Spiritual distress

Carpenito (1993) includes some 120 different nursing diagnosis headings on a general level. Very few could not be helped via aromatherapy. Nursing diagnosis represents a situation that is the primary responsibility of the nurse. Nurses may also indicate collaborative problems in their nursing diagnosis, which would indicate that both medical and nursing interventions are required, and they can pinpoint potential complications that might be collaborative problems or straightforward nursing problems.

For example, a patient with pneumonia would have potential complications within the collaborative area of septic shock, paralytic ileus, and respiratory insufficiency. The nursing diagnosis would be as follows:

Activity intolerance due to compromised respiration, high risk of fluid balance deficit due to fever and hyperventilation
Ineffective airway clearance due to pain and tracheobronchial secretions
Altered comfort related to hyperthermia, malaise, and pulmonary pathology
High risk for ineffective management of therapeutic regimen

These diagnoses would be related to nutritional needs, home-care needs, restrictions, signs and symptoms of complications, and follow-up care. With the specification of precise needs for nursing it is easier to see those areas where aromatherapy could be used. These would be in the nursing diagnosis of altered comfort and ineffective airway clearance. I shall consider the first of these as a separate issue.

Nursing Diagnosis of Altered Comfort

In this case the cause of the altered comfort is listed as follows:

Hyperthermia

Malaise

Pulmonary pathology

This means anything that is going to alleviate those causes could help enhance the comfort level of the patient. Malaise might respond to an essential oil with calming and soothing properties such as lavender, frankincense, sandalwood,or ylang ylang. Hyperthermia might be helped with a spritzer containing lavender and peppermint. Chest problems and infections might respond to an essential oil known to be bronchodilating, like eucalyptus or ravansara, which also have antibacterial or antiviral properties. A nurse could use a mixture of several essential oils to address the three problems.

Gordon (1990) developed an 11-area system for organizing the assessment of the functional health pattern of a patient:

Activity and exercise

Coping and stress

Elimination

Health management

Nutrition and metabolism

Perception

Relationships

Self-perception

Sexuality

Sleep and rest

Values and beliefs

It is easy to see that aromatherapy could fit fairly readily into most of these categories. This kind of data enables nurses to make judgments on which the nursing diagnosis will be based. As the care plan will be based on the nursing diagnosis, careful analysis of the outcomes is necessary. Care plans are blueprints to enable a continuous, consistent quality of care. They contain a diagnostic statement, desired-nursing-outcome criteria, nursing interventions, and an evaluation of the outcome.

The following case studies are true and were each carried out by a nurse in a clinical setting.

CASE STUDY   **1**   ALTERATION IN COMFORT LEVEL: MALAISE, HERPES

Outcome Criteria
>Reduction of pain of lesion
>Reduction of size of lesion
>Increase time between outbreaks

Mrs. E was a 42-year-old female with a herpetic lesion on her nasal septum. She had a history of cold sores and genital herpes. The nurse described an intervention using aromatherapy, and the patient gave her informed consent to aromatherapy. The nurse offered two essential oils, Eucalyptus globulus and tea tree. The patient liked the aroma of eucalyptus and said it reminded her of Vicks Vapor Rub. She was patch tested using a 100% dilution of Eucalyptus globulus on her forearm. No irritation or sensitization was observed after 24 hours.

A 25% solution of *Eucalyptus globulus* in aloe vera gel was given to the patient who applied it to the lesion using a cotton swab. The patient observed there was an initial "slight burning sensation, which felt healing" immediately after the first application. The application was repeated every 2 hours by the patient. Within 2 days the lesion had decreased in size. The pustular lesion gradually dried. The pain was reduced from an 8 to a 4 on a visual analog scale of 0-10 within 4 hours. Within 6 days the lesion had healed completely. The usual time-frame for lesions to heal for this patient was 10 days. Following this procedure the patient reapplied eucalyptus to lesions as they occurred. Follow-up revealed the outbreaks appeared less frequently over a period of 1 year.

Note: The clinical aromatherapy objective to alter level of comfort was measured (by visual analogue) and achieved.

Choice of Essential Oil
Eucalyptus has a well-earned reputation for being a good all-around antimicrobial agent. Hmamouchi et al (1990) and Saeed and Sabir (1995) found *Eucalyptus globulus* effective against all bacteria tested, and Benouda et al (1988) found the action to be comparable to orthodox antibiotics. Eucalyptus was also found to help the action of conventional antibiotics (Kufferath & Mundualgo 1954). Used topically, it has analgesic (Weyers & Brodbeck 1989) and antiinflammatory properties (Moscolo et al 1987). It is antifungal and is effective against *Cryptococcus neoformans,* a common infection in immune-compromised patients (Viollon & Chaumont 1994). It is antitumoral as well (Takasaki et al 1995). Aqueous extracts of eucalyptus have been found to be antiviral (Takechi et al 1985), and anecdotal evidence indicates eucalyptus essential oil is very useful in treating herpes and shingles.

CASE STUDY | 2 | ALTERATION OF LEVEL OF COMFORT:
MALAISE, PSORIASIS

Outcome Criteria
Reduce itching and cracking lesions
Reduce scaliness of lesions
Improve comfort level of patient

Mr. A, a 51-year-old male with psoriasis, was offered aromatherapy to enhance comfort levels. He had classic, raised, white, scaly skin patches with red borders. These intermittent, itchy skin lesions occurred on the skin surface with predominance over the joints, resulting in cracked skin. Discomfort level was a 7 on a scale of 0-10. A history of allergies and sensitivity was taken. The patient liked the aroma of lavender. Informed consent to aromatherapy was given. A patch test of 4% lavender was applied on the upper, inner arm. No sensitivity was recorded after 24 hours. A 2% solution (2 drops lavender to 5 ml cold-pressed vegetable oil) was applied to one lesion twice a day. As 2 days passed, the redness, scaliness, and size of the lesion decreased, but the itching remained unchanged. The lavender solution was applied to all the lesions of the same leg. Within 7 days there was marked improvement in the size, redness, and scaliness of the lesions to the extent that aromatherapy was discontinued on that leg. Discomfort was now a 0 on a scale of 0-10 for those areas. The lesions on other parts of the body that did not receive aromatherapy remained the same.

Note: The clinical aromatherapy objective to alter level of comfort was measured (by visual analogue) and achieved.

Choice of Essential Oil
Lavender is a classic essential oil for skin problems. It was used for wound cleaning in World War I and was approved by the French Academy of Medicine. As well as proven antibacterial action against many pathogenic organisms including methicillin-resistant *Staphylococcus aureus* (Nelson 1997), lavender has local-anesthetic effects (Ghelardini et al 1999) and is skin regenerative (Valnet 1990). Lavender inhibits histamine release in immediate-type allergic reactions in mice and rats (Hyung-Min & Seong-Hoon 1999) and may be useful in allergic skin problems linked to immune deficiency. Lavender was also found to be a mood elevator by Corner et al (1995) and a sedative by (Elisabtsky et al 1995). Nachi (1990) reported on the calming effects of lavender with patients undergoing magnetic resonance imaging. Saeki (2000) found lavender to be relaxing, and Itai et al (2000) reported on the antidepressant properties of lavender with chronic hemodialysis patients. Many patients with psoriasis (though not necessarily the one in this case study) have stress-related depression, which is another reason lavender can be beneficial. Lavender also enhances the sedative effects of conventional pharmaceuticals (Stanassova-Shopova et al 1972), and lavender is readily absorbed through the skin (Jager et al 1992).

CASE STUDY **3** ALTERATION OF COMFORT/CHRONIC LOW
SELF-ESTEEM: VAGINAL YEAST INFECTION

Outcome Criteria

Reduce discomfort
Remove vaginal yeast infection
Improve self-esteem

Miss C was a 21-year-old woman with diabetes. Her blood sugar was
around 130. Her diabetes was stabilized with diet and insulin injections.
She had a recurrent vaginal yeast infection and had previously used conventional antifungal drugs (Terazol and Femstat). These gave temporary relief, but
only after 5 days of treatment. She was frustrated and unable to cope with the
recurrent infections, which were impacting her self-esteem. Her discomfort was
8 on a numerical scale of 0-10. The patient inhaled the aroma of tea tree and
commented it didn't smell wonderful, but she just wanted some relief from the
itching. Informed consent was given and a patch test of 4% tea tree oil was carried out. No irritation or sensitization was observed after 24 hours. The patient
was directed to dilute tea tree to the correct solution and apply it to a tampon.
She was told to apply it vaginally three times a day, each time with a fresh solution of 2% tea tree oil (two drops of tea tree in 5 ml cold-pressed sweet almond
oil). She said after insertion the tea tree tampon felt pleasantly tingly, rather like
the effect of toothpaste while cleaning her teeth. She carried out the treatment
and reported all evidence of vaginal yeast infection disappeared after 3 days, and
on a numerical scale the discomfort was a 0. On follow-up, 6 months later the
infection had not reappeared. She felt empowered and happy to look after her
own vaginal comfort. Her level of self-esteem was enhanced.

Note: The clinical aromatherapy objective to alter level of comfort was measured (by visual analogue) and achieved.

Choice of Essential Oil

Melaleuca alternifolia (tea tree) is one of the classic aromatherapy choices for
treating infection and is safe to use vaginally (Northrupp 1995). Tea tree is useful for either bacterial infections such as abscesses, acne (Carson & Riley 1994),
or fungal infections including athlete's foot, tinea (Tong et al 1992), impetigo or
viral infections such as cold sores and herpes (Hammer et al 1996). Pena (1962)
showed its effectiveness for yeast infection, trichomoniasis, and anaerobic infections (Blackwell 1991). For vaginal infection, dilute the essential oil in a cold-
pressed vegetable oil (for example sweet almond) and apply on a tampon. Mix
two drops of tea tree in one teaspoonful of carrier oil. Roll a tampon in the
mixture and insert into vagina. Repeat with fresh tampon every 4 hours and
leave in overnight. Relief should occur within 3 days. Vaginal thrush is unlikely
to reoccur (Buckle 2001).

The next case study discusses using aromatherapy during extubation (the process of removing an endotracheal tube when a patient is capable of breathing without artificial help). This is a common task within the remit of an intensive-care nurse. Yang & Tobin (1991) state there is "no one method of weaning which has clear superiority." However, weaning requires patient physical and psychological preparedness (Logan & Jenny 1990). Extubation is a skilled nursing maneuver because patients must be alert enough to breathe on their own, but not so alert that the endotracheal tube is causing distress and they are fighting the ventilator.

CASE STUDY   DYSFUNCTIONAL VENTILATORY WEANING RESPONSE

Outcome Criteria
   Achieve weaning goals
   Remain extubated
   Not be exhausted by the process of weaning

The nursing intervention consisted of the following.
   Determined readiness for weaning
   Asked if patient liked the smell of an essential oil such as lavender
   Asked for permission to touch the patient
   Explained the weaning process and demonstrated hand "m" technique using
      lavender
   Explained patient's role in the process of weaning
   Enhanced patient's feelings of self-esteem through encouragement
   Promoted trust through conversation and touch
   Reduced negative effects of anxiety and fatigue through the use of aro-
      matherapy
   Created a positive environment with aromatherapy
   Optimized comfort status through aromatherapy
Please see patient's chart, Fig 6-1. The arrow indicates when the "m" technique was used with 2% lavender.

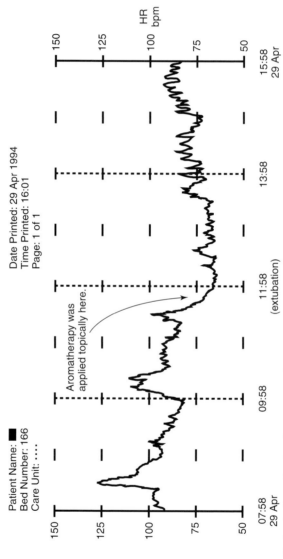
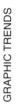

FIGURE 6-1   Patient's chart showing decrease in pulse when aromatherapy applied topically. (Courtesy Lori Mitchell)

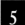 CASE STUDY **5** ALTERATIONS OF COMFORT LEVEL: CHRONIC PAIN

Outcome Criteria
Relax patient
Reduce perception of pain

Mrs. G was a 74-year-old woman with cancer and bone metastases. She was in severe pain (8 on the numeric pain intensity scale) despite having a patient-controlled analgesia of morphine. She was unable to find a comfortable position in bed and became withdrawn and depressed. Her muscles became tight from attempting to "hold" her pain. Two drops of rose essential oil were applied to a cotton hankie that was pinned on the patient's nightgown. The affect was almost instant: the patient took some deep breaths, opened her clenched fists, and smiled for the first time in many weeks. This treatment was repeated every 4 hours, and an electronic diffuser was used at night. The aroma of the garden appeared to alter the patient's perception of pain, reducing it to a 3 on the pain scale, and although the terminal nature of her disease was not affected, the quality of her life appeared to be considerably improved.

Note: The clinical aromatherapy objective to alter level of comfort was measured (by visual analogue) and achieved.

Choice of Essential Oil
Rosa damascena (rose) is the most popular and acceptable aroma in the world, recognized by almost every culture and religion. Bulgarian research indicates rose oil reduces hypertension (Kirov & Bainova 1988) and counteracts the effects of isoprenaline (Brud & Szydlowska 1991). This agrees with the historically held belief that rose strengthens and calms the heart (Lawless 1995). Rose is also an antispasmodic and a mild sedative. It has antidepressant properties (as anyone who has sat for a while in a rose garden can affirm). A Russian study on Rosalin (an ointment containing rose) showed the ointment had good antibacterial properties. This was presumably why Nostradamus used it to protect himself against the plague. Further studies indicate rose essential oil has an inhibitory effect on *Helicobacter pylori* (Boyanova & Neshev 1999). Rose has also recently shown antiviral and antiHIV activity (Mahmood et al 1996).

Rose essential oil is useful to soothe radiodermatitis and is generally helpful to all irritated skin. It is very important to use Rose otto (steam distilled) not Rose absolute (extracted with petrochemicals) and to be sure to use pure rose oil. Rose essential oil is expensive (between $1 and $2 per drop), but it is still less expensive than conventional antidepressants as only a few drops are used at a time.

Case Study 6 Spiritual Distress

Outcome Criteria

Continue spiritual practices as the patient knows them
Allow patient to express decreasing feelings of guilt and anxiety
Allow patient to express satisfaction with one's spiritual condition

Mrs. H was an 85-year-old woman with depression. Many of her friends were dead, and she lived a long way from her family who did not visit her often. She did not sleep well and was prone to hyperventilation and palpitations. She loved the smell of roses, which reminded her of a rose garden she tended with her husband when he was alive. Informed consent was given. Two drops of rose oil were inhaled on a facial tissue four times a day. In addition, two drops of rose were added to a cotton ball placed under her pillowcase. Within 1 week she was smiling, sleeping better, and discussing how she could become involved with looking after the houseplants in the facility. Staff noted she no longer hyperventilated and that she stopped complaining of palpitations. The nursing intervention consisted of the following:

Provide privacy and quiet
Be open to the patient's needs for spiritual peace
Contact the patient's spiritual leader when required
Suggest aromatherapy might enhance the patient's ability to meditate, pray, or induce a state of peacefulness
Introduce the essential oils *Boswellia carteri* (frankincense) and *Rosa damascena* (Rose)
Discuss the effects of both aromas

All people have a spiritual dimension, whether they choose to accept it or not (Dickinson 1975). Spirituality is often at the core of a person's distress, yet most people find spirituality the most difficult subject about which to communicate. During acute and chronic disease, many patients turn to their faith, lose their faith, or seek a faith where there has been none previously. Despite this, nurses commonly avoid addressing the spiritual dimension of a patient. Martin et al (1978) suggest the spiritual part of nursing involves "being with" the patient rather than "doing to" the patient. Stiles draws attention to the nurse-family spiritual relationship in cancer care (Stiles 1990).

Aromatherapy allows nurses to "be with" their patients, even while they may be "doing to," in an intimate but professional way that nurtures the relationship between the nurse and the patient. This often allows a window of inner reflection in which spiritual feelings (or needs) are verbalized. During my education as a nurse, and subsequent to it, I noticed few patients are brought up the subject of spiritual matters. Yet since I have been using aromatherapy, this sensitive area has arisen time and time again, almost as though the aromas themselves provide an atmosphere of acceptance.

Dossey (1993) writes about the need for thought to be accepted as being as genuine as any drug or surgical procedure. The thoughts generated by gentle touch and pleasing smell have a powerful effect on our psyche and on our spirituality. It is not only what nurses do for patients, but also their good intentions to "be with" them that can aid the healing process. Nursing has a curative potential. Despite the fact that 15% of nurses feel they are not prepared to provide spiritual care (Stiles 1990), they can provide spiritual support just by being there. Aromatherapy gives nurses permission to be there. A leading Buddhist teacher wrote about his own experience with his dying father, and his words are very indicative of what nurses do as part of nursing care. "There wasn't much to say. I held his hand. He was frightened. He didn't want to know about medicine. He didn't even want to talk. What mattered was that I sat there, not being afraid, not rejecting his fear and his pain, simply by holding his hand. He died after several more days" (Kornfield 2000).

CONCLUSIONS

A few case studies have been presented above as a brief argument to support the use of aromatherapy as an enhancement to nursing care. Nurses already use many over-the-counter products not prescribed by a physician, such as scented soaps and hair spray. Nurses also use synthetic sprays to mask human smells, and many of the synthetic aromas in these sprays have not been tested for long-term effect on patients. The time has come to think about what aromatherapy could mean in nursing terms: how it could enhance what nurses do and how it could enhance their job satisfaction.

One of my students said, "Aromatherapy has really changed my life; now I notice what smells good and what doesn't." She went on to say, "So much in life smells bad, doesn't it? I wonder if that is because we have made a nonsense of nature."

We are making a nonsense of nursing care if we do not allow nurses the freedom to make their patients feel as comfortable as possible. What better way than through gentle touch and the use of natural aromatics that are already part of everyday life? Even before palliative care became an accepted specialty within nursing, nurses still carried out palliative care. Then it became recognized as a distinctive and very caring form of health care. Before the first heart transplant, people thought heart transplants were not possible. Now there are countless books on surgery and cardiac nursing. Nursing as a profession is evolving as world perception changes. Nurses are already using aromatherapy in many parts of the world. They are using it because it has validity, whether one's view of nursing care is intuitive, derived through nursing diagnosis, or derived from conceptual nursing frameworks and theories.

How Aromatherapy Could be Used in Hospitals

There are many potential uses for aromatherapy in hospitals. They range from the simple mood-enhancing effects of smelling something pleasant to the specific application of an antiseptic essential oil to combat cross-infections. At present most hospitals do not smell nice, and science has shown how we feel affects how we are. If it is possible to alter our environment to make it supportive in times of need, surely this is something to be taken seriously.

Steele (1993) tested volunteers using an electroencephalogram to demonstrate changes following the inhalation of certain essential oils. He discovered changes in brain rhythms occurred within 15 seconds, and a positive change in mood took approximately the same length of time.

Patients undergoing radiotherapy or computer-assisted tomography scans are isolated in a room during treatment and have to lie absolutely still for lengthy periods of time. Many find this experience stressful. A soothing, relaxing essential oil such as lavender (*Lavandula angustifolia*), vetiver (*Vetiveria zizanoides*), or bergamot (*Citrus bergamia*) might help them. Balacs (1991) reports on research that showed 60% of patients exposed to a sweet, vanilla-like fragrance (heliotropin) experienced less anxiety than the control group.

Emergency rooms receive victims of traffic accidents, burns, and poisoning for whom immediate action is needed. Frequently relatives find it difficult to stay calm enough to explain exactly what happened, and medical professionals find it hard to maintain patience, knowing that every second is vital but needing precise information. By combining an antiseptic essential oil with a calming one, the environment is immediately made more reassuring and more hospitable.

Wards for long-term care often have unattractive smells: a mixture of incontinent patients, hospital food, and lavatory cleaner. Helen Passant, a nurse, managed to change that situation in an Oxford, England hospital when she introduced the use of aromatherapy. Her elderly patients responded to the use of touch and massage, becoming "alive" again: a situation reminiscent of the film *Beginnings*. The aromas evoked memories, and the patients began to talk about their lives and communicate their feelings. No longer isolated men and women waiting to die, the patients became an active group: talking, then singing, then dancing. In addition, the ward's drug bill was reduced by a third. The hospital rewarded her by reducing her budget by a third!

Many operating theatres have closed air conditioning. This means the same air is ventilated constantly. It is much less expensive than open air conditioning, which sucks in a constant stream of new air, warms (or cools) and filters it, then vents it back into the outside environment. Research has been carried out on airborne infections and on the prevalence of postoperative wound infections. Cruse (1980) found sufficient data to indicate postoperative wound infections, from preoperatively clean wounds, are directly related with the length of operating time. Diffused essential oils with good antibacterial and antiviral properties may reduce the cost of the additional days incurred for in-patients and for those with nosocomial (hospital-acquired) wound infections.

Some enlightened hospitals are using antibacterial essential oils in their operating rooms, with the added bonus of preventing cross-infection among medical staff. Each operating room has specific bacteria and viruses that are most prevalent, so a customized cocktail of several essential oils is employed. Use of a pleasant and uplifting essential oil, such as pine (*Pinus sylvestris*) or lemon (*Citrus limonum*) can also improve the concentration of operating staff at night.

The use of aromatherapy in hospitals in England, South Africa, Switzerland, and, more recently, in the United States shows a progressive trend toward supporting patients on a more holistic basis. Physicians and hospital managers are becoming aware that how patients feel can affect the way they respond to treatment, and therefore how quickly they recover.

Planetree Hospitals Inc. is an American group of hospitals whose staff strive to put the patient and the patient's comfort first. It had a humble beginning in 1978; Angelica Thieriot found the routine medical treatment she received in the late 1970s so dehumanizing she made it her mission to develop a new model of patient-centered care. The concept of Planetree spread nationwide, and now there are more than 40 similar hospitals and facilities throughout the United States. Patients are encouraged to take an active part in making decisions about their future, and this begins with open medical records. Patients are also invited to have a gentle massage prior to surgery and to ask their family and friends to bring in their favorite food to prepare. There is a kitchen on every floor. Gentle music fills the reception area, and nothing is too much trouble for the patient. It is no surprise patients and staff gravitate toward Planetree!

Aromatherapy is a complementary therapy much accepted by the Planetree philosophy. Desert Samaritan Hospital in Mesa, Arizona, is one of the first Planetree hospitals to have sponsored nurses not just through an 18-month clinical aromatherapy training program but to become paid instructors themselves.

Touch is known to have a dramatic effect on patients, and yet patients lying in a hospital bed are rarely touched, except for diagnostic (palpation) or procedural reasons (changing a dressing, blood-pressure recording). One method gaining popularity among nurses is the "m" technique. This method of touch is described more fully in Chapter 8 and quickly acknowledges a patient's worth as an individual. A foot or hand "m" takes only 5 minutes, but that time can totally change the way patients perceive the environment around them. Touch has also been shown to reduce blood pressure, reduce lower back pain, relieve anxiety, and alleviate depression (Montagu 1986).

Aromatherapy using touch and smell could be a complete hospital stress-management package, producing a happier and more content workforce with more secure and less anxious patients. The level of interest in aromatherapy shown by patients and nurses suggests an overwhelming desire for such integration.

Hospitals are being run like businesses. Therefore, the cost benefits of using essential oils to promote healing need to be addressed, and I hope this book will go some way toward that. There are a few ethical questions. What about consent? Is it ethical to manipulate mood? What about a patient who does not like the aromas? Yet how many patients sign a consent form approving the smell of antiseptics or air fresheners? How many nurses enter their place of work having used scented soap, hair spray, or aftershave? How many patients are allergic or sensitive to Lysol or other cleaning fluids used in hospitals? It is difficult to have one set of rules for aromatherapy if there are no rules governing other types of scent.

Another area of concern is the potential use of synthetic or adulterated essential oils that result in poor or negative results. It cannot be emphasized strongly enough that it is the quality of the essential oil that will determine the final result. Essential oils need to be judged like good wine. Good wine is expensive, and so are the best essential oils.

Perhaps one of the greatest concerns about using aromatherapy in hospitals is incorrect use due to ignorance. Contrary to media hype, aromatherapy is not the panacea for everything, a kind of "comfort-blanket" smell. Of equal importance is the quality of accompanying touch. A heavy, compressing, rapid stroke will not produce the same effect as a light, slow, gentle one. The techniques used in aromatherapy cannot be learned solely from a book; they need to be experienced.

There is an urgent need for adequate training, and reading a book is not enough. As well as learning the "m" technique, the use of essential oils in aromatherapy requires knowledge and experience. A simple name like lavender covers three completely different species, each with entirely different therapeutic effects. *Lavandula angustifolia* is a sedative, *Lavandula latifolia* is an expectorant, and *Lavandula stoechas* is effective against *Pseudomonas aeruginosa*. For Nurse Practice Acts please see www.rjbuckle.com or www.ahna.com.

Consider the following. A patient likes the smell of lemongrass and needs an essential oil with sedative effects. The patient feels isolated. A daily foot "m" technique is chosen and added to the care plan. The patient also has a fungal infection that appears to lessen following a number of foot massages with lemongrass. Although lemongrass had not been used ostensibly for its antifungal properties, it cannot stop itself from being antifungal. But what if a health professional without prescriptive powers had known about the antifungal properties and had chosen lemongrass primarily because of them? Would he or she have crossed the boundaries? The International Council of Nurses states that nurses' "fundamental responsibility is to conserve life, to alleviate suffering and to promote health." Using aromatherapy in this way could be seen to be alleviating suffering. However if the targeted outcome of an essential oil is changed to one outside the jurisdiction of the provider, a different protocol might be required.

Appendix VI is a list of hospitals using aromatherapy or having sponsored nurse's training in aromatherapy.

REFERENCES

Abdellah F, Levine E. 1965. Better Patient Care Through Nursing Research. New York: Macmillan.

Balacs T. 1991. Fragrance relaxes. International Journal of Aromatherapy. 33(3) 8.

Bender J. 2001. Nursing shortages have hospitals sending SOS. South Florida Business Journal. Retrieved August 4, 2001 from http://www.southflorida.bcentral.com.

Benouda A, Hassar M, Benjilali B. 1988. The antiseptic properties of essential oils in vitro, tested against pathogenic germs found in hospitals. Fitoterapia. 59(2) 115-119.

Blackwell R. 1991. Teatree oil and anaerobic vaginosis. Lancet. 337(8736) 300.

Boyanova L, Neshev G. 1999. Inhibitory effect of rose oil on *Helicobacter pylori* growth in vitro: preliminary report. Journal of Medical Microbiology. 48(7) 705-706.

Brud W, Szydlowska I. 1991. Bulgarian rose oil. International Journal of Aromatherapy. 2(3) 18-19.

Buckle J. 2000. The 'm' technique. Massage and Bodywork. (Feb/March) 52-68.

Buckle J. 2001. The role of aromatherapy in nursing care. Nursing Clinics of North America. 36(1) 57-72.

Bulechek G, McCloskey J. 1985. Nursing Interventions: Treatment for Nursing Diagnosis. Philadelphia: WB Saunders.

Carpenito L. 1993. Nursing Diagnosis: Applications to Clinical Practice, 5th ed. Mickleton, NJ: JB Lippincott.

Carson C, Riley T. 1994. Susceptibility of *Propionibacterium* acne to the essential oil of *Melaleuca alternifolia*. Letters Applied Microbiology. 19(1) 24-25.

Corner J, Cawley N, Hildebrand S. 1995. An evaluation of the use of essential oils on the well-being of cancer patients. International Journal Palliative Nursing. 1(2) 67-73

Crow K. 2001. Healing and burnout, 12 hours at a stretch. New York Times. Sunday June 24. 15.2-15.3.

Cruse P. 1980. The epidemiology of wound infection: a ten-year prospective study of 69,939 wounds. Surgery Clinics of North America. 60, 27-40.

DeMetro R. 2001. Medical stripmining and the new nursing shortage. Retrieved August 4, 2001 from http://www.califnurses.org.

Dickinson C. 1975. The search for spiritual meaning. American Journal of Nursing. 75, 1789–1793.

Dossey L. 1993. Healing Words. San Francisco, CA: HarperCollins.

Elisabtsky E, Coelho de Souza G, Dos Santos M et al. 1995. Sedative properties of linalool. Fitoterapia. 66(5) 407-415.

Ghelardini C, Galeotti N, Salvatore G et al. 1999. Local anesthetic activity of essential oil of *Lavandula angustifolia*. Planta Medica. 65(8) 700-703.

Gordon M. 1990. Towards theory-based diagnostic categories. Nursing Diagnosis. 1(1) 5-11.

Hammer K, Carson C, Riley T. 1996. Susceptibility of transient and commensal skin flora to the essential oil of *Melaleuca alternifolia*. Australasian Journal of Infection Control. 24(3) 186-189.

Hmamouchi M, Tantaoui-Elaraki A, Es-Safi N et al. 1990. Illustration of antibacterial and antifungal properties of *Eucalyptus* essential oils. Plantes Medicinales et Phytotherapie. 24(4) 278-289.

Hyung-Min K, Seong-Hoon C. 1999. Lavender oil inhibits immediate-type allergic reaction in mice and rats. Journal of Pharmacy and Pharmacology. 51, 221-226.

Itai T, Amauadu H, Kuribayashi M et al. 2000. Psychological effects of aromatherapy on chronic hemodialysis patients. Psychiatric and Clinical Neurosciences. 54(4) 393-397.

Jacob J. 2001. AMA house goes after nursing shortage issue. Retrieved August 4, 2001 from http://www.ama-assn.org.

Jager W, Buchbauer G, Jirovetz L et al. 1992. Percutaneous absorption of lavender oil from a massage oil. Journal of the Society of Cosmetic Chemists. 43(1) 49-54.

Kirov A, Bainova M. 1988. Rose oil: acute and subacute oral toxicity. Medico Biologic Information. 3:8-14.

Kornfield J. 2000. After the Ecstasy, the Laundry. Woodacre, CA: Rider.

Kufferath F, Mundualgo G. 1954. The activity of some preparations containing essential oils in Tuberculosis. Fitoterapia. 25:483-485.

Lawless J.1995. Rose Oil. London: Thorsons, 20.

Leddy S, Pepper J. 1993. Conceptual bases of professional nursing. Mickleton, NJ: JB Lippincott.

Logan J, Jenny J. 1990. Deriving a new nursing diagnosis through qualitative research: dysfunctional ventilatory response. Nursing Diagnosis. 1, 37-43.

Mahmood N, Piacente S, Pizza C et al. 1996. The anti-HIV activity and mechanisms of action of pure compounds isolated from *Rosa damascena*. Biochemical and Biophysical Research Communications. 229(1) 73-79.

Martin C, Burrow C, Pomilio J. 1978. Spiritual needs of patients' surveys. In Fish S, Shelly J (eds.), Spiritual Care: The Nurse's Role. Downers Grove, IL: InterVarsity Press.

McNeese-Smith D. 1999. A content analysis of staff nurse descriptions of job satisfaction and dissatisfaction. Journal of Advanced Nursing. 29(6) 1332-1341.

Montagu A. 1986. Touching. New York: Harper & Row.

Moscolo N, Autore G, Capasso F et al. 1987. Biological screening of Italian medicinal plants for anti-inflammatory activity. Phytotherapy Research. 1(1) 28-31.

Nachi K. 1990. Aromachology: the psychic effects of fragrances. The Futurist. 24, 49-50.

Nelson R. 1997. In vitro activities of five plant essential oils against MRSA and VREF. Journal of Antimicrobial Chemotherapeutics. 40, 305-306.

Nevidjon B, Erickson, J. 2001. The nursing shortage: solutions for the short and long term. Online Journal of Issues in Nursing. Retrieved August 4, 2001 from http://www.nursingworld.org/ojin/topic14/tpc14_4.htm.

Northrupp C. 1995. Women' Bodies, Women's Minds. London: Piatkus.

Pena E. 1962. *Melaleuca alternifolia* oil: Its use for trichomonal vaginitis and other vaginal infection. Obstetrics & Gynecology. 19(6) 793-795.

Reid J. 2001.Getting the massage across. Nursing Times. 97(15) 26-27.

Saeed M, Sabir A. 1995. Antimicrobial studies of the constituents of Pakistani eucalyptus oils. Journal of Faculty of Pharmacy of Gazi University. 12(2) 129-140.

Saeki Y. 2000. The effect of foot bath with or without the essential oil of lavender on the autonomic nervous system: a randomized trial. Complementary Therapies in Medicine. 8(1) 2-7.

Short L. 2001. Nurse was an angel at accident scene. Albany Times Union. Sunday July 8, B4.

Stanassova-Shopova S, Roussinov K, Boycheva I. 1973. On certain central neurotropic effects of lavender essential oil. II. Communication: Studies of the effects of linalool and terpineol. Bulletin of the Institute of Physiology. 15:149-156.

Steele J. 1993. The fragrant hospital. In Aroma 93 Conference Proceedings. Brighton, UK: Aromatherapy Publications, 22-29.

Stiles M. 1990. The shining stranger: nurse-family spiritual relationship. Cancer Nursing. 13, 235-256.

Swansea Hospital Department of Genito-Urinary Medicine, Swansea, UK. 1991. Teatree oil and anaerobic vaginosis. Lancet. 337(8736) 300.

Takasaki M, Konoshima T, Kozuka M et al. 1995. Anti-tumor promoting activities of euglabols from eucalyptus plants. Biological and Pharmaceutical Bulletin. 18(3) 435-438.

Takechi M, Tanaka Y, Takehara M et al. 1985. Structure and antiherpetic activity among the tannins. Phytochemistry. 24(10) 2245-2250.

Thompson C. 2001. Oil on troubled water. Nursing Times. 97(15) 24-26.

Tong M, Altman P, Barnetson R. 1992. Teatree oil in the treatment of Tinea Pedis. Australasian Journal of Dermatology. 33(30) 145-149.

Valnet J. 1990. The Practice of Aromatherapy. Saffron Walden, UK: CW Daniels.

Viollon C, Chaumont J. 1994. Antifungal properties of essential oils and their main components against *Cryptococcus neoformans*. Mycopathologia. 128(3) 151-153.

Weyers W, Brodbeck R. 1989. Skin absorption of volatile oils. Pharmacokinetics. Pharm Unserer Zeit. 18(3) 82-86.

Yang K, Tobin M. 1991. A prospective study of indexes predicting outcomes of trials of weaning from mechanical ventilation. New England Journal of Medicine. 324, 1445-1451.

7

ORAL AND INTERNAL USE
OF AROMATHERAPY*

Science and myth are one; the natural world is but a manifestation of thoughts and impulses all occurring on endless metaphysical planes, all enveloped by the mind of the healer.

Wade Davis
One River

THE TOPIC of oral and internal use of essential oils is controversial and confusing. Much of the confusion is due to lack of knowledge and cultural misconceptions because the oral and internal uses of essential oils are not taught in most aromatherapy training programs in the United States or United Kingdom.

There are three probable reasons for this omission.

1. Many training programs are intended for the lay public, not licensed health professionals (LHPs).
2. Most adverse interactions with conventional medications are associated with the oral use of essential oils.
3. There is a fear that oral use of essential oils may lead to poisoning.

However, this book is intended for LHPs who may wish (or need) to know about the oral and internal use of essential oils so they can decide for themselves. Ultimately, LHPs will need to decide if giving essential oils either orally or internally is within their license. The views in this chapter are mine, and this chapter is intended to open a dialogue not provide an answer.

*I am greatly indebted to the aromatic medicine courses I took with Penoel, Franchomme, Schnaubelt, Price, Harris, and Guba for this section. It is strongly recommended that the reader undertake a professional course in aromatic medicine before using essential oils orally or in high concentrations, as these methods are not covered in most aromatherapy courses.

The sale and use of essential oils, much like herbal remedies, is not controlled in the United States (or England or France). Essential oils can be purchased by anyone and used in any way. If, however, LHPs are using essential oils to enhance care, they will need to decide if this use fits within the parameters of their licenses.

Broadly speaking, LHPs can be divided into those who have prescriptive powers and those who do not. Those who have prescriptive license may feel more comfortable using the oral route of aromatherapy than those who do not. This does not mean only those who have prescriptive license may use the oral route, only that they may feel more comfortable doing so. Whatever the kind of license a health professional has, he or she has accountability. Therefore the treatment offered should be based on training received.

There are several anomalies in the practice of aromatherapy in the United States (and England). The first is over-the-counter herbal remedies and essential oils are freely available, and many people self-medicate.

The second anomaly is that although aromatherapy uses different methods: topical, inhalation, and oral, two major organizations in the United Kingdom voted against the oral use of essential oils. This is important as the United States has tended to look to the United Kingdom for aromatherapy guidelines. The Aromatherapy Registration Council (AOC), the lead aromatherapy body in the United Kingdom, stated the oral use of essential oils was not acceptable. The Royal College of Nursing (RCN) in London (which decides what a nurse may practice) also stated the oral use of essential oils lay outside the boundaries of nursing care. The AOC may well have based its decision on the fact that the majority of aromatherapy practitioners in the United Kingdom are lay people. The RCN may have made its decision because using the oral route of aromatherapy is comparable to taking medicine, and nurses are not allowed to give medicines without a prescription.

The third anomaly is the majority of aromatherapy courses focus on esthetics or stress, where internal and oral methods would not be relevant. So the idea has permeated the aromatherapy community that the oral route of essential oils is somehow out of bounds. This is understandable, but it has never been formally challenged or accepted. However, courses that are clinically oriented and intended for LHPs need to address the oral and internal use of aromatherapy because these methods could be very relevant.

The fourth anomaly is confusion between oral and internal use. The two words are not synonymous. One includes the digestive process and the other does not. The oral process involves taking essential oils by mouth, either in capsules or diluted and swallowed. Very small amounts of essential oils are used in foods and candy, such as peppermint and wintergreen, therefore thousands of people take essential oils orally every day. The internal use of essential oils includes putting them into any orifice: mouth, ear, nose, anus, or vagina. However, in this case, the essential oil is not swallowed. A clear example of this is a mouthwash. Several proprietary mouthwashes state on their labels "do not swallow." Clearly there is an established, recognizable difference between oral and internal use. Ear drops, nasal irrigation, and vaginal douches and creams can be applied to the internal skin of the body and absorbed that way. They are not digested. However, all routes, including the rectal one, are excellent ways of getting oils into the system while bypassing the liver (Schnaubelt 1998). Several products that utilize the internal skin and include essential oils are available at drug stores and health-food stores.

The fifth anomaly is the dilution or the amount of essential oil used. The standard dilution for topically applied essential oils taught in aromatherapy training is between 1% and 5%. This is suitable for stress management and esthetics and may be very effective for some clinical conditions. However in the case of an infection, considerably higher percentages might be required. Some over-the-counter remedies contain high percentages of essential oil components. For example, Bengay analgesic cream contains 15% methyl salicylate (found in wintergreen) and 10% menthol (found in peppermint). Higher percentages, and in some cases, undiluted essential oils may be required to treat chronic or acute infection. The original concept of prescription medicine was to protect the public from themselves. An extension of the Hippocratic oath, "first do no harm" is "keep them from harming themselves," which includes instructions for safe use. For aromatherapy, this would mean knowing the maximum amount of essential oil that could be used safely.

The sixth anomaly is in other parts of the world, where aromatherapy is not regulated, essential oils are frequently given orally by licensed and nonlicensed practitioners.

The seventh anomaly is the size of a drop of an essential oil can vary considerably. Much depends on whether the dropper is an integral one or a pipette. The integral droppers produce approximately 20 drops per milliliter. The pipettes produce closer to 40 drops per milliliter. This becomes very important when the maximum amount for a particular essential oil is measured in drops per day.

THE ORAL ROUTE

There is a long history in the United States of nurses and physicians giving essential oils orally to their patients prior to the advent of modern pharmaceuticals. Several essential oils such as cinnamon, clove, peppermint, sandalwood, and eucalyptus are actually listed in the 8th edition of *Useful Drugs*, a handbook published by the American Medical Association in 1930. Sandalwood was classically given for urinary infections. The majority of animal studies on this oil have included the oral route, and there is a great deal of information on toxicity.

One of the main reasons for using the oral method at all is to treat the intestinal tract, as almost every other system can be reached by the topical or inhaled route. The oral method is perfectly safe and nontoxic, provided the giver is trained in this method and appropriate dosages are not exceeded. However, not all essential oils are safe to use orally. Burfield (2000) cautions that certain essential oils such as hyssop, wormwood, and wintergreen should never be taken orally.

Essential oils that are high in phenols should be diluted and contained in gelatin capsules to avoid mucous irritation when administered orally.

Most insurance companies that cover aromatherapy exclude the oral use of essential oils. However this route is a valid option, and there are several excellent training courses available. I believe the fear of using essential oils orally is really based on a lack of knowledge. Again, as always, education is the key. As essential oils are very concentrated, doses are usually described in the number of drops given. However, drop sizes vary (Olleveant et al 1999). Therefore it is more accurate (and safer) to measure the amount of essential oil used in milliliters. Brinker (2000), a naturopath, suggests the safe range for oral use is 0.5-1.0 ml/day, although cautions apply for amounts greater than 0.5ml/day.

Method of Oral Use

Essential oils can be given orally in gelatin capsules, disper, activated charcoal, or Vitamin C tablets. Some essential oils can be taken in honey for occasional use, but not all therapists recommend this method. However some alcohol-rich essential oils (such as palma-rosa) in honey can be excellent for a sore throat.

Gelatin Capsules

Size 00 capsules are filled with an essential oil or oils diluted in a vegetable oil. The solution is made up first (up to 20% strength), then poured into the capsules and the capsules are taken like ordinary medicines. Each capsule holds approximately 0.75 ml. The process of filling the capsules is time consuming, but this is an excellent way to treat the small and large intestine. Guba (2002) suggests clove bud and cinnamon oil for diarrhea and recommends 12 drops per day of each. However, the Australian drop size may be smaller than the US drop size, so closer to six drops per day of each may be all that is required.

Disper

Disper is a lecithin-based emulsifier that holds the essential oils in a stable dispersion. This emulsifier is rapidly absorbed by the stomach and is therefore useful for acute and chronic infections. Disper can be combined with herbal tinctures and is available from several aromatherapy supply companies. The recommended proportion is one part essential oils to nine parts disper. If 1 ml of essential oil (containing 20 US drops or 40 French drops) is added to 9 ml of disper, there will be approximately 200 drops. Ten drops of the mixture will contain two drops of essential oil. The disper mixture is then diluted in water and drunk. The taste will depend on the essential oil but should not be too bitter or overwhelming. This method is very simple to use.

Activated-Charcoal Tablets

Activated-charcoal tablets are available in many health-food stores. Two hundred-milligram charcoal tablets are useful as a simple, effective base for carrying essential oils to the gastrointestinal tract. Each tablet will hold different amounts of an essential oil. Some essential oils dissolve the binders that hold the tablet together so tablets should not be premixed. Charcoal tablets are not recommended for long-term use as they can be constipating, but they can be useful for short-term use of up to 1 week.

Vitamin C Lozenges

Guba (2002) suggests Vitamin C lozenges are also a good way of introducing an essential oil orally. Place a few drops of the essential oil on the lozenge and wait until it is absorbed. The lozenge can then be chewed and swallowed with water.

Honey

Essential oils can be blended with honey water. Mix the drops of essential oil in a teaspoon of honey, add warm water, and drink. Rose is an excellent antiviral oil to use in this way.

Enteric-Coated Gelatin Capsules

Enteric-coated gelatin capsules do not release the essential oil until they are in the small intestine (an environment of pH 6.8 or higher). This can be useful for irritable bowel syndrome.

Human Studies on Oral or Internal Use

Kline et al (2001) used enteric-coated gelatin capsules containing peppermint oil in the treatment of irritable bowel syndrome symptoms. Fifty children took part in a controlled, multicentered study. Between one capsule (187 mg) and two capsules was given three times a day. During the study eight children withdrew for various reasons. However, 76% of the peppermint group showed significant reduction in symptoms compared to the placebo group (43%). No side effects were reported, and there was no change in stool consistency.

Gravett (2001) prescribed a mixture of essential oils in honey water for patients with nausea, colicky pain, anorexia, and diarrhea who were undergoing high-dose chemotherapy and stem-cell rescue. Eight patients took part in the study. They took a daily dose of 15 drops of geranium, 10 drops of German chamomile, 10 drops of patchouli, and 10 drops of turmeric (infused oil) in honey water. The mixture was divided into three batches and taken orally at equal intervals throughout the day. His patients had no ill effects from the essential oils and felt better than members of the control group, who were using conventional antiemetics. The cost of the aromatherapy treatment (28 pence = 40 cents) was substantially less than the conventional treatment (138 pence = almost $2).

Belaiche (1985) carried out a double-blind study to examine the effectiveness of *Melaleuca alternifolia* (tea tree) in the treatment of chronic cystitis. There were 26 participants in the study. The experimental group was given 24 mg of tea tree divided into three doses of 8 mg each in enteric-coated gelatin capsules. The control group was given a placebo that had the odor of tea tree. After 6 months no one in the control group showed any improvement, but 7 of the 13 women in the experimental group were completely cured (60%). During the 6 months of testing, liver functions also were monitored. There were no liver problems, and no side effects to the treatment.

Holmes (1995) describes a case study of a 23-month-old girl he treated for cellulitis from an infected bite and a concurrent upper-respiratory viral infection (tonsillitis). One drop each of tea tree, lavender, and calendula oils were added to a small feeding bottle containing fruit juice, and the mixture was given to the child to take orally, three times a day. The child also received a 20% solution of lavender, Moroccan blue chamomile (*Tanacetum annum*), and calendula as a topical treatment applied directly to the bite up to six times a day, as well as a 10% dilution of tea tree, lavender, and calendula oils massaged into the chest and back each morning and night. The fever subsided after the first day, and 4 days later the cellulitis and tonsillitis were gone. It is difficult to extrapolate whether the oral method would have worked on its own.

SUPPOSITORIES

A suppository is another method of using essential oils not taught in many aromatherapy classes, but it has a place in clinical training. This internal method is simple to use and very effective for treating many different systemic conditions.

The usual concentrations are 10% essential oil per suppository. This works out to approximately 300 mg of essential oil per 3-g suppository. For children, one drop of essential oil in a 25-mg suppository is appropriate. While molds are available, the standard 00-size gelatin capsule is just as effective. However, diluting the essential oil in vegetable oil may result in leakage, so use cocoa butter, which is solid but dissolves at body temperature. Melt the cocoa butter, mix in the essential oils, then fill the suppository mold. Store in refrigerator. Avoid using only phenol-rich essential oils in rectal suppositories as this would produce irritation as the suppository dissolves.

De la Motte et al (1997) used German chamomile in the form of an enema and/or suppository to control noncomplicated diarrhea in children. Other essential oils that could have been used to control diarrhea are geranium and turmeric. Geranium was shown to have antidiarrhea properties in animal studies (Ofuji et al 1998), and turmeric was found to alleviate upper-abdominal pain due to biliary dysfunction (Niederau & Opfert 1999). The rectal route is particularly suitable for children, for those with gastric ulcers or gastritis, or when essential oils are not tolerated via the oral route.

LICENSES, PRESCRIPTIONS, AND ESSENTIAL OILS

A dilemma may occur when oral or internal essential oils are used by an LHP who does not have prescriptive privileges. I think nurses should know about the oral uses of essential oils, but when they are practicing with their nursing license, the oral route should be avoided. This was made clear when the Massachusetts Board of Nursing voted to accept aromatherapy as part of nursing care but did not include herbal remedies, as herbal medicines are taken orally. However, nurse practitioners, physicians, and others with diagnostic skills and prescriptive privileges may wish to learn to use essential oils in this way and use them to great effect. In some states, if a lay person was to "prescribe" an essential oil to another person, he or she could be accused of practicing medicine without a license.

Conventional medicine is not accustomed to a single medicine having several different therapeutic effects. But essential oils clearly do have several different therapeutic effects. They have multiple medicinal properties, but they also give pleasure and help people relax. The *Webster's Dictionary* definition of a medicine is "any substance used in the treatment of disease." The word *medicinal* is defined by the *Oxford Dictionary* as "something having healing properties." According to several studies, prayer has a healing effect. Does this mean only a doctor can pray? Does it mean when a rotation diet works, it is medicine and therefore should be prescribed by a physician only? The idea is clearly absurd. Yet there is something similar, but in reverse, happening in aromatherapy. To give an example: when an essential oil is used for relaxation, it is not a medicine, but if that essential oil is used for its antibiotic effect, it is a medicine. How could lavender be a medicine (effective against methicillin-resistant *Staphylococcus aureus*) one moment and not a medicine (soothing and relaxing) the next? Does this mean a medicine only becomes one when the giver intends it to be one?

There is growing interest and acceptance within conventional medicine for the supplementary role of herbs in clinical practice, and some excellent studies have been published on their efficacy. The potential for interdrug reactions and toxicity issues is very small compared to the hundreds of thousands of deaths from conventional drugs or drug interaction each year. In some instances essential oils can actually enhance conventional medicines (particularly those for infection). This will become very advantageous as more pathogens become resistant to orthodox antibiotics.

It is extremely unlikely that essential oils will only be available by prescription. However, if this did occur, it would be relevant not only to physicians but also to the growing number of nonphysician clinicians (NPCs) who have prescriptive license. The next part of this section explores this option. Many of these nonphysican clinicians are referred to as doctors or physicians by state regulation or custom and are listed as such on many insurance forms. Cooper et al (1998) divides the nonphysician group into three sections. See Table 7-1 for details.

For many years, physicians held a monopoly as the main providers of health care (Cooper et al 1998). However, changes in state laws and regulations combined with an increase in the numbers of practitioners in training means the number of nonphysician clinicians is growing rapidly. As a consequence of this growth, several NPC disciplines will soon be as large as the major specialties in medicine (Cooper et al 1998). In 2005, it is estimated the number of NPCs in clinical practice will be equal to the number of family physicians (Weiner 1994).

Table 7-1 ❧ *Types of Nonphysician Clinicians in the United States*

Conventional Medicine	Alternative Practitioners	Specialty Groups
Nurse practitioners (NPs)	Chiropractors	Optometrists
Certified nurse midwives (CNMs)	Acupuncturists	Podiatrists
Physician assistants (PAs)	Naturopaths	Clinical nurse specialists (CNRs)
	Medical herbalists	Certified registered nurse anesthetists (CRNAs)

A great number of NPC practices are involved with wellness clinics and the treatment of uncomplicated acute and chronic conditions. These types of conditions make up 50%-75% of office visits to primary-care physicians. Cooper et al (1998) made projections as to the way each discipline would expand in 5 years. See Table 7-2 for their estimates on the number of graduates in NPC disciplines.

NPCS are growing in popularity with the public, which perceives them as providing a more caring service than conventional physicians, with more time to listen to and be with their patients (Guglielmo 2001). According to the American Academy of Nurse Practitioners, more than 25% of NPs work in doctor-run,

Table 7-2 ❧ *Projected Number of Nonphysician Clinician Graduates in the United States*

Discipline	1997	2001 (projected)
Acupuncturists	1030	2000
Certified nurse anesthetists	387	725
Certified nurse midwives	414	500
Chiropractors	4100	5200
Clinical nurse specialists	1365	2300
Naturopaths	170	350
Nurse practitioners	5350	7260
Optometrists	1235	1250
Physician assistants	2800	3400
Podiatrists	645	725

solo, or group practices. More and more health care insurance plans will begin to cover NP and other NPC services as they are less expensive than physicians'.

This chapter has covered the oral and internal use of essential oils and has also discussed the use of essential oils by LHPs who may or may not have prescriptive privileges. The hope is that this information will start a dialogue to help clinical aromatherapy become more accepted in health care practice.

REFERENCES

Belaiche P. 1985. Germicidal properties of the essential oil of *Melaleuca alternifolia* related to urinary infections and chronic ideopathic *Colibacillus*. Phytotherapie. 15:9-11.

Brinker F. 2000. The Toxicology of Botanical Medicine, 3rd ed. Sandy, OR: Eclectic Medical Publications, 202.

Burfield T. 2000. Safety of essential oils. International Journal of Aromatherapy. 10(1/2) 16-29.

Cooper R, Laud P, Dietrich C. 1998. Current and projected workforce of nonphysican clinicians. Journal of the American Medical Association. 280(9): 788-794.

Davis W. 1996. One River. New York: Simon & Schuster, 491.

De la Motte S, Bose-O'Reilly S, Heinisch M et al. 1997. Double blind comparison of an apple pectin-chamomile extract preparation with placebo in children with diarrhea. Arzneimittelforschung. 47(11) 1247-1249.

Fowler H, Fowler F (eds). 1972. Oxford English Dictionary (4th ed). Oxford, UK: Oxford University Press.

Gravett P. 2001. Treatment of gastrointestinal upset following high-dose chemotherapy. International Journal of Aromatherapy. 11(2) 84-86.

Guba R. 2002. Beyond Aromatherapy. Center for Aromatic Medicine. NSW. Australia. Notes published by Center for Aromatic Medicine.

Guglielmo W. 2001. Above and beyond just doctoring. Newsweek. 72.

Hatcher R, Eggleston C (eds). 1930. Useful Drugs. Chicago: American Medical Association.

Holmes P. 1995. Aromatherapy: applications for clinical practice. Alternative Medicine. 1(3) 177-182.

Kline R, Kline J, Di Palma J et al. 2001. Enteric coated pH dependent peppermint oil capsules for the treatment of irritable bowel syndrome in children. Journal of Pediatrics. 138: 125-128.

New Webster's Dictionary, Thesaurus, and Medical Dictionary. 1992. New York: Ottenheimer.

Niederau C, Opfert E. 1999. The effect of chelidonium and turmeric root extract on upper abdominal pain due to functional disorders of the biliary system. Results from a placebo-controlled, double-blind study. Medizinische Klinik. 94(8) 425-430.

Ofuji K, Hara H, Sukamoto T et al. 1998. Effects of antidiarrheal containing an extract from geranium herb on astringent action and short-circuit current actions across jejunal mucosa. Nippon Yakurigaku Zasshi. 111(4) 265-246.

Olleveant N, Humphris F, Roe B. 1999. How big is a drop? A volumetric assay of essential oils. Journal of Clinical Nursing. 8(3) 299-304.

Schnaubelt K. 1998. Medical Aromatherapy. Berkeley, CA: Frog, 223.

Weiner J. 1994. Forecasting the effects of health reform on US physician workforce requirements. Journal of the American Medical Association. 272:222-230.

8

Manual Therapies

And I realized that all the world wants to be held in spite of it all.

Jack Kornfield
After the Ecstasy, the Laundry

HIPPOCRATES DESCRIBED the importance of touch in the 5th century BC and declared it his favorite of all health essentials. Aromatherapy is already being used in many manual therapies. This chapter is to encourage therapists to use it in a clinical way. The chapter has been divided into three sections: massage therapy, chiropractic, and the "m" technique. These three sections have been subdivided into common ailments as examples of how aromatherapy could be used in each of these modalities.

Touch is a basic need. In times of crisis the need becomes overwhelming. One of the most moving images of September 11, 2001 was of two firefighters holding each other. Scores of massage therapists in New York and Maryland (and many others from across the nation) rushed to the devastated areas. They worked around the clock to treat rescue crewmembers who were stretched to their physical and emotional limits (Schwanz 2001). They treated emotionally traumatized workers, many of whom had never had a massage (Pasquale 2001). Their compassionate and much-needed gift was huge, and the impact of touch was there for the whole world to see.

MASSAGE THERAPY

In Florida, the definition of massage therapy was officially changed from manipulation of superficial tissue to manipulation of soft tissue by Governor Jeb Bush on July 19, 2001 (McGillicuddy 2001). Massage therapy has grown in acceptance dramatically throughout the last 10 years and is now the norm at sports events worldwide, including the Olympics (Swantz 2001). In a recent survey, 17% of Americans said they had received a massage in the past year. Thirty-five percent of those were for medical reasons and 25% for stress relief and relaxation (Schwanz 2001). Forty-two percent of Americans feel massage is a complementary therapy rather than just a beauty treatment, and medical practitioners ranked massage therapy as the highest (74%) in terms of effectiveness over eleven other modalities, including acupuncture (Anonymous 2001). Consumers spend $4 to $6 billion annually on massage therapy. At Boeing and Reebok, headaches, back strain, and fatigue have declined substantially since both companies began offering massage therapy to employees (Underwood 1998). Education requirements for a massage-therapy license vary from state to state. Texas requires 250 hours plus 50 intern hours, Oregon requires 330 classroom hours, and Nebraska requires 1000 classroom hours. These figures were accurate in 1997 when only 22 states required licensing. Recently, New York and Washington states increased the number of hours required for licensing to 1000 hours.

The physical effects of massage have been well documented throughout the last 10 years. Much of massage's new-found respectability began in 1986 with Tiffany Field, PhD, who found preterm babies who received massage therapy slept better, took more milk, gained weight, and could leave hospital earlier, at a savings of thousands of dollars per day, than their nonmassaged counterparts. She also found massage reduced depression (Field et al 1996) and enhanced wound healing (Field et al 1998). Research has also indicated massage enhances immune function (Harrison et al 1992), reduces perception of pain (Nixon et al), and enhances sleep (Menehan 1997; Richards 1998). Massage, once a traditional component of nursing in the 1940s, is now returning to nursing (Mower 1997) with the beginning of the National Association of Nurse Massage Therapists. Many massage therapists are interested in adding aromatherapy as an enhancement to their profession (Enteen 2001).

In the state of Washington, insurance reimbursement covers whiplash injury, provided the claim is filed within 3 years. This is often covered under personal injury protection, which is usually part of vehicle insurance. The value is between $10,000 and $20,000. As part of this coverage, massage therapy will be covered for 8 weeks, when necessary. Treatment can be biweekly and may be extended at the discretion of the therapist. A payment of $85 is allowed per treatment, and if hydrotherapy (hot packs) is also used, a further $15 is allowed. The patient is reimbursed directly by the insurance company. Hypertension and osteoarthritis are also conditions eligible for health-insurance reimbursement for massage therapy costs.

FIBROMYALGIA SYNDROME

Fibromyalgia syndrome (FMS) is the most common cause of pain seen by medical practitioners (Bennett 1995) and affects 3 to 6 million Americans, 73%-88% of which are female and 92%-100% of which are Caucasian (Muir 1999). The symptoms are widespread pain for more than 3 months with at least 11 of 18 specific points painful to palpation. There appear to be two different types of fibromyalgia—one involving myofascial pain and one more akin to chronic fatigue syndrome—although both may appear in the same patient, and there is controversy as to whether both are the same thing (Buchwald & Garrity 1994). Some patients with chronic fatigue syndrome have been wrongly diagnosed. In one study of 68 patients with chronic fatigue, 68% had been wrongly given a psychiatric label in the past (Deale & Wessley 2000).

There are many theories about FMS. Serotonin, a neurotransmitter in the central nervous system that carries signals between nerve cells and interacts with many other receptors such as dopamine, controls slow-wave sleep, and affects perception of pain, is significantly lower in those with FMS (Muir 1999). On the other hand, levels of substance P, the chemical necessary for transmission of pain, are three times higher (Russell 1994). Certain studies indicate fibromyalgia may be the result of a deficiency of relaxin, a neuropeptide with hemodynamic actions (Geddes & Summerlee 1995). Relaxin is produced by the corpus luteum in the ovary and until recently was thought to be involved only with labor (Alexander 2000). Other studies question the possibility of FMS being caused by a disorder of the limbic system or exposure to a virus (Mountz & Bradley 1995).

FMS patients also complain of insomnia, depression, fatigue, and frequent fluid retention in the morning. Whatever the cause, aromatherapy can help either by affecting the limbic system, alleviating muscle fatigue or other specific symptoms, or fighting a viral infection. For a more in-depth discussion on symptoms please consult Chapters 5, 9, and 12 on psychology, viral infection, and pain, respectively.

Maija Grace (2001) reports on a controlled, crossover study of 20 patients using Fibromix, a commercial blend of nine essential oils diluted in carrier oil (see Table 8-1 for details). Fibromix has been marketed in Finland for 3 years and was

Table 8-1   *Essential Oils in Fibromix*

Common Name	Botanical Name
Ylang ylang	*Cananga odorata*
Roman chamomile	*Chamomelum nobile*
Neroli	*Citrus aurantium*
Bergamot	*Citrus bergamia*
Melissa	*Melissa officinalis*
Black pepper	*Pipe nigrum*
Ravansara	*Ravansara aromatica*
Sandalwood	*Santalum album*
Ginger	*Zingiber officinalis*

formulated by the Maija Grace. The study was so successful in reducing FMS symptoms that a second study followed with 14 women comparing Fibromix with *Chamomelum nobile* (Roman chamomile) essential oil. The average age of the test subjects was 52 years. Treatments consisted of weekly massage sessions for 6 to 8 weeks. One of the drawbacks to using just one essential oil was that patients and therapists tired of it. However, sleep, pain, and stress all appeared to be positively affected.

Lofgren (1998) investigated the use of antiviral essential oils (see Table 8-2 for details) for FMS using a single-case-study design. The study lasted 3 months and included two treatments a week, producing 19 massage-therapy sessions. Pain, sleep, and energy were measured using a visual analog (0-10). Although the pain did not appear to change, the patient commented she had less pain in the morning and improved mobility. She also said the cycles of pain were shortened to hours instead of days. She also commented she no longer bruised so easily.

Lucas (1997) investigated the effects of a lemongrass, ginger, rosemary, and Roman chamomile mix on three patients with FMS. Treatment was weekly massage with aromatherapy and daily baths with aromatherapy. The first patient (59 years old) was diagnosed with FMS 2 years previously, although she believed the symptoms had been present for many years before that. She believed her pain was helped by the treatments, but it was difficult to assess whether the daily bath or the aromatherapy caused the improvement. The second patient (73 years old) had also been diagnosed with FMS 2 years earlier. She had previously tried massage but found "it didn't help." She found the baths not helpful (her bathtub was small and uncomfortable, which may have been the cause), but the massage with essential oils did seem to help a bit. The third patient (43 years old) had recently been diagnosed with FMS. She was taking Klonopin regularly to sleep and said massage usually helped her symptoms. She stopped taking the baths and used the inhaled essential oils at night instead. The essential oils helped her sleep, and she stopped taking sleep medication. Lucas used the "m" technique on this patient instead of massage, as the patient requested something very gentle.

Hester (1999) used four essential oils in a jojoba carrier oil (see Table 8-3 for details) for her study on four women who had each been diagnosed with FMS for 6 to 10 years. She measured pain perception, sleep, fatigue, and foggy thinking using a visual analog (0-10) for each condition throughout 4 weeks. Baseline mea-

Table 8-2 ❧ *Essential-Oil Mix Used by Lofgren (1998)*

Common Name	Botanical Name	Drops per Ounce Carrier Oil
Bergamot	*Citrus bergamia*	5
Palma rosa	*Cymbopogon martini*	9
Tea tree	*Melaleuca alternifolia*	3
Ravensara	*Ravensara aromatica*	3

Table 8-3 🦢 *Essential Oils Used by Hester (1990)*

Common Name	Botanical Name	Percentage
Lemongrass	*Cymbopogon citratus*	3%
German chamomile	*Matricaria recutita*	1%
Lavandin	*Lavandula intermedia*	2%
Rosemary	*Rosmarinus officinalis*	2%

surements were taken before the study. Two people had 80% improvement in pain; two had 50% improvement. Clearer thinking received the lowest score with an average of 35% improvement. Fatigue was improved by an average of 62.5%; sleep was improved by an average of 72.5%. While these figures are encouraging, the patients may have been biased to please the therapist!

CHIROPRACTIC

Chiropractic is growing exponentially—faster than massage, acupuncture, or herbal medicine (Kessler et al 2001). The importance of massage was emphasized at the 2001 Florida Chiropractic Convention where 150 massage therapists mingled with 1800 chiropractors and discussion topics included myofascial release and neuromuscular therapy (Solien-Wolfe & McGillicuddy 2001). Many chiropractors either employ or actively refer patients to licensed massage therapists. Many use massage techniques themselves to warm up the body prior to manipulation. While some physicians still claim that they do not know for sure if chiropractic does more good than harm (Ernst 1998), the public is voting with its feet. Stano and Smith (1996) studied 6183 patients via 2 years of insurance data and found chiropractors were given higher satisfaction and quality ratings from patients than were medical practitioners, and they had lower costs as the initial-contact provider. Shekelle et al (1995) found chiropractors were the primary-care providers for 40% of back pain and had more patient visits than orthopedic physicians did but at less cost.

Low-Back Pain

Eighty percent of adults suffer at least one episode of low-back pain in their lives (Bigos et al 1994). Among patients who use alternative medicine, back problems are the most frequently reported medical condition (Eisenberg et al 1993). In the workforce, the cost of an average back-injury claim in 1989 was $8000 and accounted for one third of worker's compensation costs (Webster & Snook 1994). The estimated national bill for the care of low-back pain per year is $38-$50 billion (Atlas & Deyo 2001). Seventy-five to 90% of patients with low-back pain report improvement within 1 month, but 50% of patients have repeat episodes within 1 year (Carey et al 1999). Since 1999, four major, randomized, controlled studies and one metaanalysis have indicated massage is beneficial for low-back pain (Crownfield 2001). A 2001 study involving 263 patients (Cherkin et al 2001) found those receiving massage needed less medication and fewer days in bed than those receiving acupuncture.

Essential oils can be used by chiropractors to reduce muscle spasm before manipulation, to reduce inflammation, and to reduce pain. Costa (1997), a massage therapist who works with a chiropractor, conducted a small study on the use of aromatherapy prior to chiropractic manipulation. She used 3% *Lavandula angustifolia* in vegetable oil massaged into the backs of six patients for 20 minutes prior to manipulation. The chiropractor assessed the ease of manipulation on a scale of 1-10, with 10 being the easiest to manipulate. The members of the experimental group were aged 16-49 and included both men and women. Twelve treatments were given to each of the six patients. Figures indicate the lavender massage had made manipulation easier than plain massage. Further essential oils were tested, and aromatherapy is currently used by the chiropractor's office.

Although efficacy can be achieved with 1-5% essential oil solutions, some therapists use up to 40% concentrations. Do not dilute the essential oil in a petroleum- or mineral-based medium as this will prevent it from being absorbed through the skin. There are specific analgesic, antiinflammatory, and antispasmodic essential oils that can help low-back pain. The oils need to be applied topically.

Commonly used and effective antiinflammatory essential oils for acute low-back pain are listed in Table 8-4 and include an essential oil that has a long history of use in Australia but is just becoming known in the United States (Webb 2000). Table 8-5 lists essential oils with analgesic qualities suitable for treating low-back pain.

In a survey on management of rheumatic-disease symptoms in aromatherapy practices in the United Kingdom, 55% therapists said they had patients referred to them by conventional medicine (Osborn et al 2001). Musculoskeletal complaints were the second most common condition treated by aromatherapists in the United Kingdom, after stress. Aromatherapy in the United Kingdom is nearly always used with massage.

Zivitz (2000) carried out a small pilot study on six women with low-back pain. The subjects' ages ranged between 24 and 73 years. Zivitz compared the effects of *Boswellia carteri* (frankincense) and *Cymbopogon citratus* (lemongrass) in two separate 4% solutions, each diluted with sweet-almond oil. The control group received a massage with plain vegetable oil. Each participant had experienced low-back pain for a minimum of 2½ years. A visual analog was used to rate pain (0-10). Participants completed the pain scale immediately before treatment, immediately after treatment, and 1 and 2 hours later. Despite favorable comments from the participants, data analysis did not show any alteration in pain perception beyond the control group (who received straight carrier oil with their massage), although everyone enjoyed the aroma.

Table 8-4 🌿 *Antiinflammatory Essential Oils for Acute Low-Back Pain*

Common Name	Botanical Name	Reference
Juniper	*Juniperus communis*	Mascolo et al 1987
Fennel (sweet)	*Foeniculum vulgare*	Mascolo et al 1987
Coriander	*Coriandrum sativum*	Mascolo et al 1987
Roman chamomile	*Anthemis nobilis*	Rossi et al 1988
Nutmeg	*Myristica fragrans*	Benet et al 1988
Everlasting	*Helicrysum italicum*	Franchomme & Penoel 1991
Yarrow	*Achillea millefolium*	Middleton & Drzewiecki 1984
German chamomile	*Matricaria recutita*	Tubaro et al 1984
Australian blue cypress	*Callitris intratropica*	Webb 2001
Lemongrass	*Cymbopogon citratus*	Seth et al 1975
Clove	*Syzygium aromaticum*	Guillleman et al 1989
Lavender	*Lavandula angustifolia*	Ghelardini et al 1999

Soltis (2000) compared the effects of *Piper nigrum* (black pepper) and *Origanum majorana* (sweet marjoram) on patients with low-back pain. Again the sample was small, six participants. There were four women and two men. This time each essential oil (2%) was self-applied twice a day for 1 week. Most participants thought the black pepper was warming and this helped the pain, although two participants did not like the aroma. Most participants believed sweet marjoram helped, and one stopped taking Motrin for pain relief. However, there were many

Table 8-5 🌿 *Analgesic Essential Oils for Acute Low-Back Pain*

Common name	Botanical name	Reference
Peppermint	*Mentha piperita*	Krall & Krause 1993
Lemongrass	*Cymbopogon citratus*	Viana et al 2000
Lavender	*Lavandula angustifolia*	Ghelardini et al 1999
Not known	*Artemesia caerulescens*	Moran et al 1989
Myrrh	*Commiphora molmol*	Dolara et al 2000
Spike lavender	*Lavandula latifolia*	Von Frohilche 1968
Clary sage	*Salvia sclarea*	Moretti 1997

variables, and it is difficult to come to any conclusion with such a small number of participants.

Port (1999) conducted a small, controlled study on the effects of lavender and black pepper on osteoarthritis. Participants were seven women and one man. All participants used analgesics and antiinflammatory medication, and several took them daily. The participants were randomly allocated to two groups. The experimental group received 20 ml of 3% black pepper and lavender oils in sweet almond oil. The control group received 20 ml of plain carrier oil. Both groups were instructed to rub the mixture into the painful joint once in the morning and once at night for 7 days. At the end of this time they were to stop the treatment and evaluate their pain and stiffness using a visual analog (0-10).

The control group did not have any measurable effect from this process. The experimental group did experience a reduction in stiffness and pain. One woman stopped taking her antiinflammatory medicine, but when the study was finished her stiffness and pain returned, and she started taking her medicine again. Two participants had significant improvement in their range of motion. One person was able to make a fist for the first time in years. This is a very small study but is encouraging to those of us who are getting older!

THE "M" TECHNIQUE

The "m" technique is a registered method of touch suitable for the very fragile or when massage is inappropriate (either because the receiver is too fragile or because the giver is not trained in massage). The "m" technique is a series of stroking movements performed in a set sequence. Each movement, identified with a mnemonic name (a name that acts as a "hook" to enable the giver to remember it), is repeated a set number of times. Because the technique is structured in terms of strokes, sequence, number, and pressure, it is completely reproducible and therefore useful in research. The "m" is so gentle and soothing that a physician has called it "physical hypnotherapy" (Merrill 1999).

The "m" first arrived in the United States in 1994 when I began teaching in Florida and Georgia. The "m" technique was registered by the United States Patent and Trademark Office in March 1998. Since 1994, the technique has been taught in universities, nursing colleges, and massage schools across America. Students have even created a new verb and talk about "m"-ing their patients! Currently more than 1000 people have learned the "m" technique, and the word is spreading. The "m" was devised as a simple, easy to learn method of touch (one weekend) that would allow a patient to feel relaxed as quickly as possible. Created initially for nurses not wanting to train in massage but wanting to touch their patients, the "m" technique is used by many other licensed health professionals.

The "m" technique is quite different from massage as it follows a set structure that never changes. Each movement and sequence is done in a distinctive pattern that is not modified. Each stroke within each movement is repeated three times, so a group of practitioners carrying out the technique would all be doing exactly the same stroke at the same time. The rationale for this set form of repetition is simple: to build confidence and remove anxiety in the receiver. The first time patients experience an "m"-technique stroke, they will pay attention. The second time they feel the same stroke, they will recognize it. By the third time, the receiver knows what is going to happen and will begin to relax. By experiencing each stroke a set number of times, the receiver learns what is going to happen and is lulled into a deep state of relaxation in a very short period of time. The "m" technique also uses a set pressure. If pressure was measured on a scale of 0-10, with 0 as no pressure and 10 as crushing pressure, the "m" technique 's pressure should always be a 3. Conventional massage alters the pressure depending on the situation.

Many massage therapists are learning this technique to use in their practice alongside conventional massage therapy. Sharon Gibson, a massage therapist in New Jersey, says normally 65% of her clients go to sleep on the table during a massage. However, with the "m" technique, 100% fall asleep within the first 10 minutes. Lori Mitchell, a critical care nurse in Kalispell, Montana, used the "m" technique in critical care and said it brought rapid and prolonged relaxation to her patients, some of whom had not responded to orthodox sedation. Aurora Ocampo, RN, a clinical nurse specialist at Beth Israel Hospital in New York City uses the "m" technique to relax patients prior to surgery.

In 1996 the "m" technique was used in the research laboratory at Columbia Presbyterian Medical Center in New York City. The "m" technique was applied to the feet of medical students and a measurable effect on their parasympathetic nervous systems was recorded using an 8-lead electrocardiogram machine attached to a heart-variation monitor. Slater (2001) measured the effects of the "m" technique in a study on muscle tension, relaxation, and mood with 14 participants. Slater compared the effect of the "m" technique applied with and without lavender essential oil. Data were entered into a database program and analyzed using a two-sample t-test, assuming equal variances. The effects of the "m" technique were statistically significant without the lavender ($p = <0.005$). However, with lavendar, the effects were increased substantially ($p = <0.00004$). Limitations of the study were lack of randomization, small study size, and dominance of female participants.

Miller (2000), a critical care nurse at Desert Samaritan Hospital in Mesa, Arizona, used the "m" technique on her patients. The first was a female patient with a history of multiple sclerosis who was ventilator dependent and very apprehensive about her caregiver. Postoperatively (tracheostomy) the patient was pulling on the ventilator tubing constantly and complaining of discomfort. The "m" was used on her legs and feet. She fell asleep before the treatment was completed (less than 10 minutes) and slept for 2 hours. She was much calmer upon awakening. A second patient was a 37-year-old female with cancer metastasized to the bones and now affecting her brain. Diagnosed 4 years previously, she had been treated with chemotherapy and radiation. She was ventilator dependent. She wanted to stay alert so she could "say good bye to her family in a dignified way."

She chose rosemary essential oil to accompany her "m" technique, as she remembered using it before. The "m" was used on her feet and legs. Her need for narcotics decreased from every 2 hours to every 6 hours. Four of those hours she was asleep. The third patient was a 72-year-old female who just had abdominal surgery. She was very fragile, weak, and afraid. Pain medication was given every 2 hours. After the "m" to her hands, the patient slept for 3 hours and did not request any further pain medication for 2 more hours. The fourth patient was a 76-year-old male who just had abdominal surgery. He rated his pain as a 7. After the "m" to his feet, he belched and passed flatulence, which greatly relieved his pain. He slept without analgesics and later rated his pain as a 1 or 2. The following day he was still thanking Miller for using the "m" technique on him. Miller noted that as well as physical responses of facial expressions in her patients, often there was a significant drop in heart rate of 5-10 beats per minute.

The "m" is simple enough for a 5-year-old child to do and can be shared with family members. It is empowering for the giver and beneficial for the receiver. The chaplain of Mercy Hospice in Scranton, Pennsylvania, learned the "m" technique to "give physical comfort at a soul level." A hand or foot "m" takes only 5 minutes and has far-reaching effects. I have found teaching the "m" technique to be one of the most satisfying aspects of my career. Details of training programs and an instructional video can be found at www.rjbuckle.com.

REFERENCES

Alexander M. 2000. How Aromatherapy Works, Vol 1. Odessa, FL : Whole Spectrum.

Anonymous. 2001. Post Legislative Mandate: two-thirds of group health clinician respondents view CAM as effective. Integrator for the Business of Alternative Medicine. (April).

Atlas S, Deyo R. 2001. Evaluating and managing acute low back pain in the primary care setting. Journal of General Internal Medicine. 16, 120-131.

Benet A, Stamford F, Tavares I. 1988. The biological activity of eugenol, a major constituent of nutmeg: studies on prostaglandins, the intestine and other tissues. Phytotherapy Research. 2, 125-129.

Bennett R. 1995. Fibromyalgia: the commonest cause of widespread pain. Alternative & Complementary Therapies. 21(6) 269-275.

Bigos S, Bowyer O, Braen G et al. 1994. Acute low back pain in adults. In Clinical Practice Guidelines, No 14. Rockville, MD: Agency for Healthcare Policy and Research, US Dept of Health & Human Services, available www.spinehealth.com.

Buchwald D, Garrity D. 1994. Comparison of patients with chronic fatigue syndrome, fibromyalgia and chemical sensitivities. Archives of Internal Medicine. 154, 2049-2053.

Carey T, Garrett J, Jackman A et al. 1999. Recurrence and care seeking after acute back pain: results of a long-term follow-up study. Medical Care. 37, 157-164.

Cherkin D, Eisenberg D, Sherman K et al. 2001. Trial comparing Chinese medical acupuncture, therapeutic massage, and self care. Archives of Internal Medicine 161(8) 1081-1088.

Costa D. 1997. Lavender eases chiropractic manipulation. Unpublished dissertation, Hunter, New York: RJ Buckle Associates.

Crownfield P. 2001. Massage for back pain: let's look at the research. Massage Today. 1(9) 1, 16-17.

Deale A, Wessley S. 2000. Diagnosis of psychiatric disorder in clinical evaluation of chronic fatigue syndrome. Journal of the Royal Society of Medicine. 93, 310-312.

Dolara P, Luceri C, Ghelardi C et al. 2000. Analgesic effect of myrrh. Nature. 376, 29.

Eisenberg D, Kessler R, Foster C et al. 1993. Unconventional medicine in the United States. New England Journal of Medicine. 328, 246-252.

Enteen S. 2001. Inside aromatherapy: how to recognize and offer high-quality aromatherapy. Massage Today. 1(7) 1, 8, 11.

Ernst E. 1998. Chiropractic for low back pain. British Medical Journal. 317:160-160.

Field T, Grizzle N, Scafidi F et al. 1996. Massage and relaxation therapy effects on depressed adolescent mothers. Adolescence. 31, 903-911.

Field T, Peck M, Krugman S et al. 1998. Burn injuries benefit from massage therapy. Journal of Burn Care & Rehabilitation. 19, 241-244.

Franchomme P, Penoel D. 1991. Aromatherapie Exactement. Limoges, France: Jollois.

Geddes B, Summerlee A. 1995. The emerging concept of relaxin as a centrally acting peptide hormone with hemodynamic action. Journal of Neuroendocrinology. 7:511-517.

Ghelardini C, Galeotti N, Salvatore G et al. 1999. Local anesthetic activity of essential oil of *Lavandula angustifolia*. Planta Medica. 65(8) 700-703.

Guillemain J, Rouseeau A, Delaveau P. 1989. Effects neurodepresseurs de l'huile essentielle de *Lavandula angustifolia*. Annales Pharmaceutiques Francaises 47:337-343.

Harrison L, Groer M, Modricin-McCarthy M et al. 1992. Effect of gentle human touch on pre-term infants. Research in Nursing and Health 23:435-446.

Hester G. 1990. The effects of aromatherapy for the treatment of fibromyalgia. Unpublished dissertation, Hunter, New York, RJ Buckle Associates.

Jakovlev V, Isaac O, Thiemer K et al. 1979. Pharmacological investigations with compounds of chamomile. II. New investigations on the antiphlogistic effects of a bisabolol and bisabolol oxide. Planta Medica. 35, 125-140.

Kessler R, Davies R, Foster D et al. 2001. Long-term trends in the use of complementary and alternative medical therapies in the USA. Annals of Internal Medicine. 135, 262-268.

Khanna T, Zaidi FA. 1993. CNS and analgesic studies on *Nigella sativa*. Fitoterapia. 64(5) 407-410.

Kornfield J. 2000. After the Ecstasy, the Laundry. London: Rider, 223.

Krall B, Krause W. 1993. Efficacy and tolerance of *Mentha arvensis aethoeroleum*. Paper presented at 24th International Symposium on Essential Oils. Berlin, July 21-24, 1993, Germany.

Lofgren J. 1998. Aromatherapy and fibromyalgia: an antiviral approach. Unpublished dissertation, Hunter, New York, RJ Buckle Associates.

Lucas M. 1997. Fibromyalgia and essential oils. Unpublished dissertation, Hunter, New York, RJ Buckle Associates.

Maija Grace U. 2001. Treating fibromyalgia syndrome with essential oils. International Journal of Aromatherapy. 11(1) 20-25.

Mascolo N, Autore G, Capasso F. 1987. Biological screening of Italian medicinal plants for anti-inflammatory activity. Phytotherapy Research. 1(1) 28-31.

McGillicuddy M. 2001.New legislation expands definition of massage. Massage Today. 1(8) 1, 8.

Menehan K. 1997. Massage laws nationwide. Massage Magazine. Sept/Oct 67 125.

Merrell W. 1999. Personal communication.

Middleton E, Drzewiecki G. 1984. Flavanoid inhibition of human basophil histamine release stimulated by various agents. Biochemical Pharmacology. 33, 3333-3338.

Moran A, Martin N, Montero MJ. 1989. Analgesic, antipyretic and anti-inflammatory activity of essential oil of *Artemisia caerulescens* subsp. *gallica*. Journal of Ethnopharmacology. 27(3) 307-317.

Moretti M, Peana A. 1997. A study on the anti-inflammatory and peripheral analgesic action of salvia sclarea oil and its main components. J Essent Oil Research. 9:199-204.

Mountz J, Bradley L. 1995. Fibromyalgia in women. Arthritis & Rheumatism. 38(7) 926-938.

Mower M. 1997. Massage returns to nursing. Massage Magazine. Sept/Oct 67. 47-50.

Muir M. 1999. Fibromyalgia syndrome. Alternative & Complementary Therapies. 5(2) 79-84.

Nixon M, Teschendorff J, Finney J et al. Expanding the nursing repertoire: the effect of massage on post-operative pain. Australian Journal of Advanced Nursing. 14(3) 21-26.

Osborn C, Barlas P, Baxter G et al. 2001. Aromatherapy: a survey of current practice in the management of rheumatic disease symptoms. Complementary Therapies in Medicine. 9:62-67.

Pasquale S. 2001. Bringing relief to the World Trade Center rescue workers. Massage Today. 1(11) 1.

Port M. 1999. Lavender and black pepper for osteoarthritis. Unpublished disseration, Hunter, New York: RJ Buckle Associates.

Richards K. 1998. Effects of back massage and relaxation intervention on sleep in critically ill patients. American Journal of Critical Care. 7, 288-299.

Rossi T, Melegari M et al. 1988. Sedative, anti-inflammatory and anti-diuretic effects induced in rats by essential oils of varieties of *Anthemis nobilis:* a comparative study. Pharmacological Research Communications. 20(Suppl.) 71-74.

Russell I. 1994. Biochemical abnormalities in fibromyalgia syndrome. Journal of Musculoskeletal Pain. 2(3) 101-115.

Schwanz M. 2001. MERT (Massage Emergency Response Team) aids relief of Pentagon rescue workers. Hands On. 17(6) 1,6.

Seth G, Kolate C, Varma K. 1975. Effect of essential oils of *Cymbopogon citratus* on central nervous system. Indian Journal of Experimental Biology. 14(3) 370-373.

Shekelle P, Markovich M, Louie R. 1995. Comparing the costs between provider types of episodes of back pain care. Spine. 20(2) 221-226.

Slater V. 2001. The effects of the "m" technique with and without *Lavandula angustifolia.* Unpublished dissertation, Hunter, New York, RJ Buckle Associates.

Slater V. 2001. The "m" technique. Unpublished dissertation, Hunter, New York: RJ Buckle Associates.

Solien-Wolfe L, McGillicuddy M. 2001. Massage therapy makes presence felt at Florida Chiropractic Association's national convention. 1(10) 1, 17.

Soltis K. 2000. Black pepper and sweet marjoram for low back pain. Unpublished dissertation, Hunter, New York: RJ Buckle Associates.

Stano M, Smith M. 1996. Chiropractic and medical costs of low back care. Medical Care. 34(3) 191-134.

Swantz S. 2001. Massage at the 2002 Winter Olympics. Massage Today. 1(11) 1.

Tubaro A, Zillia C, Redaeli C et al. 1984. Evaluation of anti-inflammatory activity of chamomile extract topical application. Planta Medica. 50(4) 359-360.

Underwood A. 1998. The magic of touch. Newsweek. April 6. 71-72.

Viana G, Vale T, Pinho R et al. 2000. Antinociceptive effect of the essential oil from *Cymbopogon citratus* in mice. Journal of Ethnopharmacology. 70, 323-327.

Von Frohilche A. 1968. A review of clinical, pharmacological and bacteriological research into *Oleum spicae*. Wiener Medizinische Wochenschrift. 15:345-350.

Webb M. 2001. Australian essential oils profile: Blue cypress. Aromatherapy Today. 19:37-39.

Webster B, Snook S. 1994. The cost of 1989 compensation low back pain claims. Spine. 19, 1111-1116.

Zivitz E. 2000. Do the essential oils of frankincense and lemongrass alter perceptions of back pain? Unpublished dissertation, Hunter, New York, RJ, Buckle Associates.

SECTION II

Clinical Use of Aromatherapy

General Clinical Subsection

Specialized Departments Subsection

Introduction to Section 2

Aromatherapy is certainly viewed by many as being primarily concerned with stress management. This may be the case today, but it would be a pity if the myriad other therapeutic properties of essential oils were ignored now and in the future. This section of the book is an exploration of how aromatherapy could be used clinically, and is divided into two subsections: a general section and a specialized section.

In the general clinical section, I have focused on the broad-ranging problems of infection, insomnia, nausea and vomiting, pain, and stress management. The first four of these areas have far-reaching effects on the quality and cost of healthcare, and are of interest to a wide range of readers. While the role of aromatherapy in stress management has been covered by other authors, I have attempted to place the role of stress management within a clinical context.

The ability of Western medicine to contain the increasing demands of healthcare users is reaching a breaking point. Essential oils might provide a little more elasticity because essential oils are much cheaper than conventional medicines. Just compare the use of peppermint with Zofran in the treatment of nausea. While there may be many incidences when Zofran is needed and the only drug that will work, there are also many instances when peppermint will work and it could be offered first. So it is in the interest of healthcare providers to be conversant regarding what essential oils could achieve in a clinical setting.

The chapter on infection was an exciting one for me to write, as I feel there is tremendous potential for essential oil to be used against emerging drug-resistant pathogens. In vitro and animal studies indicating antimicrobial activity do not prove that essential oils will necessarily be effective in a human, but such studies are an encouraging beginning, particularly when the power of synthetic antibiotics is waning.

The specialized subsection focuses on a handful of specific problems within each clinical specialty and how aromatherapy might help those problems, again with reference to published research, my clinical experience, and case studies and small pilot studies. The aim in writing Chapters 14–25 is to make licensed healthcare professionals (LHP) aware of the clinical potential of aromatherapy within specific departments. References have been given where possible although many of them are in-vitro or animal studies. But at least it is a beginning. Where the studies have been on whole herbs rather than essential oils, this fact is indicated. There is a separate treatment of the oral use of essential oils back in Chapter 7. This specialized, updated clinical section includes new chapters on OB/GYN and psychiatric care. The chapter on immunology has been much expanded and the number of references to this section has been doubled.

Obviously there will be some overlap among chapters, and the reader is advised to refer to the general index at the back of the book to find other areas in the book where the symptom will be addressed.

I am grateful for the input of many reviewers in this section whose help and advice was most appreciated. The reviewers include: Ann Adams BSN, Ben Evans MSN, Claire Everson BSN, Diana Guthrie RN, PhD, Susan Hageness MSN, Dorathy Larkin RN, PhD, Lori Mitchell BSN, Gayle Newsham PhD, Mary Poolos RN, PhD, Ganson Purcell MD, Scottie Purol-Hershey RN, PhD, Linda Scaz RN, PhD, Neil Schultz MD, Kay Soltis MSN, Brenda Talley RN, PhD, and Mark Warner, MD.

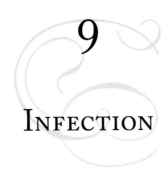

9

INFECTION

The use of perfumes, and especially that of lavender, is a more certain and pleasant means of combating diseases and hindering the spread of epidemics.

Rene-Maurice Gattefosse (1948)

HOSPITAL-ACQUIRED INFECTIONS

Infectious diseases were, until recently, the most common cause of death (Mac-Sween & Whaley 1992). Despite an improvement in living conditions among the technically advanced countries of the world, infections such as the common cold and influenza are major causes of working days lost. Smallpox may have been irradicated and the incidence of diphtheria greatly reduced, but viral infections and mutated or newly discovered bacteria are on the increase. Since September 11, 2001, anthrax and other bacteria that could be potential biological weapons have gained publicity. Three essential oils, palma rosa, basil, and black cumin, are moderately effective in vitro against anthrax. However, aromatic medicine has been for the most part ignored as a possibility for combating the pathogen. Tuberculosis (TB) is also on the increase and will infect 8.4 million people this year and kill 2 million (Reichman & Tanne 2001). Several essential oils are effective against TB in vitro and others augment the effect of conventional medicines.

Animals are also falling prey to new infections or infestations. Of wild honeybees, 90% have been killed following an infestation of mites. The mites, which had become resistant to conventional pesticides, were thought to have been brought into the United States with illegally imported bees several years ago. Bob Noel, a farmer in Cumberland, Maryland, tried fighting the mites using wintergreen essential oil mixed with shortening and sugar placed directly in the hive. It killed all the mites but did not harm the bees. Peppermint, lavender, pennyroyal, spearmint, and patchouli were also successful in killing mites, and the results were posted on the Internet (Amrine 1996).

However, of greatest concern to all health professionals are the infections acquired by patients as a direct result of being in a hospital (Ward 1993). Infection is caused by organisms such as bacteria, viruses, fungi, protozoa, and parasites. Gascoigne (1993), a British physician, suggests these organisms can be spread by the methods listed in Table 9-1.

Being a hospital patient brings with it the threat of infection (Fig. 9-1). Every year almost 2 million American patients acquire an infection in a hospital, and of those 2 million patients, 80,000 die (Fisher 1994). Urinary-tract infections increased the duration of hospitalization by 5.1 days. Rubinstein et al (1982) found wound infections increased the period of hospitalization by 12.9 days, a heavy price for a hospital budget.

Table 9-1 ✹ *Spread of Infections*

Spread by:	Results in:
Droplet infection	Common cold, influenza
Implantation	*Streptococcus, Staphylococcus*
Direct contact	Scabies, sexually transmitted diseases
Food or water contamination	Cholera, *Listeria*
Injection, human or insect	HIV virus, hepatitis, yellow fever, malaria

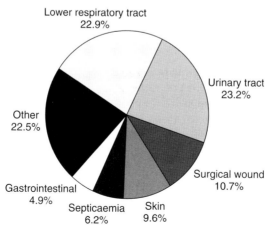

FIGURE 9-1   The frequency of different types of hospital-acquired infection. From Wilson J. 2001. Infection Control in Clinical Practice, 2nd ed. London: Elsevier Science.

The most common hospital-acquired infections (HAI) are *Campylobacter enteritis, Pseudomonas aeruginosa,* methicillin-resistant *Staphylococcus aureus* (MRSA), and vancomycin-resistant enterococci. HAI (nosocomial) can be acquired from an outside source, such as poor hygiene standards of the hospital staff, equipment, or even visitors, or as a result of self-infection. Sometimes infection can be due to the enforced relocation of a commensal. A commensal is a bacterium symbiotic to the health of the host, such as *Escherichia coli* in the gut. However, when the commensal is transplanted to another part of the body, an infection ensues. A common example is *E. coli,* which, when transported from the gut to the urinary tract, causes cystitis.

Common Forms of Hospital-Acquired Infection

Campylobacter enteritis

According to Sleigh et al (1992), *C. enteritis* causes one of the most common forms of infective diarrhea. This form of diarrhea is caused by organisms that affect the digestive tract, many of which have not yet been identified or are totally new.

Pseudomonas aeruginosa

P. aeruginosa has become more common in hospitals. A strictly aerobic, gram-negative bacillus, *P. aeruginosa* flourishes in water and aqueous solutions. The organism produces a pigment called pyocyanin, as well as fluorescein, and these compounds together create the characteristic blue, offensive pus seen in *P. aeruginosa* infections (MacSween & Whaley 1992). *Pseudomonas* is rapidly becoming resistant to antibiotics. Nearly 70% of people with cystic fibrosis are chronically infected with this bacterium.

Methicillin-Resistant Staphylococcus aureus

MRSA has been responsible for global outbreaks of infection. *Staphylococcus* infections tend to remain localized, possibly because of the production of coagulase, which clots fibronogen (MacSween & Whaley 1992). Some essential oils such as peppermint, thyme, lavender, tea tree, and juniper have been found effective against MRSA in vitro (Nelson 1997). Hospital-acquired *S. aureus* bacteremia continues to be a frequent and serious complication of hospitalization worldwide (Jensen et al 1999).

Multiple-Resistant Serratia marcescens and Klebsiella

Serratia marcescens and *Klebsiella* were the cause of an epidemic involving four hospitals in the 1970s. The spread of infection was finally linked to the lack of hand washing by personnel who worked in all four hospitals. By the time the infection was brought under control, 400 patients had been infected, and 17 patients had died (Fisher 1994).

S. marcescens is a gram-negative bacillus that occurs naturally in soil and water and produces a red pigment at room temperature. It is associated with urinary and respiratory infections, endocarditis, osteomyelitis, septicemia, wound infections, eye infections, and meningitis. Transmission is by direct contact. Droplets of *S. marcescens* have been found growing on catheters and in supposedly sterile solutions. Most strains are resistant to several antibiotics. Between 1951 and 1952 the US Army conducted a study called Operation Sea-Spray to study wind-currents that might carry biological weapons. They filled balloons with *S. marcescens* and burst them over San Francisco. Shortly afterwards, doctors noted a dramatic increase in pneumonia and urinary-tract infections (www.sunysccc.edu/academic/mst/microbes/23smarc.htm). Recently the Azerbaijan Medical Association announced on their Web site (http://azma.org) that *S. marascens* was killed in 30 minutes in vitro by essential oil of *Nepata transcaucasica* (an aromatic herb that grows wild in the Absheron region of Azerbaijan).

Streptococcus

Group A *Streptococcus* (GAS) is a bacterium found in the throat and on the skin. Many people carry it with no symptoms. Most GAS infections are mild, such as strep throat and impetigo. However, life-threatening GAS infections can occur when the bacterium gets into a part of the body where it is not normally found, resulting in necrotising fasciitis (flesh-eating bacteria) and strep toxic shock syndrome. Of patients with necrotising fasciitis, 20% die; more than 50% of patients with strep toxic shock die. Approximately 10% to 15% of patients with other forms of invasive GAS infections die. In 1999, there were 9400 cases of invasive GAS in the United States. According to the Centers for Disease Control and Prevention, people with chronic illnesses, those taking steriods, or those who have low immune function are most at risk for this type infection (www.cdc.gov/ncidod/dbmd/diseaseinfo/groupastreptococcal_g.htm).

Vancomycin-resistant enteroccoci

Vancomycin-resistant enteroccoci (VRE) were first isolated in 1987. In some hospitals, VRE are responsible for 20% of enteroccoccal infections (Leclercq et al 1988). VRE are directly related to the dramatic increase in vancomycin use in hospitals in the early 1980s and 1990s (Ena et al 1993). A metaanalysis of 420 published reports and 98 conference reports confirms this view (Carmeli et al 1999).

Each of the bacteria mentioned previously are becoming more common in hospitals, but there is a whole range of pathogenic organisms that surround us every day. These common causes of HAI can be resistant to orthodox medication. However, in-vitro studies suggest these pathogens are sensitive to the antibacterial action of specific essential oils. Pathologists who are experts in the use of essential oils as antibacterial agents stress that the "terrain" of the patient can affect the efficacy of the antibacterial action of an essential oil, and an individual aromatogram is required. However, the standard aromatograms described here give a general idea as to which essential oils might be efficacious in a particular patient.

Following a brief classification of bacteria, there is a description of some the published research into the antimicrobial effects of essential oils. This research suggests essential oils could be used to enhance antibacterial/antifungal/antiviral drug therapy or to treat infections on their own.

BACTERIAL CLASSIFICATION

Although the following information may seem elementary, it may be helpful to have the basics reiterated to provide context for the information on essential oils. Bacteria are first classified according to their shape (Fig. 9-2). The two main groups of bacteria are cocci and bacilli (Hope et al 1993). These two groups are then subdivided into gram-positive and gram-negative bacteria. (Gram was the microbiologist who devised the staining method.) Gram staining uses a mixture of violet dye and iodine to stain the magnesium ribonucleate found in some bacteria deep purple. The purple stain cannot be washed out by alcohol. Bacteria that can be stained purple are said to be gram-positive. Bacteria that do not contain magnesium ribonucleate do not retain the purple stain and are described as gram-negative (Ward 1993). *Mycobacterium* (the cause of TB and leprosy) is not revealed by the gram-stain method and instead is stained with an acid-fast method

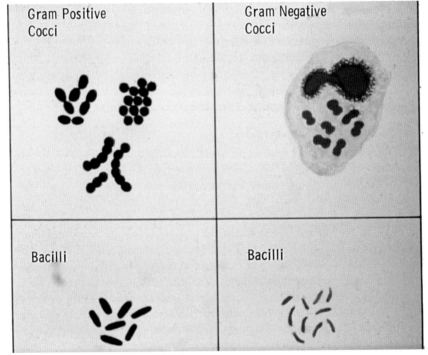

FIGURE 9-2   Four main groups of bacteria: Clockwise from top left: Gram-positive cocci, gram-negative cocci, gram-negative bacilli (rods), gram-positive bacilli.   From Wilson J. 2001. Infection Control in Clinical Practice, 2nd ed. London: Elsevier Science.

called the Ziehl-Nielsen method (MacSsween & Whaley 1992). A second sub-division of bacteria is between aerobic organisms, which need air to survive, and anaerobic organisms, which do not require air. An increasingly common anaero-bic bacterium causes vaginitis. In optimum in vitro conditions, bacteria divide ap-proximately every 20 minutes (MacSween & Whaley 1992).

Coccus Bacteria

The cocci bacteria include *Staphylococcus,* named for the Greek word *staphyl,* meaning grapes, because, seen under a microscope, the bacteria have this charac-teristic shape. *Staphylococcus* is the cause of many skin infections. *Streptococcus* is named after the Greek word *streptos,* meaning twisted, because the bacteria re-semble twisted chains. *Streptococcus* often causes throat infections. Other members of the coccus family include *Pneumococcus,* which causes pneumonia, and *Neisse-ria,* which causes gonorrhea. *Streptococcus* can be further classified into A, B, or nonhaemolytic types and aerobic or anaerobic types.

Bacillus Bacteria

The bacillius group includes Enterobacteriaceae such as *E. coli* and *Salmonella,* both of which can cause diarrhea. It also includes *Proteus mirabilis* and *Bacillus anthracis,* which cause proteus and anthrax, respectively. Other bacteria in the bacillus group include *Corynebacterium diphtheriae,* which causes diphtheria, *Pseudomonas aeruginosa,* and *M. tuberculosis,* which causes TB. Anaerobic bacilli include *Clostridium tetani,* which causes tetanus, and *C. difficile,* which causes pseudomembranous colitis.

In addition to the two main groups, there are the spirochete group and a fur-ther group of organisms that are neither viruses nor bacteria, but something in be-tween. This group includes *Rickettsia,* which causes typhus fever, and *Chlamydia trachomatis,* which causes genitourinary infections (Hope et al 1993). A classifi-cation of pathogens is shown in Fig. 9-3.

ANTIBIOTICS

The antibiotics industry has seen huge growth in the last 30 years, with sales in-creasing from $94 million in 1971 to $8 billion in 1994 (Fisher 1994). Antibiotics (which, roughly translated, means "against life") are secondary metabolites of mi-croorganisms and, at high dilutions, are inhibitory to most other microorganisms. An antibiotic is capable of inhibiting the growth of a microorganism or destroy-ing it (Tamm 1971). It does this by inhibiting the synthesis of the bacteria's cell wall, protein or nucleic acid production, or by reducing the permeability of the cy-toplasmic membrane. This prevents the bacteria from reproducing so rapidly and enables the host to work toward eliminating the organism (Lewis & Lewis 1977).

Although many antibiotics are synthetic, most are derived from natural sub-stances. The most commonly used type is a broad-spectrum antibiotic that is nonselective. Laboratory testing of a swab or blood sample indicates which

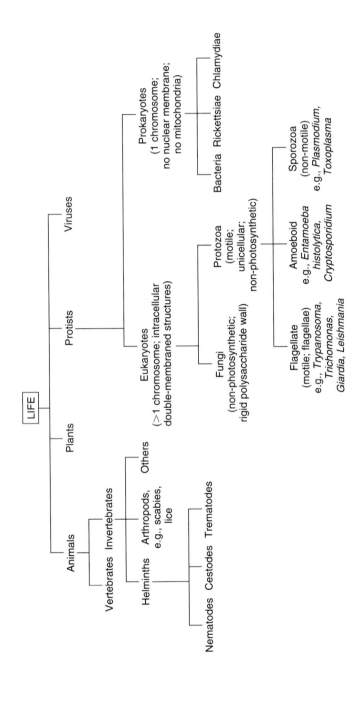

FIGURE 9-3   Classification of pathogens.   From Hope R, Longmore J, Hodgetts T et al. 1993. Oxford Handbook of Clinical Medicine. Oxford, UK: Oxford University Press, p. 172.

antibiotic is appropriate, but this method of testing has largely been abandoned in favor of broad-spectrum antibiotics, mainly because of cost and time, but also because physicians are under intense pressure to prescribe immediately. Broad-spectrum antibiotics do not always succeed in killing the bacterium causing the disease. Despite this, broad-spectrum antibiotics remain very popular and are usually the first line of defense. Broad-spectrum antibiotics usually destroy almost every other "friendly" gut bacterium as well. As a result, a great many people now support colonies of fungi that have taken the place of the friendly digestive bacteria. *Candidiasis,* the existence of which was once denied by the medical profession, is thriving in the gut of millions of people who have taken broad-spectrum antibiotics and have not replaced their friendly bowel flora.

The majority of antibiotics are (or have been until recently) active against gram-positive microorganisms (such as *Staphylococcus* and *Streptococcus*). Although manmade antibiotics are becoming increasingly sophisticated in an attempt to compete with organisms that can mutate and thereby initiate resistant colonies, they are not as complicated as most essential oils. Essential oils have 100 or more components, so it is arguable that an organism would find it more difficult to become resistant to them. Without a doubt, synthetic antibiotics have saved lives and will continue to do so. However, the overuse and improper use of antibiotics during the last few years has led to a growing population of antibiotic-resistant bacteria (Fisher 1994).

Penicillin, the first antibiotic, was found to be effective against *Staphylococcus* but completely ineffective against *E. coli*. As early as 1942, Fleming (who discovered penicillin) was advising the medical profession of the possibility that *Staphylococcus* could become resistant to penicillin. Today, 95% of *Staphylococcus* is resistant to penicillin. Antibiotics are also listed in the group of drugs most frequently associated with adverse reactions such as nausea and gastrointestinal problems, skin rashes, and headaches (Blaschke & Bjornsson 1995). In addition, antibiotics are thought to be linked to an increase in food allergies and to chronic fatigue syndrome (Schmidt 1995). Some bacteria can be killed within a few hours with direct exposure to sunlight, and most are killed at 100° C (the boiling point of water). However, some bacteria are notoriously difficult to eradicate, especially in a person with a compromised immune system. Fig. 9-4 shows how many bacilli and cocci have become resistant to antibiotics, resulting in the development of the so-called "superbugs."

Resistance to Antibiotics

Some strains of bacteria have become resistant to antibiotics for various possible reasons, such as the following:

1. Patients have not completed the prescribed course of antibiotics. This means the bacteria are not completely eradicated and become immune to the next dose of that particular antibiotic.
2. Antibiotics have been prescribed for viral illness such as the common cold. In the United States, some 900,000 prescriptions per year are written for antibiotics to treat the common cold (Fisher 1994).

	Penicillin V/G	Flucloxacillin	Amp/Amoxycillin	Carbenicillin/Ticarcillin	Piperacillin/Azlocillin	Cefradine/Cephalothin/Cefazolin	Cefuroxime/Cephamandole/Cefotaxime	Ceftazidime	Imipenem	Erythromycin	Lincomycin/Clindamycin	Tetracyclines	Chloramphenicol	Trimethoprim	Aminoglycosides	Vancomycin	Metronidazole	Ciprofloxacin
Staphylococcus aureus (penicillin sensitive)	1	0	0	0	2	0	2	2	2R	R	2R	R	R	2	2	2	R	2
Staphylococcus aureus (penicillin resistant)	R	R	R	R	R	R	R	R	2R	R	2R	R	2R	2	R	2	R	2
Streptococcus (group A)	1	0	0	0	2	0	2	2	2R	2	R	R	R	R	0	R	R	R
Streptococcus pneumoniae	1	0	0	0	2	0	2	2	2R	2	2R	R	R	R	0	R	R	R
Enterococcus faecalis	R	R	2	R	R	R	R	R	0	R	2	R	R	2R	2R	R	0	R
Neisseria meningitidis	1	0	2	0	2	0	2	2	0	R	0	2	2	2	R	R	0	0
Listeria monocytogenes	2	0	2	0	2	0	R	R	R	0	0	2	2	2	2R	R	R	0
Haemophilus influenzae	R	1R	0	R	2	2	0	0	2	R	2R	R	1R	0	R	R	2	2
E. coli	R	R	R	R	R	2	R	R	R	R	R	R	1R	2R	R	R	2	2
Klebsiella species	R	R	R	R	R	2R	R	R	R	R	R	R	1R	2R	R	R	2	2
Serratia/Enterobacter species	R	R	R	R	R	2R	2R	R	R	R	R	R	1R	2R	R	R	2	2
Proteus species	R	1R	R	R	R	2R	R	R	R	R	R	R	1R	2R	R	R	2	2
Pseudomonas aeruginosa	R	R	R	R	R	R	R	2	R	R	R	R	R	1R	R	R	2	2
Bacteroides fragilis	R	2R	R	2R	2	R	2R	2	2	2	2R	2R	R	R	R	R	1	R
Other Bacteroides species	R	R	R	R	R	R	R	2R	R	2R	2R	2R	R	R	R	R	1	R

Key: 1 = susceptible, first choice; 2 = susceptible, second choice; R = resistance likely to be a problem; 0 = usually inappropriate.   From: Hope R, Longmore J, Hodgetts T et al. 1993. Oxford Handbook of Clinical Medicine. Oxford, UK: Oxford University Press, p. 176.

FIGURE 9-4   Susceptibility of selected bacteria to certain antibacterial drugs.

3. Antibiotics have been used prophylactically. In the United States, until 1992, a 48-hour course of antibiotics was given preoperatively to patients thought to be at risk for infection.
4. During the past 40 years, the antibiotics penicillin and tetracycline have been added to animal feed.
5. Antibiotics are regularly used by the food industry to protect fruits and vegetables and are also used in the fish industry.

Over-prescription of antibiotics has been widespread. In 1991, 240 million prescriptions for antibiotics were written in the United States, one for every person in the country (Fisher 1994). This dropped to 110 million prescriptions for antibiotics in 1995, but 50% of these are thought to be inappropriate for the disease being treated (Schmidt 1995).

Antibiotics are given to animals to increase growth: in some cases chickens fed with a broth of antibiotics have grown to three times larger than normal (Jukes 1973). Although only minute amounts of antibiotics produce this growth, animals destined for human consumption regularly contain antibiotics, leading to a potential immunity or resistance in humans to those antibiotics. This immunity first manifested itself with an outbreak of *Salmonella* in England in 1965. Normally, *Salmonella* would have been swiftly brought under control with antibiotics. However, on this occasion, investigations showed that the bacterium was resistant and six people died (Corpet 1987).

Following this outbreak, the Swann Committee (composed of microbiologists and physicians) led an intensive enquiry. Their recommendation was a ban on the use of antibiotics used in human medicine for promoting animal growth. Although England, Scandinavia, the Netherlands, and most European countries agreed to the ban, the US government never approved the ban and still allows farmers to use the same antibiotics employed in human medicine as growth stimulants for animals (Fisher 1994).

In fact, shortly after penicillin was discovered, researchers found some strains of *Staphylococcus* could manufacture an enzyme called penicillinase, which rendered penicillin inactive (Abraham & Chaine 1940). This resistant strain spread through hospitals, and by 1955 80% of patients infected with *Staphylococcus* died if penicillin was the only antibiotic used to combat the infection (Fisher 1994).

Methicillin and cephalosporin were introduced in the 1960s in an effort to control penicillin-resistant *Staphylococcus*. They appeared to be effective, but then gram-negative bacteria such as *Serratia* and *Klebsiella* began to show resistance to these new drugs. Another antibiotic, gentamycin, appeared on the market and seemed to have the situation under control until *Staphylococcus* reappeared, this time more resistant than before, the first MRSA. The pharmaceutical business regrouped and produced a new antibiotic, ciprofloxacin (Cipro), but MRSA quickly became immune. By 1980, MRSA was resistant to everything except vancomycin. Vancomycin had been held back, not only because it was toxic, but because it was feared that if MRSA became resistant to it there would be nothing else to throw at the bacterium. These fears became reality in the late 1980s when hospitals began to report vancomycin-resistant infections. Today, a growing number of pathogens are becoming resistant to conventional antibiotics.

Resistant bacteria are still often treated with cephalosporin, an antibiotic derived from a fungus. Cephalosporin was discovered by Giuseppe Brotzu, a bacteriologist from Cagliari in Sardinia (Fisher 1994). The disadvantages of the cephalosporin group of antibiotics are the hypersensitivity they cause in more than 10% of patients and their adverse effects on blood-clotting mechanisms (Hope et al 1993).

Many sexually transmitted diseases, including gonorrhea and chlamydia, now are multiple-drug resistant. *Shigella,* the cause of many fecal-contaminated gastric upsets, is multiple resistant, as are many respiratory infections. Chowdhury (1998) carried out studies on monkeys infected with mutiple-resistant *Shigella flexneri* and found oral doses of black cumin *(Nigella sativa)* essential oil (1 to 3 ml diluted in soybean oil) were very effective. The experimental group of monkeys became entirely free of infection within 2 days, whereas the control group was still infected after 6 days. According to a Web site dedicated to black cumin (www.nigella-sativa.com), the essential oil is made from the plant's seed and was found in Tutankhamen's tomb. The essential oil contains 46.8% p-cymene and 21% carvone. In addition, cumin seed essential oil was found to be effective against *E. coli, Staphylococcus aureus,* and *Streptococcus faecalis* (Jain & Purohit 1992).

ESSENTIAL OILS AS POTENTIAL ANTIBACTERIAL AGENTS

Essential oils are not just pleasant aromas. Many have specific antibiotic, antiviral, and antifungal properties and have been classified accordingly (Natural Medicines Comprehensive Database 2002). The responsibility for prescribing an antibiotic usually lies with a physician or nurse practitioner. For many other health professionals, antibiotic prescription is outside their boundaries or scope of practice and is inappropriate. However, the use of an essential oil to reduce stress caused by an infection is acceptable. What is needed is a more detailed look at essential oils' antibacterial properties. Can they be used to enhance orthodox medicine? Can they be used when antibiotics are ineffective? In a world where pathogens are mutating faster than synthetic medicines can be created to kill them, essential oils might have a very beneficial role to play. They may even turn out to be the antibiotics of the future.

There is a long history of essential oils being used against pestilence. A large number of perfumers and glovemakers appeared to survive the Black Death in Europe. This could be because glovemakers were licensed to impregnate their wares with essential oils and because perfumes were made of essential oils. Deinenger (1995) cites Schweistheimer, who wrote that the English town of Bucklesbury was spared from the plague—at the time Bucklesbury was the center of the lavender trade. Lavender has antibacterial properties and has recently been found effective against MRSA. Nostradamus was supposed to have successfully treated the plague with pills of crushed roses placed under the tongues of plague victims. Rose contains l-citronellol, geraniol, nerol, linalol, and phenylethyl alcohol (Guenther 1952). Alcohols are thought to be strong antiinfection agents with antiviral properties (Franchomme & Penoel), so the actions of Nostradamus seem to be logical.

Approximately 58% of all isolated antibiotics are produced from *Streptomyces,* a bacterium. Another 9% are derived from other bacteria, 19% from fungi, lichens, and mosses, and 14% from higher plants. Lewis writes that "the total 909 antibiotics known in 1967 represent only a fraction of those found in nature. Not a single one, used therapeutically, is from the higher plants, even though these possess the largest single group of antibiotics for which there is no known use" (Lewis & Elvin-Lewis 1977). Tamm (1971) reported on ansamycins, a group of antibiotics characterized by an aliphatic bridge linking two nonadjacent positions found in an aromatic nucleus.

Some of the plants known to have antibiotic properties include yellow cypress, wild ginger, golden seal, poplar tree, turnip, wallflower, hops, cabbage, sweet clover, common bean, cashew, black walnut, potato, corn, and garlic. Each has been tested against bacteria, fungi, viruses, or protozoa and found to be effective in vitro (Lewis & Elvin-Lewis 1977). Valnet (1990) suggests if essential oils were used to treat pathogens, the surrounding tissue would not be adversely affected. Conventional medicines can sometimes destroy the surrounding tissue along with the infection, because antibiotics typically kill bacteria by puncturing their cell walls, which allows toxins to spill out (Service 1994).

In the case of burns, in which the breakdown of tissue causes the body to re-absorb pathogenic toxins, Valnet (1990) suggests the use of essential oils could be a suitable or alternative method of treatment, because many essential oils have tissue-protecting properties that prevent putrefaction. However, essential oils with a high phenol content can cause dermal irritation and should not be used to treat burns. Please see Chapter 3 for more information about phenols and phenol-rich essential oils.

RESEARCH ON THE ANTIBACTERIAL PROPERTIES OF ESSENTIAL OILS

The primary effect of essential oils on bacteria and viruses appears to be on the cell membrane (Harris & Harris 1995) where they seem to alter the osmotic regulatory function (Savino et al 1984). Fifty years ago antibiotic researchers were investigating possible plant alternatives. The Second National Symposium on Recent Advances in Antibiotic Research was held in Washington in 1945, under the auspices of the National Institutes of Health. During the proceedings, the effects of lupulon, a lipid-soluble, antibiotic-like substance prepared from hops *(Humulus lupulus)* were discussed. Chin et al (1949) found lupulon inhibited the growth of *Staphylococcus aureus, Mycobacterium phlei,* and *Mycobacterium tuberculosis* in vitro at concentrations of 1.56, 5.0, and 25 g/mL, respectively. Combining lupulon with a 2% solution of sodium chloride increased the antibiotic activity. Hops produce an essential oil (Budavari 1996).

Maruzella and Sicurella (1960) reported on the antibacterial activity of 133 essential oils in vitro. These were tested against six pathogens, namely *E. coli, Staphylococcus aureus, B. subtilis, Streptococcus faecalis, Salmonella typhosa,* and *Mycobacterium avium.* Of the essential oils tested, 71% were shown to be effective against *M. avium,* 19% against *B. subtilis,* 14% against *Staphylococcus aureus,* 12% against *Streptococcus faecalis,* and 6% against *E. coli.* Among the most effective essential oils were lemongrass, oregano, savory, red thyme, and cinnamon. This research was conducted just 2 years after an earlier paper (Maruzella & Percival 1958) investigated the antimicrobial activity of perfume oils.

Deans and Svoboda (1987) found that marjoram *(Oregano majorana)* was effective against *Pseudomonas aeruginosa, Salmonella pullorum,* and *Yersinia enterocolitica* in vitro at a concentration of 1:10 in absolute ethanol. All three organisms are of significance in public health. Essential oils of black pepper *(Piper nigrum),* geranium *(Pelargonium graveolens),* nutmeg *(Myristica fragrans),* oregano *(Origanum vulgare),* and thyme *(Thymus vulgaris)* were tested against 25 different genera of bacteria, and each was found to exhibit considerable inhibitory effect (Dorman & Deans 2000). Peana et al (1999) found sage *(Salvia officinalis)* and clary sage *(Salvia sclarea)* effective against various bacteria including *Staphylococcus aureus, E. coli,* and *S. epidermidis.*

P. aeruginosa appears to be less susceptible to tea tree than many bacteria, and this tolerance is thought to be because of the bacteria's outer membrane. However, the addition of polymyxin B nonapeptide (PMBN) to the essential oil appears to permeabilize the outer membrane, allowing tea tree to become effective (Mann et al 2000). PMBN may also help other essential oils become effective against *P. aeruginosa.*

Zakarya et al (1993) examined the antimicrobial activity of 21 essential oils of eucalyptus. The effects of the volatile constituents of lemon gum *(Eucalyptus citriodora)* were found to be the most effective against *E. coli* (gram-negative) and *B. megaterium* and *S. aureus* (both gram-positive). Although, when the whole essential oil was used, sugargum *(Eucalyptus cladocalyx)* was most effective. This brings up the point, which has been paralleled in many other studies, that isolating the active, common constituents of essential oils will not produce the same effects as using the whole essential oil. It is interesting that *E. globulus, E. smithi,* and *E. radiata* were not among the eucalyptus types selected for testing, as they are regularly used in aromatherapy to treat infections (Penoel 1991/1992).

Ferdous et al (1992) studied the effect of black cumin *(Nigella sativa)* essential oil on the treatment of dysentery, and it was shown effective against several multiple-drug-resistant organisms, such as *Shigella, Vibrio cholera,* and *E. coli.* The activity of the oil was compared with that of ampicillin, tetracycline, cotrimoxazole, gentamycin, and nalidixic acid and was active against all of the bacterial strains tested, except for one strain of *Shigella dysenteriae* (strain 1548). Black cumin is commonly known as Roman coriander, nutmeg flower or fennel flower, although it is not in any way related to fennel. It actually belongs to the buttercup family. The French formerly used the seeds as a substitute for pepper, and in

India the seeds are commonly used in curries (Greive 1931). Lemon essential oil *(Citrus limon)* was found to completely inhibit *Vibrio cholera* in a further study by de Castillo et al (2000). *Vibrio* species also showed a high sensitivity to basil and sage essential oils in a study by Koga et al (1999).

Helichrysum picardii, a member of the everlasting flower family, was shown to be effective against gram-positive bacteria such as *Staphylococcus aureus, Bacillus subtilis, B. cereus, B. maegaterium,* and gram-negative *E. coli.* Its antibacterial activity was thought to be less potent than clove and thyme (de la Puerta et al 1993). *Helichrysum* is used as a tobacco flavorant.

Deans and Ritchie (1987) of the Department of Biochemical Sciences, at the Scottish Agricultural College in Auchincruive, Scotland, tested the effect of 50 essential oils against 25 genera of bacteria in vitro. Their research found that the most effective essential oils were bay, cinnamon, clove, thyme, marjoram, pimento, geranium, and lovage. One year later, Deans and Svoboda (1988) found French tarragon *(Artemesia dracunculus)* to be effective against *P. aeruginosa, S. aureus, S. faecalis,* and *Yersinia enterocolitica.* In this study, the whole oil was tested against several of the main chemical constituents such as eugenol, limonene, linalol, menthol, cis-ocimene, anisaldehyde, and α-pinene. This same study produced firm evidence that the constituents of essential oils change, depending on the time of their harvesting. In this instance, tarragon plants harvested midseason were the least potent of the tarragon plants tested. That the constituents of tarragon essential oil alter according to the time of harvesting is not new to aromatherapy, but this is one of the few studies that actually demonstrates this. Also of interest is the way the physical configuration of the molecule affected the essential oil (the difference between cis- and transisomers). In tarragon, the cis configuration produced a more antimicrobial plant. Tarragon is used as a flavor ingredient in many foods, as well as in alcoholic beverages and soft drinks. It is also an important ingredient of bearnaise sauce. Several hybrids (man-made cultivars) of lavender, sage, savory, and thyme were also tested against 25 bacteria in vitro. All four hybrids showed substantial antibiotic activity, but each was most potent against specific bacteria. See Table 9-2 for details.

Table 9-2   ❧   *Hybrids and Their Antibacterial Properties*

General	**Common Name**	**Bacteria Affected**
Thymus	thyme	*Moraxella* spp., *Clostridium sporogenes*
Salvia	sage	*Acinetobacter calcoacetica, Brevibacterium linens, Clostridium sporogenes, Moraxella* spp.
Satureja	savory	*Brevibacterium linens, Enterobacter aerogenes, Klebsiella pneumonia, Moraxella* spp.
Lavandula	lavender	*Brevibacterium* linens, *Clostridium sporogenes, Moraxella* spp, *Staphylococcus aureus*

In another paper Deans et al (1992) demonstrated the antibacterial properties of *Oregano officinalis* (a specially bred strain from Israel) and West Indian lemongrass *(Cymbopogon citratus)*. Other essential oils found to have antibacterial activity were tarragon, basil, sage, thyme, and celery. Among the bacteria tested were *Salmonella pullorum, E. coli, Klebsiella pneumonia, P. aeruginosa, Staphylococcus aureus, Streptococcus faecalis,* and *Proteus vulgaris*. Deans and Svoboda (1989) also found summer savory *(Satureja hortensis)* to be an effective antibacterial agent against the previously mentioned organisms.

The antibacterial properties of lemongrass were the subject of a detailed investigation by Onawunmi and Ogunlana (1986). This particular lemongrass is grown in Nigeria, where it is traditionally used for the treatment of rheumatism. German chamomile *(Matricaria recutita)*, renowned for its deep-blue color and antiinflammatory properties, also has substantial antimicrobial activity, especially against gram-positive bacteria such as *Staphylococcus aureus* and *Streptococcus faecalis*. The antibiotic component is thought to be α-bisabolol, which is more active than chamazulene (Kedzia 1991).

Balacs (1993) reviewed the antibacterial properties of the plant family Lamiacae, which includes rosemary *(Rosmarinus officinalis)*, wild basil *(Calamintha nepeta)*, thyme *(Thymus vulgaris)*, and savory *(Satureja montana)*. The effective chemical parts of these plants are thought to be carvacrol (in savory), α-pinene and 1,8-cineole (in rosemary), thymol (in thyme), and pulegone and para-cymene (in wild basil).

Benouda et al (1988) tested essential oils against hospital-pathogenic bacteria. This study examined essential oils of armoise *(Artemesia herba alba)*, oregano *(Thymus capitatus)*, and eucalyptus *(Eucalyptus globulus)* against *Staphylococcus aureus, Streptococcus* C and D, *Proteus* spp., *Klebsiella* spp., *Salmonella typhi, Haemophilus influenza*, and *P. aeruginosa* and found that the three essential oils had an action comparable to standard antibiotics. Thyme was the most effective essential oil, although none of the oils were found to have any impact on *Pseudomonas*.

A review paper by Carson and Riley (1993) found that tea tree *(Melaleuca alternifolia)* was an effective antibiotic against *Staphylococcus, Streptococcus*, and many gram-negative bacteria, and they concluded that the full therapeutic potential of tea tree had not yet been realized. In The Cowthron Report, Cooke and Cooke (1994) found manuka *(Leptospermum scoparium)* and kanuka *(Kunzea ericoides)*, New Zealand's answer to tea tree, produced impressive results. This study was supported by Maori funds and covered the effects of these two essential oils against various bacteria and fungi. Manuka appeared to be very effective against *Staphylococcus aureus* and ringworm. It was believed manuka could be a useful essential oil in cases of MRSA infection, although the paper stated that no clinical trials had been carried out.

An additional paper by Carson et al (1995) showed tea tree was effective against MRSA. It was tested against 64 methicillin-resistant and 33 mupirocin-resistant isolates of *S. aureus* and was found to be effective in all cases, using dilutions of 0.25% and 0.50%. These results were duplicated in a UK study using similar methods. The tea tree used in the UK study was chemotype terpineol greater than 30%, and the cineole content (an oxide and harsher on the mucous membrane) was less than 15%. Chan and Loudon (1998) carried out an *in vitro* study on 28 isolates of MRSA and eight clinical isolates of coagulase-negative staphylococci at Manchester Royal Infirmary in Manchester, England. The minimum inhibitory concentrations (MICs) were repeated three times and ranged from 0.25% to 0.5% tea tree. No resistant isolates were found. Many cosmetic products contain 2% to 5% tea tree. Carson found an added bonus; although tea tree inhibited MRSA, it did not inhibit CNS and therefore preserves the skin flora.

Human Studies

For skeptics who may argue the effective antimicrobial activity of an essential oil *in vitro* does not guarantee a similar action in humans, Caelli et al (2001) carried out a study on humans using 4% tea tree nasal ointment and 5% tea tree body wash against a control of 2% mupirocin nasal ointment and triclosan body wash on MRSA. The tea tree combination appeared to be better than the conventional one. However, because of the small number of patient participants (n = 30) no statistical significance could be drawn.

A study by Sherry et al (2001) indicates that essential oils can be effective in humans and may be effective when nothing else works. The authors reported on a chronic case of MRSA osteomyelitis. A 49-year-old man sustained an open fracture to his left tibia. He underwent debridement and insertion of an intramedullary nail. He underwent a free-flap procedure to the lower tibia 2 months later to reposition the nail, and a femoral-popliteal bypass graft. Debridement of the flap was done 8 months later. Debridement of an infective focus of the left tibia was performed 15 months later. He subsequently developed chronic osteomyelitis (MRSA). Long-term antibiotic therapy (oral and intravenous) of 1 gr flucloxacillin and 1 gr dicloxacillin every 6 hours had been unsuccessful. Amputation was being considered.

In December, 2000, via a 3-cm percutaneous incision, the lower tibia was drilled and washed out with 4000 ml of saline. Then it was packed with calcium sulfate pellets impregnated with lemongrass, eucalyptus, tea tree, clove, and thyme essential oils in an ethanol base. A catheter was left in situ to allow delivery of further essential oils. One ml of antiseptic essential oil mixture was administrated daily. The dilution and ratio of the essential oils was not given by the authors. The wound healed and the culture was clear within 3 months. The symptoms resolved, and a plain x-ray examination showed resolution of the infective process with incorporation of the bone graft. The authors commented that essential oils have a strong antimicrobial action, are cheap, simple to use, and can be used topically (Sherry et al 2001).

Many essential oils, at a dilution known to be safe, have also been shown effective against drug-resistant pathogens. In 1994, a workshop was given at the Royal Society of Medicine in London, England, on aromatograms and the use of essential oils as antibacterial agents. Michael Smith, a London-based pathologist who conducts aromatograms for several London hospitals, gave his analysis of the antibacterial properties of several essential oils on MRSA. Every one tested was effective. The essential oils included oregano, thymol (*Thymus vulgaris* CT3), Moroccan chamommile *(Ormenis mixta),* Dutch mill lavender (*Lavandula* x *intermedia* CT Super), Italian cypress *(Cupressus sempervirens),* peppermint *(Mentha piperita),* ravensara *(Ravensara aromatica),* juniper *(Juniperus communis),* lemon, palmarosa *(Cymbopogon martini),* eucalyptus, and gully gum *(Eucalyptus smithi).* Most of these are essential oils that are commonly used for stress management and are generally accepted as being safe. Many of them are used by health professionals in the United States. The time is right to consider using essential oils for *all* their properties.

My students have had some impressive case-study results using essential oil compresses on wound infections and infected bedsores. Swabs to indicate infectious pathogens were taken, and the relevant essential oil selected. One particularly impressive case study was conducted by a nurse practitioner. A female patient had a chronically infected bedsore. This patient had been on systemic antibiotics without effect. A wound swab showed the infection had been caused by *Clostridium.* Searching through her notes, the nurse practitioner found a reference to a paper by Ross et al (1980). After she had discussed the safety and potential efficacy of sweet marjoram *(Origanum majorana)* with the patient's physician and had shown him the monograph, he gave his consent for her to use this essential oil. The treatment was discussed with the patient and consent obtained.

A compress was applied directly to the infected site, using a 5% solution of sweet marjoram. The compress was reapplied three times a day. Within 24 hours there was a dramatic improvement, and within 5 days the wound was healed. In other case studies, essential oils with antibacterial properties have been selected without a swab being taken. Dilutions of up to 10% have been used. Not one case has shown any negative side effect to date. In most instances, the infection has healed very rapidly. For more information on wounds and protocols please see Chapter 15 on care of the elderly.

Further research is required. Animal testing has already been done for potential toxicity of essential oils; atoxicity studies on human tissue have indicated a safe level at which essential oils can be used. What is needed now is a series of controlled trials to explore the antimicrobial efficacy of essential oils in humans. As Peter Mansfield, MD, (1996) writes, "Science is really a method for answering questions. If we ask stupid questions, scientific methods will faithfully produce for us a stupid answer." It is not stupid to ask questions relating to aromatherapy and stress, but it is perhaps stupid *not* to ask questions about aromatherapy and infection. Just because these oils are natural does not mean they are not powerful. Norman Farnsworth, Director of Pharmacognosy at the University of Illinois College of Pharmacy is quoted as saying,: "There is not a dime's bit of difference between chemicals in plants and synthetics" (Sears 1995).

THE AROMATOGRAM

Just like synthetic antibiotics, many essential oils are effective against particular pathogens. The skill lies in knowing which essential oil to use for which infection. Conventional medicine regularly takes wound or throat swabs, or urine or blood samples to cultivate and identify a pathogen.

Gattefosse used exactly the same principle of this process, which is called an antibiogram, in France and renamed it an aromatogram. The only difference in the procedure is with an aromatogram an essential oil is added to the Petri dish instead of an antibiotic. A hypothetical example of an aromatogram is shown in Fig. 9-5.

The Petri dish is lined with a culture medium such as agar-agar. A culture broth of the pathogen is spread across the plate. Several small paper circles, each impregnated with different essential oil, are placed on the agar-agar, and the Petri dish is incubated for 24 hours. If the essential oil is the correct antidote, an area of inhibition occurs in a circle around the impregnated paper. Sometimes an essential oil not effective on its own is effective when it is close to a second essential oil. Sometimes two essential oils together give a large area of inhibition but individually produce no area of inhibition. Aromatograms are used in France and England and could be of great use in the United States. So far I have been unable

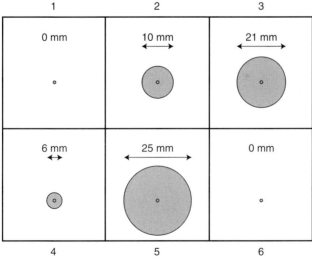

FIGURE 9-5   Hypothetical example of an aromatogram. Six different essential oils, here identified only by number, are being tested against one bacterial culture from the body of a patient. The shaded area in each square is known as the "area of inhibition" and shows how effective each oil is against the bacteria. In this case essential oils 3 and 5 would be used to treat the patient.   From Tisserand R. 1988. Aromatherapy for Everyone. Harmondsworth, UK: Penguin Books.

to find a laboratory in the United States prepared to conduct an aromatogram, but this is obviously the way of the future. Belaiche (1979), a French doctor, has created many tables illustrating the specific uses of essential oils against specific bacteria and their effects.

In England, Deans and Ritchie (1987) used the aromatogram technique in a comprehensive and impressive study that examined 25 genera of bacteria and 50 essential oils. This kind of sensitivity testing for essential oils in the treatment of bacterial infections is being carried out by several London hospitals, and there is active campaigning to increase the understanding of how aromatograms work (Blackwell & Smith 1995). It is hoped that this scientific method of selecting essential oils in sensitivity testing will become more widespread as it becomes better understood. However, a new microdilution method using the redox dye Resazurin has also been developed for determining the MIC of an essential oil (Mann & Markham 1998). This method overcomes the problem of adequate contact between an essential oil and the test bacteria and obviates the need for a chemical emulsifier.

Blackwell and Smith (1995) and Valnet (1990) both emphasize that standard organisms do not respond in exactly the same way as a host organism. Even though a pathogen is known and named, it may not respond in an identical way; the host must be taken into consideration. To illustrate this, Valnet writes that a colibacillus in one patient may respond to the essential oil of pine, whereas in another patient it may respond to the essential oil of lavender or thyme. This is quite different from the Western approach in which everyone is given the same antibiotic (usually broad-spectrum). However, the selection of essential oils for testing via an aromatogram is based on the antibacterial properties reported in the literature.

VIRUSES

A virus is different than any other pathogen because it is a coiled strand of nucleic acid protected by a protein coat, which can only survive and reproduce inside a host cell (Roberts 1986). Because viruses are so small, their biology was not understood for many years until electron microscopy revealed what they looked like. Many biologists still do not classify them as living organisms in their own right but only when they are inside a host cell. There are basically two types of virus: those that attack bacteria and those that attack the cells of other living organisms, such as animals and humans. The basic structure of a virus is illustrated in Fig. 9-6.

Viruses are classified as either DNA viruses or RNA viruses. The DNA viruses are subdivided into single-strand and double-strand viruses. RNA viruses also occur as single or double strands, with retroviruses, such as AIDS, in the single-strand group. A retrovirus contains an enzyme called reverse transcriptase that allows the RNA in the virus to be reverse-transcribed into DNA. Drugs such as zidovudine (AZT) and zalcitabine (HIVID) are designed to inhibit production of reverse transcriptase. Resistance acquired by viruses during antiviral therapy

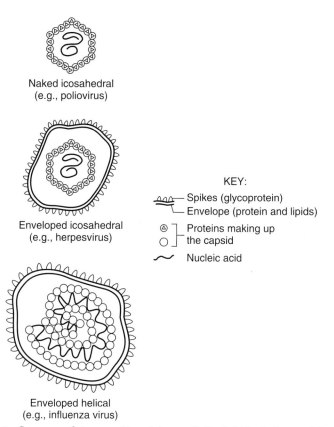

Naked icosahedral
(e.g., poliovirus)

Enveloped icosahedral
(e.g., herpesvirus)

KEY:

Spikes (glycoprotein)
Envelope (protein and lipids)

Proteins making up
the capsid

Nucleic acid

Enveloped helical
(e.g., influenza virus)

FIGURE 9-6   Structure of viruses.   From Ackerman B, Dunk-Richards G. 1991. Microbiology: An Introduction for the Health Sciences. Australia: WB Saunders.

has been well documented and usually occurs when the virus mutates (MacSween & Whaley 1992).

Viruses that cause glandular fever, hepatitis, influenza, warts, the common cold, mumps, and measles are well known; less common is the rabies virus. More recent viruses are herpes and Lassa fever. Of these viruses, only smallpox has been eradicated through immunization. A compulsory immunization program in the West has controlled mumps and measles, although they remain potential killers in developing countries. Patients with immune deficiency (or dysfunction), both primary and secondary, are more vulnerable to infections of any kind than persons with intact immune systems.

SYNTHETIC ANTIVIRALS

Geoffrey Carr (1996) of *The Economist* wrote, "No viral epidemic has ever been stopped by drugs." Synthetic viricides are difficult to manufacture, and none of them appear to be totally effective to date. Most have moderate to severe side effects. They work in one of three ways: through immunological control, through stimulation of the natural resistance mechanism of the host, or through chemotherapy. One of the most successful, AZT, stops the phosphate linkage from being formed. This means the virus cannot manufacture DNA (Craig & Stitzel 1994). Other synthetic antivirals include acyclovir (Zovirax), famcyclovir (Famvir), Vidarabine (Vira-A), and rimantadine (Flumadine).

Highly active antiretrovial therapy (HAART) is a powerful weapon that has greatly affected the AIDS epidemic—an epidemic that may well turn out to be more devastating than the plague itself. AIDS/HIV has killed three times more Americans than the Vietnam war (Sullivan 1995). Unfortunately HAART drugs also have potent side effects and it is difficult for patients to completely adhere to the treatment regimen.

ANTIVIRAL PROPERTIES OF ESSENTIAL OILS

Many plants and their aqueous extracts have been tested for antiviral activity. Interestingly, when the essential oil from the plant is used, it too seems to have an antiviral effect, although the essential oil has a different chemistry than the aqueous extract. Therefore a good pointer is to study the published research on the aqueous extracts.

An investigation supported by the National Institutes of Health showed an aqueous extract of lemon balm *(Melissa officinalis)* had antiviral properties (Kucera & Herrmann 1967). The aqueous extract was tested on embryonic eggs and in tissue culture infected with Semliki forest (a mouse brain disease), Newcastle disease, vaccinia, and herpes simplex. The results showed lemon balm protected the embryonic eggs against the lethal action of all viruses tested. It is thought that the antiviral action was produced by the tannin-like polyphenol. This activity is thought to be unrelated to that of tea tannins, although they are known antivirals and effective on influenza A (Cohen et al 1964). Kucera and Herrmann (1967) also explored the antiviral effects of the aqueous extract of lemon balm against influenza A and B, mumps, and three different strains of parainfluenza (1, 2, and 3). The results showed that lemon balm had an antiviral effect on mumps and the three parainfluenza strains, but had no effect on influenza A and B. Extract of lemon balm is sold in commercial antiviral preparations in Germany (Foster & Duke 1960). I have found lemon balm essential oil (5-25%) to be effective against herpes simplex 1 and 2.

Penoel (1991/1992) writes that essential oil of gully gum has strong viricidal action and suggests the antiviral properties are due to 1,8-cineole (sometimes also called eucalyptol). 1,8-cineole is found in several essential oils such as bay laurel *(Laurus nobilis)*, ravensara, spike lavender *(Lavandula latifolia)*, rosemary, Spanish sage *(Salvia lavendulaefolia)*, and cardamom *(Elettaria cardamomum)*. Penoel (1991/1992) suggests that limonene and α-pinene reinforce the antiviral action of 1,8-cineole, whereas alcohols strengthen its antiviral action. I have found gully gum, ravensara, spike lavender, and rosemary all effective against both herpes and the cold virus. I have not tested them against influenza.

Cariel and Jean (1990) tested cypress *(Cupressus sempervirens)* for viricidal properties and then applied for a patent. Lemon gum was found to be an effective antiviral by Mendes et al (1990). This eucalyptus was also studied for its anti-HIV activities, together with eight other medicinal plants from Zaire (Muanza et al 1995). May and Willuhn (1978) found eucalyptus had antiviral properties. This is of particular interest to patients with HIV/AIDS as eucalyptus is also known to enhance the activity of streptomycin, isoniazid, and sulfetrone in TB, a common opportunistic infection among those with AIDS (Kufferath & Mundualgo 1954). Extract of eucalyptus was also found effective against herpes simplex I (Takechi & Tanaka 1985). Extract of sweet marjoram was found to work as an antiviral in a study by Kucera and Herrmann (1967). Sweet marjoram is a safe essential oil to use on the skin.

Duke (1985) writes that ceylon cinnamon *(Cinnamomum verum)* and clove *(Syzygium aromaticum)* have antiviral properties. Takechi and Tanaka (1981) suggest the actual antiviral substance from the bud is eugeniin. Clove bud oil, which is used in baking, perfumes, lipsticks, soaps, and dentistry, has caused hand dermatitis (Lovell 1993), although clove bud essential oil is thought to be safe for use at up to 5% dilution (Opdyke 1979).

Cinnamon produces two essential oils: one from the leaf and one from the bark. The leaf essential oil contains less than 7% cinnamic aldehyde (a known skin irritant), but the essential oil obtained from the bark contains up to 90% cinnamic aldehyde (Lovell 1993). The latter is therefore contraindicated for topical applications, as even at such low dilutions as 0.01%, positive reactions have been found in patch testing (Mathias 1980).

May and Willuhn (1979) tested 178 species of medicinal plants belonging to 69 families for their virustatic properties. In total, 75 aqueous extracts appeared to have antiviral properties. These were tested against polio, influenza, and herpes viruses. Bay laurel, oregano, rosemary, and sage were the most effective of the Lamiaceae family against all three viruses. Juniper also showed substantial antiviral action against herpes and influenza. Bay laurel should perhaps be avoided because it can cause contact dermatitis, although the Research Institute for Fragrance Materials (RIFM) monographs report in three separate tests there were no reactions on human volunteers (Tisserand & Balacs 1995). Oregano is high in phenols and known as a skin irritant so is best avoided (Opdyke 1979). However, oregano can be used in aromatic medicine for acute and chronic infections when taken by mouth, diluted in gelatin capsules. Please see section of Chapter 7 on oral use. Juniper is a good choice for topical use because it contains mainly terpenes and has a very astringent action.

Essential oil of sandalwood was found to have antiviral activity in a study by Benencia and Courreges (1999). Their study focused on herpes simplex 1 and 2 and was carried out on the kidney cells of monkeys. Sandalwood was most effective against herpes simplex 1. Benencia and Courreges speculated the antiviral effect could be due to sandalwood's modulatory influence on cellular glutathione S-transferase activity.

Isoborneol, a monoterpenic component of several essential oils, was found to have viricidal activity against herpes simplex virus 1. Isoborneol inactivated the virus within 30 minutes of exposure at a concentration of 0.06%, and completely inhibited viral replication without affecting viral adsorption (Armaka et al 1999). Isoborneol did not show significant cytotoxicity when tested against human cell lines at 0.16%. Therefore essential oils containing major proportions of isoborneol might be useful in treating herpes.

A lesser-known essential oil, chameleon *(Houttynia cordata),* was tested against herpes simplex, influenza, and HIV-1 in a Japanese study by Kyoko et al (1994). This oil showed remarkable effects, although it was not effective against the polio and coxsackie virus. The research showed that essential oils have the potential to interfere with the virus envelope, which results in the loss of infectivity of the virus, because the attachment to the cell surface must necessarily involve viral-surface glycoproteins present in the envelope.

Garlic has been used against infections for centuries and is the subject of almost 1000 research papers. Recent research has shown garlic to be effective against herpes virus types 1 and 2, parainfluenza virus type 3, vaccinia virus (cowpox), and human rhinovirus type 2 (a common cold virus). The active ingredients, allicin and ajoene, are thought to attack the virus inside the cell, possibly in the cell membrane (Weber 1992). Although garlic essential oil is available, it is unlikely to be used in a clinical setting because of its strong, pervasive odor.

Franchomme and Penoel (1990) list three chemotypes of *Thymus vulgaris* (CT thymol, geraniol, and linalol) as antivirals. Sweet marjoram, lemon balm, cypress, eucalyptus, and juniper essential oil are all safe to use for treating herpes simplex 1 and 2. Essential oils that contain a high 1,8-cineole content should be used with caution in high dilutions on irritated mucous membrane, because they may cause skin sensitivity. Essential oils that contain 1,8-cineole include gully gum, bay laurel, ravensara, spike lavender, rosemary, Spanish sage, and cardamom. Essential oil of eucalyptus is my first choice against herpes simplex 1 and 2. Essential oils can play an important role in the treatment of viral illness. For more information about the treatment of herpes, including protocols, please see Chapter 20 on immunology.

FUNGAL INFECTIONS

Some of the most deadly infections come from fungi in the air we breathe; when a healthy immune system is in place, the fungi have no effect (Richardson 2000). A fungus is a primitive organism classified as neither a plant nor an animal. Only a few fungi are pathogenic to man, and most cause superficial, mild lesions (MacSween & Whaley 1992). Fungi are divided into three categories: superficial, subcutaneous, and systemic. All can be environmental in origin. Fungal infection is caused by airborne allergens, elaborating toxins, or direct infection. A disease, or infection, caused by fungi is called a mycosis (Parish 1991). With an airborne allergen (such as tinea, or ringworm) the spores, or hyphae, of the fungus infiltrate the outer layers of the skin and cause destruction of the epidermis. With mycetoma, a localized infection occurs that may slowly spread, although with *candidiasis* and *cryptococcosis* the infection can become systemic.

Cryptococcosis

Cryptococcosis is a yeast infection that is spread by bird droppings and begins as a sporadic disease manifesting with lung infestation. From the lungs, yeast cells migrate to the CNS. Techically there is a blood-brain barrier (BBB) but this barrier is not 100% leakproof and under certain conditions, such as immune deficiency, the BBB is compromised and CNS infection can occur. Standard treatments are fluconazole, itroconazole, or amphotericin B encapsulated in liposomes (Cordonnier 1993). This treatment is still in use (Evans 2000). However, clinical resistance occurs fairly quickly.

Aspergillosis

Spores of this *Aspergillosis* are present in the atmosphere, and many species are infectious to man. The most common is *Aspergillus fumigatus.* Although the effect of this fungus is not as rapid as that of *Cryptococcus,* the possible resulting bronchial asthma can be debilitating. The fungus may colonize a bronchial cavity and can result in necrotizing pneumonia. This tends to occur only in immunocompromised patients.

Candida albicans

Candida is normally present in the mouth, intestinal tract, vagina, and on moist skin and does not pose a problem. However, in certain circumstances, the fungus begins a mucocutaneous, or systemic, invasion. The mucosal infection occurs when an alteration in the pH of the body tissue produces an alkaline medium that allows the yeast fungus to proliferate. From the mucosa, *Candida* can invade surrounding surfaces such as nail beds, producing chronic, granulomatous inflammation of the underlying tissue. It can also spread throughout the body, invading the heart valves, lungs, liver, and kidneys with multiple, small abscesses containing the fungus (MacSween & Whaley 1992). The symptoms of mucosal infestation are severe itching, with creamy, curd-like deposits. *Candida* is the major fungal pathogen of immunocompromised patients (Kwon-Chung & Bennett 1992) but is also common in diabetes, pregnancy, antibiotic therapy, and after radiation and chemotherapy. Recently, *Candida* has become resistant to many conventional drugs and metabolic inhibitors that have no commonality (Goldway et al 1995).

The incidence of *Candida* overgrowth has increased dramatically during the preceding few years and is thought to be related to immune supression, the use of the contraceptive pill, and the overuse of antibiotics (Zarno 1994).

SYNTHETIC ANTIFUNGALS

It is more difficult to treat fungal infections than bacterial infections, because many fungal infections occur in tissues with poor (if any) blood supply. Examples of infection sites are the nails, hair, and skin. However, fungal infections are thought to be less difficult to treat than viral diseases by orthodox medicine. The drug of choice for fungal infections is fluconazole (Diflucan) or mycostatin (Nyastatin). Although topical application may keep the fungal infection at bay, systemic treatment is often given to reduce the incidence of recurrence following multiple infections. Fluconazole can affect kidney function. Of the other drugs used to treat fungal infection, many cause nausea and induce skin rashes, and a few can cause liver damage (Parish 1991). More recently developed antifungals like itraconazole or Lamasil do cause liver damage (Newsham 2002).

ANTIFUNGAL PROPERTIES OF ESSENTIAL OILS

Essential oils appear to have an antisporulating and respiration-inhibitory effect on fungi (Inouye et al 1998). In 1927 Myers published some of the earliest research on the antifungal properties of essential oils. He was prompted to investigate the fungicidal properties of essential oils following successful treatment of a lesion with a diluted solution of cinnamon oil, which caused immediate relief of symptoms and rapid healing. He observed that thymol, carvacrol, and oil of lemon destroyed yeast in less than a minute. His research involved nine yeast-like organisms, which were isolated from infections in humans, including two lung infections, two tongue infections, one infection involving a nail lesion, and various other cutaneous ulcerations. Each infection rapidly became yeast-negative and was resolved with no recurrence. Laboratory work has shown that volatile oils exhibit antifungal activity at very low concentrations in growth medium. One example is 1 to 10 μL^{-1} of marjoram reduced the growth of filamentous fungiby up to 89% (Deans & Svoboda 1990). Electrical or battery-operated diffusers and nebulizers are the most effective ways of getting essential oils into the lungs. Nebulizers are a very suitable method of treatment for lung infestations by yeast, fungi, or bacteria as they fill the air with an extremely fine mist of micromolecules of essential oil. Nebulizers can be programmed to come on and off at specific times.

Cryptococcosis

Viollon and Chaumont (1994) tested the susceptibility of a strain of *Cryptococcus neoformans* isolated from the blood of a patient with AIDS to 25 essential oils and 17 separate chemical constituents found in essential oils. Many of the essential oils used showed good fungistatic action. The best effects were from palma rosa, geranium, savory, sandalwood, thyme, marjoram, and lavender. Pattnaik et al (1996) reported that lemongrass, eucalyptus, palma rosa, and peppermint were the most effective essential oils tested against *Cryptococcus*. Basil and thyme were not included in this study. (Lemongrass in low dilutions was effective not only against *Cryptococcus* but against all 11 other fungi tested.) MIC for each of the four essential oils against *Cryptococcus* was 5 μL^{-1}.

In another paper, Pattnaik et al (1997a) found complete essential oils were more effective against *Cryptococcus* than their isolated, active components. Lemongrass was the exception. The effectiveness of lemongrass was equal to the isolated parts of citral and geranial. Larrondo and Calvo (1991) compared the topical and inhaled action of citral against the systemic effects of clotrimazole. Although the actual way essential oils work as fungicides is not completely clear, it seems metabolism and growth of the fungus is inhibited, often with a break-down in the lipid part of the membrane, resulting in increased permeability or rupture (Larrondo et al 1995).

Soliman et al (1994) found rosemary and Mehrotra and Rawat (1993) found *Artemisia parviflora* (a member of the Indian tarragon family) to be effective against *Cryptococcus*. Although this *Artemisia* is not in common use, rosemary is used topically for muscle tension and is inhaled for its antispasmodic effect on coughs (Price & Price 1995). Viollon and Chaumont (1994) suggest geranium, palma rosa, savory, and thyme might also be good choices for *Cryptococcus*. If the rosemary is a ketone chemotype, avoid using it for extended periods of time (Tisserand & Balacs 1995).

Aspergillosis

Onawunmi (1989) found West Indian lemongrass *(Cymbopogon citratus)* and Garg and Dengre (1988) found cumin *(Cuminum cyminum)* effective against aspergillosis. Tisserand & Balacs (1995) suggest that because cumin has a strong photosensitizing action, it should not be used topically on patients who will be exposed to ultraviolet light within 12 hours, and dilutions should be kept to 0.04%. Other effective essential oils include tarragon *(Artemisia dracunculus)* (Mehrotra & Rawat 1993) and lemon gum (Hmamouchi et al 1990). Of these, perhaps lemongrass and lemon gum are most commonly used. Neither of these essential oils has any known adverse reactions at dilutions of 1% to 5 % (Opdyke 1976). Inoye et al (2000) found that just the vapor of lavender and tea tree stopped the apical growth of hyphae of *Aspergillus* in closed containers.

West Indian lemongrass was found effective against *Aspergillus fumigatus*, various isolates of *Candida*, and *Trichophyton mentagrophytes* by Onawunmi (1989). The most active component of lemongrass is citral (70% to 80%), which is thought to be responsible for the antifungal activity of this plant. In another study, lemongrass was found to be effective against 15 fungi, including *Aspergillus terreus, A. flavus, A. ochraceus, A. parasiticus, A. fumigatus, A. ustus, A. niger, Penicillin nigricans, P. melin, P. chrysogenum, P. brevicompactum, Fusarium moniliforme,* and *F. oxysporum* (Agarwal et al 1980). Other plants with a high citral content are lemon grass, citronella, lemon verbena, and lemon gum. Pattnaik (1999) confirmed the antifungal acitivty of most *Cymbopogon* spp. Camphor *(Cinnamomum camphora)* was found to be as effective as Ceresan, copper oxychloride, and

Thiovit (all synthetic, commonly used antifungal agents) against *Aspergillus flavus,* a common spoiler of stored food. However, essential oils of both brown and yellow camphor are contraindicated in human use because they contain safrole, which is thought to be carcinogenic.

Candida albicans

Specific essential oils effective against *Candida* include tea tree (Belaiche 1985), lemon grass (Larrondo & Calvo 1991), and lemon gum (Hmamouchi et al 1990).

Much has been reported about the antifungal effects of tea tree from Australia (Belaiche 1985a; Shemesh 1991), and certainly this is one of the safest and most effective essential oils to use, particularly in the vagina. However, many other essential oils have antifungal properties. Caraway, clove, geranium, lavender, lemon, lemongrass, neroli, peppermint, petitgrain, spearmint, coriander, and sweet orange leaf are all effective to varying degrees (Galal et al 1973). Coriander is one of the flavorants of the liqueurs Chartreuse and Benedictine (Lawless 1992). Cuong (1994) found cajuput *(Melaleuca cajuputi)* effective against *Candida albicans.* The cajuput tree grows to a height of 45 feet, and its resilience has made it something of an unwanted visitor in some parts of the Far East, where it appears to resist burning and cutting. The principal constituent of the oil is 1,8-cineole. Traditionally, cajuput has been used in Vietnamese medicine to treat skin diseases, lice, and fleas (Guenther 1952).

Research from India shows that many Indian essential oils have antifungal properties (Satinder & Sinha 1991). Although not in common use, these essential oils can be specially ordered from some of the leading essential-oil distributors. Some of the Indian essential oils mentioned by Guenther (1952) are as follows:

Long pepper *(Piper longum)* is a climbing shrub with heart-shaped leaves and berries that fuse together to form spike-like cylindrical cones. The essential oil is pale green with an odor somewhere between that of black pepper and ginger. It is effective against *Candida albicans.*

Holy basil *(Ocimum sanctum)* has a strong odor of cloves and contains 71% eugenol, which has antifungal properties.

Ajowan *(Trachyspermum ammi),* which resembles the parsley plant although it has a totally different smell, is used in India to treat intestinal problems. The essential oil has a high thymol content and is used in Indian medicine to treat cholera as well as fungal infections

Deans and Svoboda (1990) found sweet marjoram effective against *Aspergillus niger* and, to a lesser extent, against *A. flavus, A. ochraceus, A. parasiticus,* and *Trichoderma viride. Candida albicans* was also inhibited by 21 different *Eucalyptus* species in a study by Faouzia et al (1993).

Lippia alba, which grows widely in Central and South America, has been shown to have strong antifungal activity against *Trichophyton mentagrophytes* var. *interdigitale* and *Candida albicans.* Several chemotypes of the plant exist, so the essential oil from Aruba was thought to be most suitable because it contains 64% citral (Fun & Svendsen 1990). Lemon verbena *(Lippia citriodora)* contains 30% to 35% citral.

Tea tree has been shown to be extremely effective in the treatment of *C. albicans* (Belaiche 1985a) in deep nail infections. These infections, which are usually notoriously difficult to treat, responded well to tea tree. In all eight patients treated, mycosic degeneration stopped. In two of the cases, the infected nail fell off but the regrowth was healthy. In the other six cases the nail changed color. This effect disappeared as the regrowth progressed. Belaiche noted that this has not been observed with any other antifungal agents. Another important facet of the study was that the treatment was pain free, and the skin appeared to be very tolerant of this method.

Tea tree mouthwashes were effective against oral thrush in a young man who had a bone-marrow transplant. He had a patch of white and green with some yellow on his tongue and had been treated for several months with Nystatin with no success. However, after just 4 days of using a mouthwash with 2% tee tree, his tongue was clear (Ogden 2001).

Clove *(Eugenia caryophyllata)* was shown to have fungicidal action at 0.4% dilution against *C. albicans* in a study published by Briozzo et al (1989). Dube et al (1989) found 22 species of fungi, including *Aspergillus,* were inhibited by the essential oil of basil *(Ocimum basilicum).* Larrondo et al (1991) found lemon balm to be 100% effective against *C. albicans.* Lemon balm contains 30% citral and 39% citronella (Wagner 1984). Celery *(Apium graveolens)* and cumin used together were effective in inhibiting the growth of 29 fungi tested, including *A. flavus* and *A. parasiticus.* Nenoff et al (1996) reported on the antifungal activity of a component of tea tree, γ terpinene. Jedlickova et al (1992) found terpinene-4-ol enhanced antibiotic (ticarcillin) effects against *P. aeruginosa.* Terpinene-4-ol is also an effective antifungal agent. The functional groups of alcohol and terpene are safe to use on the mucous membrane.

These are just a few examples of the hundreds of research studies (most of them conducted *in vitro*) carried out over the last few years indicating the antifungal properties of essential oils. Many of these essential oils are currently being used only for stress management, not for their antifungal properties, because their antifungal properties are not appreciated.

Plant oils are also being investigated for agricultural use. The *New York Times* reported in 1999 that benzaldehyde, the compound that gives peaches their aroma, also kills *Fusarium oxysporum, Rhizoctania solani, Pythium aphanidermatum,* and *Sclerotinia minor,*which are all common fungi found in soil. Benzaldehyde could be a potential replacement for methyl bromide, a widely used pesticide that is toxic to people and also damages the planet's protective ozone layer (Cushman 1999).

Parasites

A mainly temperate country such as the United States does not have as much of a problem with parasites as do countries farther south, where bilharzia and malaria can be endemic. However, with international travel, West Nile virus has arrived in the United States and epidemiologists theorize it is only a question of time before malaria and yellow fever follow. Bilharzia may not be common in the United States but scabies, *Trichomonas vaginalis,* lice, ticks, and fleas are common parasites, and infestations by hookworm and roundworm can be found.

SYNTHETIC ANTIPARASITES

The antiparasitic drug market is worth $3 billion worldwide. The first modern anthelmintic (after mercury and arsenic), Thiabendazole, was developed in 1960. Since then pentamidine (Diamidine) and nitroheterocyclic antiprotozoal drugs such as metronidazole have been developed. The major problem with treating parasites with drugs is that the patient may become infected again almost immediately. Many parasites, including malaria-carrying mosquitoes, are becoming drug resistant, particularly in Africa and Asia where there are no effective drugs left. The World Health Organization suggests that mefloquine should only be used for treating the most difficult, drug-resistant cases of malaria. Currently, there are no effective drugs for *Cryptosporidia,* which infects the lining of the gut and causes diarrhea, or *Pneumocystis,* which infects the lungs.

ANTIPARASITIC PROPERTIES OF ESSENTIAL OILS

Malaria

There are approximately 300 to 500 million cases of malaria a year, resulting in 1.75 to 2.5 million deaths (Kayser et al 2002). The reemergence of malaria as a major health problem, particularly in Africa, is due to the resistance of the plasmodium-bearing mosquito to quinine, chloroquine, pyrimethamine, cycloguanil, and mefloquine.

Essential oils from plants such as lemon grass, Palma rosa, and citronella *(Cymbopogon nardus)* have a long history of repelling mosquitoes (Ansari & Razdan 1995) and are as effective as the chemical insect repellent N,N-diethyl-meta-toluamide (DEET) (Rutledge et al 1983). Neem *(Azadirachta indica)* and tumeric are also effective (Ansari & Razdan 1995). Watanabe et al (1993) found *Eucalyptus camaldulensis* effective, Chokechaijaroenporn et al (1994) found basil effective, and Mwaiko (1992) found lemon and orange peel oils effective. Studies my students and I carried out have confirmed the ability of basil, palma rosa, and eucalyptus essential oils to deter mosquitos in human subjects.

Massoud and Labib (2000) studied the effect of extract of myrrh *(Commiphora molmol)* against mosquito larvae. Microscopic examination showed great pathologic effect on mosquitos' fat, muscle, gut, and nervous tissue. Currently, clinical trials are being completed on *Artemisia annua* (Juteau et al 2002). *In vitro* trials using isolated, biologically active substances (artemisinin and quinghaosu) obtained from this species of *Artemisia,* have shown it to have pronounced antimalarial properties (Klayman et al 1985; Cubukcu et al 1990; Liu et al 1992; Chalchat et al 1994). Artemisinin and quinghaosu are not found in the essential oil but may be the precursors, similar to matricin and chamazulene.

Scabies

Scabies *(Sarcoptes scabii)* produces a papular, intensely itchy rash with burrows in the finger clefts (Hope et al 1993). Larvae, nymphal instars, and adult mites were all were killed within 3 hours after applying 5% tea tree in vitro (Walton et al 2000).

Bilharziasis

Bilharziasis is endemic in 76 countries and affects approximately 200 million people worldwide (Marston & Hostettmann 1991). It is spread by larvae, which penetrate the host skin and are carried by the blood to the liver. In the liver they mature, mate, and relocate to the veins around the small intestine where they lay eggs. Conventional medication is Praziquantel, which kills the worms *in situ.* Unfortunately the dead worms may still be carried back to the liver and cause intense inflammation. By interrupting the infectious process at the level of the intermediate host, this is avoided. Lahlou and Berrada (2001) tested 28 essential oils from Moroccan aromatic plants against the molluscan intermediate host of the urinary parasite *Bulinus truncatus,* which causes bilharziasis. Of the essential oils tested, 75% had molluscicidal acitvity. The most effective were *Citrus aurantium* L. var. *valencia* and *Origanum compactum.* These were effective within 24 hours and at low concentrations (0.21 to 0.38 parts per million). Fringed rue *(Ruta chalepensis),* wormseed *(Chenopodium ambrosioides),* and Roman chamomile were also effective.

Other Parasites

Trichomonas vaginalis is a flagellate parasite that causes vaginitis, and there are other amoebas that cause dysentery-like symptoms. Perhaps more common in the West are infestations by worms (both roundworms and tapeworms), lice, ticks, and fleas. Although several aromatherapy books suggest that various essential oils have anthelmintic properties (which would make them suitable for removing intestinal worms), very little research data are available. To treat the gastrointestinal tract, essential oils need to be taken orally. Parasites that live on or just under the skin can be effectively treated with topically applied essential oils. Several of my students in Florida have used essential oils topically to kill sea-lice and remove the itching and erythema that accompany infestations of this kind. The essential oil they used was true lavender, either undiluted or at 5% dilution. The effect was "almost instant."

Lemon gum has been found to be antiparasitic both for amoeba and for worms (Gilbert & Mors 1972; De Blasi & Debrot 1990). Eucalyptus has also been found effective against certain amoeba.

American wormseed *(Chenopodium ambrosioides* L. var. *anthelminticum)* has a long history of use by North American Indians, who used it to dispel worms and parasites from the intestine. (They take the herb orally.) Sometimes called Jerusalem oak, the seeds from this plant produce an essential oil that has been used for hundreds of years that appears to be safe enough for children (Erichsen-Brown 1979). Grieve (1931) found this variety of *Chenopodium* an effective remedy for hookworm and roundworm, and it was listed in the official *American Pharmacopoeia.* However, there is often confusion between the herbs *Chenopodium ambrosioides* L. var. *anthelminticum* and *Chenopodium botrys* L., which contains a much higher percentage of ascaridole and can cause fatalities.

Wormseed lavant *(Artemisia cina)* also has a long history of use dating back to Dioscorides. Its anthelmintic action is thought to be caused by santonin, which accumulates in the flower heads. It is an effective agent against roundworms and, to a lesser extent, against threadworms but has no effect on tapeworms. However the side effects include vision disturbances that add a yellow tinge to everything the patient sees. Santonin is not found in the essential oil but may be in the CO_2 extract. There are three wormwoods (common, sea, and Roman), which belong to the genus *Artemisia,* which also includes tarragon, thought to be an anthelmintic itself (Lawless 1992). All three herbs *(Artemisia absinthium, Artemisia maritima,* and *Artemisia pontica)* possess anthelmintic properties.

Indian Pinkroot *(Spigelia marilandica)* is another North American plant that has been used as a vermifuge by the American Indians (Lewis & Elvin-Lewis 1977). However, Duke (1995) suggests that if used, its extract should be followed by a saline aperient because the herb is toxic and has effects similar to those of strychnine. It is used homeopathically for mania and strabismus.

Tea tree and lavender (either *Lavandula latifolia* or *L. angustifolia*) are common essential oils used to treat lice, ticks, and fleas. *L. angustifolia* can also be safely used on children and animals. Grosjean (1992) suggests geranium, sage, or lavender for lice. Marigold *(Tagetes minuta)* was reported to have anthelmintic properties by Lawless (1992). Tisserand (1989) suggests the use of bergamot, chamomile, camphor, eucalyptus, fennel, hyssop, lavender, lemon balm, or peppermint. Valnet (1990) suggests all of these, plus cajuput, caraway, cinnamon, clove, lemon, niaouli, savory, tarragon, and thyme. For the treatment of ticks, Lawless (1992) suggests sweet marjoram, and for lice she suggests cinnamon, eucalyptus (blue gum), geranium, spike lavender, Scotch pine, rosemary, or thyme.

Although some of these essential oils are difficult to obtain and their use may be controversial, essential oils or CO_2 extracts appear to have potential as antiparasitic agents. In the tropics or developing countries where orthodox drugs are expensive and difficult to obtain, essential oils might make economic sense. However, although the information provided here suggests that the essential oils discussed could have antiparasitic effects, there is no guarantee. Clinical trials are needed.

CROSS-INFECTION

No discussion of infection is complete without mentioning cross-infection. Although this might come under the heading of hospital-acquired infections, cross-infection can occur anywhere outside a hospital. It can become rampant in institutions or buildings, especially those that have a closed air-conditioning system. Cross-infection includes bacterial, viral, fungal, or protozoan infections.

Bardeau (1976) investigated which essential oils can purify and deodorize the air. Vaporized essential oils were tested for their capacity to destroy bacteria such as *Proteus*, *Staphylococcus aureus*, and *Streptococcus pyogenes*. Within 3 hours, 90% of microbes were destroyed. The oils found to be most effective were clove, lavender, lemon, marjoram, mint, niaouli, pine, rosemary, and thyme. Kazarinova et al (2001) published an abstract of their research on using essential oils to "clear" a hospital surgical unit of unspecified bacteria. The surgical rooms were routinely irradiated with UV light from 5 PM to 9 AM, after surgery hours. Essential oils of *Organum vulgare* and *Origanum tyttanthum* (two types of oregano) were sprayed inside the rooms at 2 PM, the time at which the maximum number of microbes was observed. The antimicrobial effect of the *Organum vulgare* and *Origanum tyttanthum* diffused in the air lasted 1 to 4 hours. As a result of this study, the Russian Federation is confirming a patent.

Benouda et al (1988) tested six essential oils, including tarragon, *Coridothymus capitatus*, and eucalyptus, against 16 drug-resistant bacteria, with excellent results.

Research is ongoing as more and more pathogens become resistant to conventional drugs. Hammer et al (1999) tested 52 plant oils and extracts against *Enterococcus faecalis*, *Escherichia coli*, *Klebsiella pneumoniae*, *Pseudomonas aeruginosa*, *Salmonella enterica* subsp. *enterica* serotype *typhimurium*, *Serratia marcescens*, and *Staphylococcus aureus* using an agar dilution method. Lemon grass, bay, and oregano inhibited all oganisms at concentrations of less than or equal to 2%. Twenty of the oils were effective against *Candida*. Vetiver was effective against *Staphylococcus aureus* at 0.008%. The authors concluded that essential oils "have a role as pharmaceuticals." Essential oils could be important for maintaining antisepsis in operating theaters and for protecting health-care professionals. They are simple to use, considerably less expensive than conventional drugs, have thousands of years of use, have been tested for toxicologic effect, have far fewer side effects than conventional drugs, and they smell great!

REFERENCES

Abraham E, Chaine E. 1940. An enzyme from bacteria able to destroy penicillin. Nature. 3713, 837-838.

Ackerman, B, Dunk-Richards G 1991. Microbiology: An Introduction for the Health Sciences. Sydney: Harcourt Brace Jovanovich.

Agarwal I, Kharwal H, Methela C. 1980. Chemical study and antimicrobial properties of essential oil of *Cymbopogon citratus*. Bulletin of Medico-Ethnobotanical Research. 1, 401-407.

Amrine J. 1996. Oils might help beekeepers save hives. The New Mexican, E5.

Ansari M, Razdan R. 1995. Relative efficacy of various oils in repelling mosquitoes. Indian Journal of Malariology. 32:104-111.

Armaka M, Papanikolaou E, Sivropoulou A et al. 1999. Antiviral properties of isoborneol, a potent inhibitor of herpes simplex virus. Antiviral Research. 43(2) 79-92.

Balacs T. 1993. Antimicrobial Lamiaceae. In Research Reports, International Journal of Aromatherapy. 5(4) 34.

Bardeau F. 1976. The use of essential oils to purify and deodorise the air. Chirugien-Dentiste de France (Paris). 46(319) 53.

Belaiche P. 1979. Traite de phytotherapie et d'aromatherapie, Tome 1: L'aromatogramme. Paris: Maloine.

Belaiche P. 1985. Treatment of vaginal infections of *Candida albicans* with essential oils of *Melaleuca alternifolia*. Phytotherapy. 15:13-14.

Belaiche P. 1985a. Treatment of skin infections with essential oils *of Melaleuca alternifolia*. Phytotherapy. 15:15-17.

Benencia F, Courreges M. 1999. Antiviral activity of sandalwood oil against herpes simplex viruses 1 and 2. Phytomedicine. 6(2) 119-123.

Benouda A, Hassar M Benjilali B. 1988. In vitro antibacterial properties of essential oils tested against hospital pathogenic bacteria. Fitoterapia. 59(2) 115-119.

Blackwell R, Smith M. 1995. Aromatograms. International Journal of Aromatherapy. 7(1) 22-27.

Blaschke T, Bjornsson T. 1995. Pharmacokinetics and pharmacoepidemiology. Scientific American. 8:1-14.

Briozzo J, Nunez L, Chirife J et al. 1989. Antimicrobial activity of clove oil. Journal of Applied Bacteriology. 66(1) 69-75.

Budavari S (ed.). 1996. Merck Index, 12th ed. Whitehouse Station, NJ: Merck Co. Inc.

Caelli M, Porteous J, Carson C et al. 2001. Tea tree oil as an alternative topical decolonization for methicillin-resistant Staphylococcus aureus. Journal of Hospital Infection. 46(3) 236-237.

Cariel L, Jean D. 1990. Antiviral compositions containing proanthocyanidols.

Carmeli Y, Samore M, Huskins C. 1999. The association between antecedent vancomycin treatment and hospital acquired vancomycin resistant enterococci. Archives of Internal Medicine. 159(20) 2461-2468.

Carr G. 1996. The profit and loss of AIDS. The Economist. 340:85-86.

Carson C, Riley T. 1993. Antimicrobial activity of essential oil of *Melaleuca alternifolia*. Letters in Applied Microbiology. 16:49-55.

Carson C, Cookson B, Farrelly H et al. 1995. Susceptibility of methicillin-resistant *Staphylococcus aureus* to the essential oil of *Melaleuca alternifolia*. Journal of Antimicrobial Chemotherapy. 35(3) 421-424.

Chalchat J, Garry R, Lamy J. 1994. Influence of harvest time and composition of *Artemisia annua*. Journal of Essential Oil Research. 6:261-268.

Chan C, Loudon K. 1998. Activity of tea tree oil on methicillin-resistant *Staphylococus aureus* (MRSA). Journal of Hospital Infection. 39(3) 244-245.

Chin Y, Chang N, Anderson H. 1949. Factors influencing the antibiotic activity of lupulon. Paper presented at the Second National Symposium on Recent Advances in Antibiotic Research, 11-12 April. Washington, DC: National Institutes of Health.

Chokechaijaroenporn O, Bunyapraphatsara N, Kongchuensin S. 1994. Mosquito repellent activities of *Ocimum* volatile oils. Phytomedicine. 1/2:135-139.

Chowdhury A. 1998. Therapeutic potential of the volatile oils of *Nigella sativa* in monkey model with experimental Shigellosis. Physiotherapy Research. 12(5) 361-363.

Cohen R, Kucera L, Herrmann E. 1964. Antiviral activity of *Melissa officinalis.* Proceedings of the Society for Experimental Biology and Medicine. 117:431-434.

Cooke A, Cooke M. 1994. Cawthron Report Number 263: An investigation into the antimicrobial properties of manuka and kanuka oil. Nelson, New Zealand: Cawthron.

Cordonnier C. 1993. Les traitment preventifs et curatifs des mycoses en oncohematologie. In Euromedicine 1993. Monpelier-Le Corum. 9emes Rencontres internationals de recherches et de technologies medicales et pharmaceutiques. (Conference.) Paris: 10-13 Nov 1993.

Corpet D. 1987. Antibiotic residues and drug resistance in human intestinal flora. Antimicrobial Agents and Chemotherapy. 31(4) 587-593.

Craig C, Stitzel R. 1994. Modern Pharmacology, 4th ed. Boston: Little, Brown & Co.

Cubukcu B, Bray D, Warhurst D. 1990. In vitro antimalarial activity of crude extracts and compounds from *Artemisia abrotanum.* Phytotherapy Research. 4:203-204.

Cuong N. 1994. Antibacterial properties of Vietnamese cajuput oil. Journal of Essential Oil Research. 6:63-67.

Cushman J. 1999. Peach oil may work as a pesticide. New York Times. Sunday, March 14, 18.

De Blasi V, Debrot S. 1990. Amoebicidal effect of essential oils in vitro. Journal of Clinical Toxicology and Experimental Therapeutics. 10:351-373.

de Castillo M, de Allori C, de Gutierrez R et al. 2000. Bactericidal activity of lemon juice and lemon derivatives against *Vibrio.* Biological & Pharmaceutical Bulletin. 23(10) 1235-1238.

de la Puerta R, Saenz M, Garcia M. 1993. Cytostatic activity against HEp-2 cells and antibacterial activity of essential oils from *Helichrysum picardii.* Phytotherapy Research. 1:378-380.

Deans S, Ritchie G. 1987. Antibacterial properties of plant essential oils. International Journal of Food Microbiology. 5:165-180.

Deans S, Svoboda K. 1988. Antibacterial activity of French tarragon *(Artemisia dracunculus)* essential oil and its constituents during ontogeny. Journal of Horticultural Science. 63(3) 503-508.

Deans S, Svoboda K. 1989. Antibacterial activity of summer savory *(Satureja hortensis)* essential oil and its constituents. Journal Of Horticultural Science. 64(2) 205-210.

Deans S, Svoboda K. 1990. The antimicrobial properties of *marjoram (Origanum majoranum)* oil. Flavour and Fragrance Journal. 5:187-190.

Deans S, Svoboda K et al. 1992. Essential oil profiles of several temperate and tropical aromatic plants: Their antimicrobial and antioxidant activities. Acta Horticulturae. 306:229-233.

Deinenger E. 1995. The spectrum of activity of plant drugs containing essential oils. In Conference Proceedings, Holistic Aromatherapy. San Francisco: Pacific Institute of Aromatherapy, 15-43.

Dolara P, Corte B. Ghelardini C et al. 2000. Local anesthetic, antibacterial and antifungal properties of sesquiterpenes. Planta Medica. 66(4) 356-358.

Dorman H, Deans S. 2000. Antimicrobial agents from plants: Antibacterial activity of plant volatile oils. Journal of Applied Microbiology. 88(2) 308-316.

Dube S, Upadihay P, Tripathi S. 1989. Antifungal, physiochemical and insect-repelling activity of the essential oil of *Ocimum basilicum.* Canadian Journal of Botany. 67(7) 2085-2087.

Duke J. 1985. Handbook of Medicinal Herbs. Boca Raton, FL: CRC Press.

Ena J, Dick R, Wenzel R. 1993. The epidemiology of intravenous vancomycin usage in a university hospital: A ten-year study. Journal of the American Medical Association. 269(5) 598-602.

Erichsen-Brown C. 1979. Medicinal and Other Uses of North American Plants. New York: Dover.

Faouzia H, Fkih-Tetouani S, Tantaoui-Elaraki A. 1993. Antimicrobial activity of twenty-one *Eucalyptus* essential oils. Fitoterapia. 64:1.

Ferdous A, Islam S, Ahsan M. 1992. In vitro antibacterial activity of the volatile oil of *Nigella sativa* seeds against multiple drug-resistant isolates of *Shigella* spp. and isolates of *Vibrio cholerae* and *E. coli.* Phytotherapy Research. 6:137-140.

Fields H. 1997. Pain: Anatomy and physiology. Journal of Alternative & Complementary Medicine. 3(Suppl 1) S41-S46.

Fisher J. 1994. The Plague Makers. New York: Simon & Schuster.

Foster S, Duke J. 1960. A Field Guide to Medicinal Plants (Eastern/Central). New York: Houghton Mifflin Co.

Franchomme P, Penoel D. 1990. L'aromatherapie. Limoges, France: Jollois.

Franchomme P, Penoel D. 1991. L'aromatherapie Exactement. Limoges, France: Jollois.

Fun C, Svendsen A. 1990. The essential oils of *Lippia alba.* Journal of Essential Oil Research. 2(5) 265-267.

Galal E, Adel M, El-Sherif S. 1973. Evaluation of certain volatile oils for their antifungal properties. Journal of Drug Research. 5(2) 235-245.

Garg S, Dengre S. 1988. Antifungal activity of some essential oils. Pharmacie. 43(2) 141-142.

Gascoigne S. 1993. Manual of Conventional Medicine for Alternative Practitioners, Vol. 1. Richmond, VA: Jigme Press.

Gattefosse R. 1948. French lavender: Production and economics. Perfumery and Essential Oil Record. 39:318-319.

Gilbert B, Mors W. 1972. Anthelmintic activity of essential oils and their constituents. Anais da Academia Brasileira de Ciencias. 44:423-428.

Goldway G, Teff D, Schmidt R et al. 1995. Multidrug resistance in *Candida albicans:* Disruption of the BEN gene. Antimicrobial Agents and Chemotherapy. 39(2) 422-426.

Grieve M. 1931. A Modern Herbal. Harmondsworth, UK: Penguin Books.

Grosjean N. 1992. Aromatherapy from Provence. Saffron Walden, UK: CW Daniels.

Guenther E. 1952. The Essential Oils. Malabar, FL: Krieger.

Hammer K, Carson C, Riley T. 1999. Antimicrobial activity of essential oils and other plant extracts. Journal of Applied Microbiology. 86(6) 985-990.

Harris B, Harris R. 1995. Essential oils as antifungal agents. Aromatherapy Quarterly. 44:25-27.

Hawkes N. 2001. Oxygen cuts infections by half. The Times. Wednesday June 27, 5.

Hmamouchi M, Tantaoui-Elaraki A, Es-Safi N et al. 1990. Illustrations of antibacterial and antifungal properties of *Eucalyptus* essential oils. Plantes Medicinales et Phytotherapie. 24(4) 278-279.

Hope R, Longmore J, Hodgetts T et al. 1993. Oxford Handbook of Clinical Medicine, 3rd ed. Oxford, UK: Oxford University Press, 217.

Inouye S, Watanabe M, Nishiuyama Y et al. 1998. Antisporulating and respiration-inhibitory effect on filamentous fungi. Mycoses. 41(9-10) 403-410.

Inoye S, Tsuruoka T, Watanabe M et al. 2000. Inhibitory effect of essential oils on apical growth of *Aspergillus fumigatus* by vapor contact. Mycoses. 43(1-2) 17-23.

Jain S, Purohit M. 1992. Pharmacological evaluation of *Cuminum cyminum*. Fitoterapia. 6314:291-294.

Jedlickova Z, Mottl O, Sery V. 1992. Antibacterial properties of the Vietnamese Cajeput oil and Ocomum oil in combination with antibacterial agents. Journal of Hygiene, Epidemiology, Microbiology and Immunology. 36(3) 303-309.

Jensen A, Wachmann C, Poulsen K et al. 1999. Risk factors for hospital acquired *Staphylococcus aureus* bacteremia. Archives of Internal Medicine. 159(13) 1437-1444.

Jukes T. 1973. Public health significance of feeding low levels of antibiotics to animals. Advances in Applied Microbiology. 16:1-29.

Juteau F, Masotti V, Bessieve V. Antibacterial and antioxidant activiy of Artemesia annua essential oil. 2002. Fitoterapia. 73 (6) 532-535.

Kayser O, Kiderlen A, Croft S. 2002. Natural products as potential antiparasitic drugs. Freie Universitat Berlin. Berlin, Germany.

Kazarinova N, Tkachenko K, Shurgaja A. 2001. Essential oils of *Origanum vulgare* and *Origanum tyttanthum* Gontsch as the remedy of struggle against intrahospital infections. Botanical Institute, Russian Academy of Sciences. St. Petersburg, Russia.

Kedzia B. 1991. Antimicrobial activity of oils of *chamomile* and its components. Herba Polonica. 37(1) 29-38.

Klayman D. 1985. Qunghaosu (artemisin): An antimalarial drug from China. Science. 228(4703) 1049-1055.

Koga T, Hirota N, Takumi K. 1999. Bactericidal activities of essential oils of basil and sage against a range of bacteria and the effect of these essential oils on *Vibrio parahaemolyticus*. Microbiological Research. 154(93) 267-273.

Kole C. 1997. Antibacterial and antifungal activity of aromatic constituents of essential oils. Microbios (Cambridge). 89:39-46.

Kucera L, Herrmann E. 1967. Antiviral substances in plants of the mint family (Labiatae). 1. Tannin of *Melissa officinalis*. Proceedings of the Society for Experimental Biology and Medicine. 124:865, 874.

Kufferath F, Mundualgo G. 1954. The activity of some preparations containing essential oils in TB. Fitoterapia. 25:483-485.

Kwon-Chung K, Bennett J. 1992. Medical Mycology. Philadelphia: Lea & Febiger, 280-336.

Kyoko H, Kamiya M, Hayashi T. 1994. Viricidal effects of the steam distillate from *Houttynia cordata* and its components on HSV-1, influenza virus and HIV. Planta Medica. 61(3) 237-241.

Lahlou M, Berrada R. 2001. Potential of essential oils in schistosomiasis control in Morocco. International Journal of Aromatherapy. 11(2) 87-96.

Larrondo J, Calvo M. 1991. Effects of essential oils on *Candida albicans:* A scanning electron microscope study. Biomedical Letters. 46(184) 269-272.

Larrondo J, Agut M, Calvo-Torres M. 1995. Antimicrobial activity of essences from labiates. Microbios. 82:171-172.

Larrondo J, Calvo M. 1991. Effect of essential oils on *Candida albicans:* A scanning electron microscope study. Biomedical Letters. 46(184) 269-272.

Lawless J. 1992. Encyclopedia of Essential Oils. Shaftesbury, UK: Element Books.

Leclercq R, Derlot E, Duval J et al. 1988. Plasmid-mediated resistance to vancomycin and teicoplanin in *Enterococcus faecium.* New England Journal of Medicine. 319(3) 157-161.

Lewis W, Elvin-Lewis M. 1977. Medical Botany. New York: Wiley Interscience.

MacSween R, Whaley K (eds.). 1992. Muir's Textbook of Pathology, 13th ed. London: Edward Arnold.

Liu K, Yang S, Roberts M. 1992. Antimalarial activity of *Artemisia annua* flavonoids from whole plants and cell cultures. Plant Cell Reports. 11(12) 637-640.

Lovell C. 1993. Plants and the Skin. Oxford, UK: Blackwell Scientific Publications.

Mann C, Cox S, Markham J. 2000. The outer membrane of *Pseudomonas aeruginosa* NCTC 6740 contributes to its tolerance to the essential oil of *Melaleuca alternifolia.* Letters in Applied Microbiology. 30(4) 294-297.

Mann C, Markham J. 1998. A new method for determining the minimum inhibitory concentration of essential oils. Journal of Applied Microbiology. 84(4) 538-544.

Mansfield P. 1996. Animal experiments are an obstacle to health. Holistic Health. 50:4-7.

Marston A, Hostettmann K. 1991. Assay for molluscicidal, cercaricidal, schistosomicidal and piscicidal activities. Methods in Plant Biochemistry. 6:153-178.

Maruzella J, Percival H. 1958. Antimicrobial activity of perfume oils. Journal of the American Pharmaceutical Association. XLVII, 471-476.

Maruzella J, Sicurella N. 1960. Antibacterial activity of essential oil vapors. Journal of the American Pharmaceutical Association (Scientific Edition). 49(11) 693-695.

Massoud A, Labib I. 2000. Larvicidal activity of *Commiphora momol* against *Culex pipiens* and *Aedes caspius* larvae. Journal of the Egyptian Society of Parasitology. 30(1) 101-115.

Mathias C. 1980. Contact urticaria from cinnamic aldehyde. Archives of Dermatology. 116(1) 74-76.

May G, Willuhn G. 1979. Antiviral activity of aqueous extracts from medicinal plants in tissue cultures. Arzneimittel-Forschung Drug Research. 28(1) 1-7.

Mehrotra S, Rawat A. 1993. Antimicrobial activity of the essential oils of some Indian *Artemisia* species. Fitoterapia. 14:65-68.

Mendes N, Araujo N, De Souza C et al. 1990. Molluscicidal and carcaricidal activity of different species of *Eucalyptus.* Revista Societe Brasilia Medicinale Tropicale. 23(4) 197-199.

Muanza D, Euler K, Williams L et al. 1995. Screening for antitumor and anti-HIV activities of nine medicinal plants from Zaire. International Journal of Pharmacology. 33(2) 98-105.

Mwaiko G. 1992. Citrus peel oil extracts of mosquito larvae. Insecticides. 69(4) 223-226.

Myers H. 1927. An unappreciated fungicidal action of certain volatile oils. Journal of the American Medical Association. 1834-1836.

Natural Medicines Comprehensive Database 2002, 4th ed. Stockton, CA: Therapeutic Research Faculty.

Nelson R. 1997. In vitro activities of five plant essential oils against methicillin-resistant *Staphylococcus aureus* and vancomycin-resistant *Entericoccus faecium*. Journal of Antimicrobial Chemotherapy. 40(2) 305-306.

Nenoff P, Haustein U, Brndt W. 1996. Anifungal activity of *Melaleuca alternifolia* (teatree oil) aginst pathogenic fungi in vitro. Skin Pharmacology and Applied Skin Physiology. 9:388-394.

Newsham G. 2002. Personal communication.

Onawunmi G. 1989. Evaluation of the antifungal activity of lemongrass oil. International Journal of Crude Drug Research. 27(2) 121-126.

Onawunmi G, Ogunlana E. 1986. A study of the antibacterial activity of essential oil of lemongrass. International Journal of Crude Drug Research. 24(2) 64-68.

Opdyke D. 1976. Inhibition of sensitization reactions induced by certain aldehydes. Food and Cosmetics Toxicology. 14(3) 197-198.

Opdyke D (ed.). 1979. Monographs on Fragrance Raw Materials. Oxford, UK: Pergamon Press.

Parish P. 1991. Medical Treatments: The Benefits and the Risks. Harmondsworth, UK: Penguin Books.

Pattnaik S, Subramanyam V, Kole C. 1996. Antibacterial and antifungal activity of essential oils in vitro. Microbios. 86(349) 237-246.

Pattnaik S, Subramanyam V, Bapaji M et al. 1997. Antibacterial and antifungal activity of aromatic constituents of essential oils. Microbios. 89(358) 39-46.

Peana A, Moretti M, Juliano C. 1999. Chemical composition and antimicrobial action of the essential oils of *Slavia desoleana* and *Salvia sclarea*. Planta Medica. 65(8) 752-754.

Reichman L, Tanne J. 2001. Timebomb: The Global Epidemic of Multi-Drug-Resistant Tubercuolosis. New York: McGraw-Hill.

Penoel D. 1991/1992. *Eucalyptus smithi* essential oil and its use in aromatic medicine. British Journal of Phytotherapy. 2(4) 154-159.

Price S. 1995. Aromatherapy for Health Professionals. London: Churchill Livingstone.

Richardson K. 2000. www.organicessentialoils.com/articles/kenrichardson/html.

Roberts M. 1986. Biology: A Functional Approach, 4th ed. Walton on Thames, UK: Nelson.

Ross S, El-Keltawi N, Megella, S. 1980. Antimicrobial activity of some Egyptian aromatic plants. Fitoterapia. 51(4) 201-205.

Rubinstein E, Green M, Molan M. 1982. The effects of nosocomial infections on the length and costs of hospital stay. Journal of Antimicrobial Chemotherapy. 9(Suppl.) 93.

Rutledge L, Collister D, Meixsell V et al. 1983. Comparative sensitivity of representative mosquitos to repellents. Journal of Medical Entomology. 20(5) 506.

Satinder K, Sinha G. 1991. In vitro antifungal activity of some essential oils. Journal of Research into Ayurveda and Siddha. 12:200-205.

Savino A, Lollini M, Menghini A. 1994. Antimicrobial activity of the essential oil of *Pneumus boldus* (boldo). Aromatogram and electron microscopy observations. Bollettino di Microbiologia e Indagini Laboratorio. 14(1) 5-12.

Schmidt M. 1995. Antibiotics: The promise and the peril. In Conference Proceedings, Holistic Aromatherapy. San Francisco: Pacific Institute of Aromatherapy, 81-88.

Sears C. 1995. How to sell drugs. New Scientist. Nov 4, 37-40.

Service R. 1994. *E. coli* scare spawns therapy search. Science. 265:475-476.

Shemesh A. 1991. Australian tea-tree: A natural antiseptic and fungicidal agent. Australian Journal of Pharmacy. 12:802-803.

Sherry E, Boeck H, Warnke P. 2001. Percutaneous treatment of chronic MRSA osteomyelitis with a novel plant-derived antiseptic. BioMed Central Surgery. www.biomedcentral.com.

Sleigh J, Pennington T, Lucas S. 1992. Microbial infection. In MacSween R, Whaley K (eds.), Muir's Textbook of Pathology, 13th ed. London: Edward Arnold, 301–302.

Soliman F, El-Kashoury E, Fathy M et al. 1994. Analysis and biological activity of essential oil of *Rosmarinus officinalis*. Flavour and Fragrance Journal. 9:29-33.

Sullivan A. 1995. When plagues end. New York Times Magazine. Nov 10, 52-84.

Takechi M, Tanaka Y. 1981. Purification and characterisation of antiviral substance eugenin from the bud of *Syzygium aromatica aromaticum*. Planta Medica. 42:69-71.

Takechi M, Tanaka Y, Takehara M et al. 1985. Structure and antiherpetic activity among the tannins. Phytochemistry. 24(10) 2245-2250.

Tamm C. 1971. Recent advances in the field of antibiotics. In Wagner H, Wolffe P (eds.), New Natural Products and Plant Drugs with Pharmacological, Biological or Therapeutic Activity. Berlin, Germany: Springer-Verlag, 82-136.

Tisserand R. 1988. Aromatherapy for Everyone. Harmondsworth, UK: Penguin Books.

Tisserand R. 1989. The Art of Aromatherapy. Saffron Walden, UK: CW Daniels.

Tisserand R, Balacs T. 1995. Essential Oil Safety. London: Churchill Livingstone.

Valnet J. 1990. The Practice of Aromatherapy. Saffron Walden, UK: CW Daniels.

Viana G, Vale T, Pinho R et al. 2000. Antinociceptive effect of the essential oil of *Cymbopogon citratus* in mice. Journal of Ethnopharmacology. 70(3) 323-327.

Viollon C, Chaumont J. 1994. Antifungal properties of essential oils and their main components against *Cryptococcus neoforms*. Mycopathologia. 128(3) 151-153.

Wagner H. 1984. Plant Drug Analysis. Berlin, Germany: Springer-Verlag.

Walton S, Myerscough M, Currie B. 2000. Studies in vitro on the relative efficacy of current acaricides for *Sarcoptes scabiei* var. *hominis*. Transactions of the Royal Society of Tropical Medicine and Hygiene. 94(1) 92-96.

Ward K. 1993. Care of the person with an infection. In Hinchcliff S, Norman S (eds.), Nursing Practice and Health Care. London: Edward Arnold, 402-434.

Watanabe K, Shono Y, Kakimizu A et al. 1993. New mosquito repellent from *Eucalyptus camaldulensis*. Journal of Agriculture & Food Chemistry. 41(11) 2164-2166.

Weber N, Andersen D, North J. 1992. In vitro viricidal effects of *Allium sativum*. Planta Medica. 58(5) 417-423.

Wilson J. 2001. Infection Control in Clinical Practice, 2nd ed. London: Bailliere Tindall.

www.sunysccc.edu/academic/mst/microbes/microbes.htm. (Accessed March 16, 2003).

www.cdc.gov/ncidod/dbmd/diseaseinfo/groupastreptococcal_g.htm. (Accessed March 16, 2003).

Zakarya D, Fkih-Tetouani S, Hajji F. 1993. Antimicrobial activity of twenty-one *Eucalyptus* essential oils. Fitoterapia. 64:319-331.

Zarno V. 1994. Candidiasis. International Journal of Aromatherapy. 6(••) 20-23.

IO

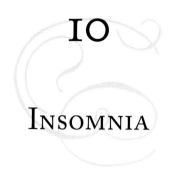

Insomnia

One sees clearly only with the heart, everything essential is invisible to the eyes.

Antoine De Saint-Exupery
The Little Prince

Insomnia

Today's society is fast-moving and achievement-oriented in which thousands of people travel daily, often across time zones. Regularity and sleep patterns are constantly disturbed as new sounds and unfamiliar surroundings compound the sense of timelessness caused by continuous movement. Sleep has become a commodity to be bought and sold.

Patients in hospitals are separated from everything that makes them relaxed and sleepy. They are in a strange bed, with a strange routine, and often have a sense of fear. It is hardly surprising that sleeping pills are almost *de rigueur*. Aromatherapy offers another alternative, especially in the case of patients in the hospital for a long stay who take sleeping tablets regularly.

Sleepless nights can affect us all at some time in our lives. Trauma, worries, and jet lag can all cause insomnia. However, repeated sleepless nights result in a poor attention span and, ultimately, in poor health, both physical and mental.

Sleep is defined by Manley (1993) as an "altered state of consciousness from which a person can be aroused by stimuli of sufficient magnitude." Why sleep is necessary is unclear, but this period of "opting out" is essential for healthy living. Going without sleep produces varying degrees of symptoms, ranging from feeling irritable to psychosis. For a patient in the hospital, sleep deprivation is just one more stressor.

Sleep occurs in two modes: rapid eye movement (REM) sleep, when dreaming occurs, and orthodox sleep. Both types of sleep are important. Sleep is thought to be controlled by a natural chemical called melatonin, which is secreted by the pineal gland. It is possible to buy this compound over the counter as a supplement, although it has recently been banned in the United Kingdom.

Insomnia is usually transitory, and after the trauma causing the insomnia has passed, normal sleep rhythms return. However, chronic insomnia threatens to destroy normal functioning. This kind of sleep problem can occur in two forms: failure to drift off to sleep or waking up after a short period. Both occur in a hospital, where strange noises and smells permeate through dreams or prevent sleep from occurring. A bedtime routine is also very difficult to maintain in the hospital.

SLEEPING TABLETS

Orthodox treatment of insomnia involves two types of drugs, sedatives (anxiolytics) and sedative-hypnotics. The most common sleeping tablet is a benzodiazepine, which is both sedative-hypnotic and anxiolytic, such as diazepam (Valium), lorazepam (Ativan), or nitrazepam (Mogadon). Dependency can occur within weeks.

Benzodiazepines

Benzodiazepines have the basic structure of a benzene ring coupled to a seven-membered, heterocyclic structure containing two nitrogen atoms (diazepine) at positions 1 and 4 (Dailey 1994). This molecule binds to specific macromolecules within the central nervous system (CNS) at receptors closely associated with γ-aminobutyric acid (GABA) transmission. GABA is the main inhibitory neurotransmitter in the brain. Research has indicated that benzodiazepines potentiate GABA transmission.

Benzodiazepines depress the CNS and in low dosages produce a feeling of calm. As the dose is increased, a feeling of drowsiness is followed by hypnosis and muscle relaxation. The interval between feeling drowsy and potential death by overdose is a large one. Because these drugs have a large therapeutic index they are extremely useful for many patients, although their long-term use can be problematic. Benzodiazepines have almost entirely replaced the previous favorite sleeping pill, the barbiturate.

Barbiturates

Barbiturates are used to treat intractable insomnia and are increasingly rarely prescribed. They, too, bind to receptors associated with GABA transmission. However, this class of drug prolongs, rather than intensifies, the GABA effect. Public awareness of the dangers of barbiturate dependence was heightened in the 1970s by novels like *Valley of the Dolls*, by Jacqueline Susann. Barbiturates have significant drug interactions. Several of the drugs they react with are in common use, for example, the contraceptive pill, digoxin, beta-blockers, and anticoagulants. Barbiturates accelerate the metabolism of these drugs, necessitating an increased dosage. In addition, if the patient is on anticoagulant therapy, when barbiturates are discontinued a dangerous reaction resulting in severe hemorrhage can occur (Dailey 1994). This type of reaction can also occur with other drugs because the induction of GABA metabolism has stopped.

ESSENTIAL OILS WITH SEDATIVE EFFECTS

"Lavender Beats Benzodiazepines" was a 1988 headline in the *International Journal of Aromatherapy* (Tisserand 1988). In this article, the use of essential oils as sedatives in a hospital setting was outlined. Of particular note were lavender, marjoram, geranium, mandarin, and cardamom.

Helen Passant, possibly the most holistic nurse after Florence Nightingale, introduced aromatherapy into the Churchill Hospital, in Oxford, England, where she was in charge of a ward for the elderly. Remarkably, Passant reduced her original drug bill by one third by gradually replacing analgesia and night sedation with essential oils. She found her patients seemed to "get off to sleep just as easily, if not better, with oils of lavender or marjoram, either vaporized or applied by massage" (Tisserand 1988). In the same article another hospital was mentioned. The Radcliffe Infirmary, also in Oxford, introduced aromatherapy into Beeson Ward at about the same time. Patients were given the option of aromatherapy instead of night sedation or analgesics. Nearly all of the patients chose aromatherapy (Tisserand 1988).

Traditionally, true lavender *(Lavandula angustifolia)* has been used in aromatherapy to promote sleep and relaxation and to relieve anxiety. In Bulgaria, Atanassova-Shopova et al (1973) found that linalol and terpineol were the active components of lavender and had a depressing effect on the CNS. Oral doses of linalool were found to be hypnotic and anticonvulsant in mice in a study by Elisabetsky et al (1995). Elisabetsky et al (1995a) also established that linalol inhibited glutamate binding in rat cortex in a way similar to phenobarbital. The glutamate binding involved all receptor subtypes investigated. A Japanese study (Yamada et al 1994) concurred that inhaled lavender had anticonvulsant effects in mice.

In France, Guillemain et al (1989) agreed that oral doses of lavender (diluted at 1:60 in olive oil) had marked sedative effects on mice and enhanced barbiturate sleep time. In Germany, Buchbauer et al (1991) in Germany found that true lavender had a sedative effect when inhaled by mice. Interestingly, the more agitated the animal (as a result of the injection of caffeine), the more effective the calming effect of true lavender. Jager et al (1992) established that lavender diluted in peanut oil was absorbed through the skin.

Henry et al (1994) carried out a study on human subjects at Newholme Hospital in Bakewell, England. The effects of nighttime diffusion of lavender in a ward of dementia patients was monitored. The trial ran for 7 weeks and showed that lavender had a statistically significant sedative effect when inhaled. Hudson (1995) also found lavender was effective for elderly patients in a long-term unit. Eight of the nine patients in the study had improved sleep at night and improved alertness during the day. Lavender straw (the byproduct of distillation) was itself found to reduce stress of pigs in transit in a study by Bradsaw et al (1998).

Jager et al (1992a) found that neroli had a sedative effect on mice. In this study, the sedative effects were observed during the first 30 minutes of exposure to the aroma. Citronellal and phenylethyl acetate (components of essential oils) were also found to have sedative properties. Citronellal is found in citronella *(Cymbopogon nardus)*, lemon gum *(Eucalyptus citriodora)*, narrow-leaved peppermint *(Eucalyptus radiata)*, lemon, rose, melissa, lemongrass, basil, and geranium. Phenylethyl acetate is found only in neroli, but phenylethyl alcohol is also found in geranium (bourbon) and rose (Sheppard-Hangar 1995).

Buchbauer et al (1992) found essential oils of passionflower *(Passiflora incarnata)* and lime blossom *(Tilia cordata)* had sedative effects. Lime blossom and its major component, benzyl alcohol, decreased the motility of animals in both normal and induced-agitation states. Interestingly, passionflower and its main components, maltol and 2-phenylethanol, only reduced motility when the animals were in an agitated state. This underscores the feeling amongst herbalists and aromatherapists that essential oils are adaptogens.

Khanna et al (1993) found black cumin *(Nigella sativa)* essential oil had a sedative effect more powerful than the drug chlorpromazine (Largactil) and was also an analgesic. The study suggested black cumin contained an opioid-like component. West and Brockman (1994) reported on how aromatherapy helped dementia patients with disturbed sleep and compulsive daytime activity. Several essential oils were used.

Weihbrecht (1999) investigated the effect of inhaled true lavender on 10 adults (3 men and 7 women) who had a history of chronic insomnia. Subjects took baseline measurements for the first 14 days and recorded difficulty getting to sleep, naps taken during the day, difficulty returning to sleep, and feeling rested in the morning. A visual analog scale of 1 to 10 was used (1 = very difficult, 10 = no difficulty). Subjects were asked not to change what they normally did and to continue their sleep medication. For days 15 to 29 of the study, 2 drops of true lavender were placed on the patients' pillows or on a tissue kept nearby at bedtime. Subjects mailed back a sleep questionnaire, and a telephone interview was completed with each of them following completion of the study. One participant pulled out of the study because she did not like the smell of lavender. Eight participants had improved sleep in 1 of the 4 areas measured, and 8 reported less difficulty in getting to sleep. One person reported that his difficulty was neither improved nor worsened by the use of lavender, but he had the flu during the experimental stage. Of all participants, 8 reported feeling more rested in the morning. The sleep aids normally used by the participants did not change.

King (2001) tested the effect of Roman chamomile *(Chamomelum nobile)* and sweet marjoram *(Origanum majorana)* on insomnia. Ten women between the ages of 36 and 59 with sleep problems took part in the study. One client had an allergy to ragweed so a patch test was completed before the study began to make sure she was not allergic to chamomile. Each subject was given a bottle containing a mixture of Roman chamomile and sweet marjoram in a ratio of 1:2. For the first 7 days, baselines were established. The second week the subjects used the aromatherapy mixture; the third week was a washout week with no aromatherapy; and the fourth week was a repeat of the second week. During week 2 and week 4 (the aromatherapy weeks), 2 drops of essential oils were put on a cotton ball and placed in the pillowcases of the subjects at bedtime. Subjects recorded time to fall asleep, number of times waking, how long it took to fall back to sleep, span of time from bedtime to getting up, and whether they felt rested in the morning. The data were entered on in spreadsheet software program so results could be compared.

Two subjects withdrew from the study because they reacted negatively to the mixture. Neither of them liked the aroma. One subject experienced nausea and headache, and the other had a severe headache. These two subjects were not entered into the analysis. The results indicated a small improvement in almost every category. Five women experienced an improvement in the time it took to go to sleep. One subject took 240 minutes to fall asleep one night because of a death in her family. The outcomes of the study were not changed to accommodate that. Six women showed a reduction in the number of times they woke up during the night. Only three women showed a reduction in the time taken to fall back to sleep. Five women felt more rested after a night's sleep with the aromatherapy mixture.

Most people enjoy the smell of roses. Rose is perhaps the most popular aroma in the world. Despite the fact that essential oil of rose is expensive, the cost may be justified where chronic insomnia is concerned. To date, there have been no clinical studies to show that rose is effective in promoting sleep in humans. However, Nacht and Ting (1921) and Rovesti and Columbo (1973) showed that rose *(Rosa damascena)* essential oil has sedative effects. Certainly my personal experience, as well as that of my students and patients, suggests that rose is a strong contender and certainly an essential oil to try for insomnia.

Finally, while conducting routine toxicity investigations of Tastromine (β-dimethylaminoethyl thymol ether), it was observed that the animals used in the study became sedated (Ashford et al 1993). Further investigation revealed that significant CNS depressant activity appeared when the basic ethers involved were derived from thymol. Isomers of thymol, namely carvacrol and isothymol, were relatively inactive. The structural requirements of morphinelike analgesics were similar to the structure of thymol ether.

REFERENCES

Ashford A, Sharpe C, Stephens F. 1993. Thymol basic ethers and related compounds: central nervous system depressant action. Nature. 4871(197) 969-971.

Atanassova-Shopova S, Roussinov K, Boycheva I. 1973. On certain central neurotropic effects of lavender essential oils. II. Communications: studies on the effects of linalol and of terpineol. Bulletin of the Institute of Physiology. 55:149-156.

Bradsaw R, Marchant J, Meredith M et al. 1998. Effects of lavender straw on stress and travel sickness in pigs. Journal of Alternative and Complementary Medicine. 4(3) 271-275.

Buchbauer G, Jirovetz L, Jager W. 1991. Aromatherapy: Evidence for sedative effects of the essential oil of lavender after inhalation. Zeitschrift fur Naturforschung 46 (11−12) 1067-1072.

Buchbauer G, Jirovetz L, Jager W. 1992. Kurzmitteilungen: Passiflora and lime-blossoms—Motility effects after inhalation of the essential oils and of some of the main constituents in animal experiments. Archiv der Pharmazie (Weinheim). 325(4) 247-248.

Dailey J. 1994. Sedative-hypnotic and anxiolytic drugs. In Craig C, Sitzel R (eds.), Modern Pharmacology, 4th ed. Boston: Little Brown & Co., 369-377.

Elisabetsky E, de Souza G, Dos Santos M et al. 1995. Sedative properties of linalool. Fitoterapia. 66(5) 407-415.

Elisabetsky E, Marschner J, Souza D. 1995a. Effects of linalool on glutamatergic system in the rat cerebral cortex. Neurochem Res. 20(4) 461-465.

Guillemain J, Rousseau A, Delaveau P. 1989. Effects neurodepresseurs de l'huile essentielle de *Lavandula angustifolia*. Annales Pharmaceutiques Francaises. 47(6) 337-343.

Henry J, Rusius C, Davies M et al. 1994. Lavender for night sedation of people with dementia. International Journal of Aromatherapy. 6(2) 28-30.

Hudson R. 1996. The value of lavender for rest and activity in the elderly patient. Complementary Therapies in Medicine. 4(1) 52-57.

Jager W, Buchbauer G, Jirovetz L, et al. 1992. Percutaneous absorption of lavender oil from a massage oil. Journal of the Society of Cosmetic Chemists. 43(1) 49-54.

Jager W, Buchbauer G, Jirovetz L. 1992a. Evidence of the sedative effect of neroli oil, citronella and phenylethyl acetate on mice. Journal of Essential Oil Research. 4(4) 387-394.

Khanna T, Zaidi F, Dandiya P. 1993. CNS and analgesic studies on *Nigella sativa*. Fitoterapia. 64(5) 407-410.

King P. 2001. An insomnia study using *Origanum majorana* and *Chamomelum nobile*. Unpublished dissertation. R J Buckle Associates, Hunter, NY.

Macht D, Ting G. 19211921. Sedative properties of some aromatic drugs and fumes. Journal of Pharmacology and Experimental Therapeutics. 18:361-372.

Manley K. 1993. Care of the acutely ill. In Hinchcliff S, Norman S, Schober J (eds.), Nursing Practice and Health Care, 2nd ed. London: Edward Arnold, 1067-1072.

Rovesti P, Columbo E. 1973. Aromatherapy and aerosols. Soap, Perfumery & Cosmetics. 46:475-477.

Sheppard-Hangar S. 1995. Aromatherapy Practitioner Reference Manual, Vol. II. Tampa, FL: Atlantic School of Aromatherapy.

Tisserand R. 1988. Lavender beats benzodiazepines. International Journal of Aromatherapy. 1(1) 1-2.

Weihbrecht L. 1999. A comparative study on the use of *Lavandula angustifolia* and its effect on insomnia. Unpublished dissertation. R J Buckle Associates, Hunter, NY.

West B, Brockman S. 1994. The calming power of aromatherapy. Journal of Dementia Care. March/April, 20-22.

Yamada K, Mimaki Y, Sashida Y et al. 1994. Anticonvulsant effects of inhaling lavender oil vapor. Biological & Pharmaceutical Bulletin. 17(2) 359-360.

II

Nausea and Vomiting

As aromatic plants bestow
No spicy fragrance while they grow;
But crushed or trodden to the ground,
Diffuse their balmy sweets around.

Oliver Goldsmith
The Captivity, Act 1.

Nausea and vomiting are symptoms that should be addressed separately, because nausea does not always lead to actual vomiting. However, the causes of nausea are similar to those of vomiting. Aromatherapy has recently been recommended by an internet-based medical consultancy, www.mdconsult.com, as being useful in nausea related to pregnancy. Vomiting is activated by the vomiting center in the brain, which triggers nerves supplying the stomach and chest muscles. Vomiting can have numerous causes.

Gastrointestinal Causes

Gastrointestinal causes of vomiting include the following:
Stomach or intestinal irritation, gastroenteritis
Appendicitis
Obstruction
Hypertrophic pyloric stenosis

Central Nervous System Causes

Central nervous system (CNS) causes of vomiting include the following:
Loss of sense of balance resulting from middle or inner ear trauma, labyrinthitis
Sensory responses in the brain activated by smell, sight, or emotion

Raised pressure in the brain (caused by tumors, hemorrhage, meningitis)
Head injury
Migraine
Psychiatric disorder
Chemoreceptor trigger areas that respond to either chemicals produced by the
body (e.g., kidney and pancreas) or to motion sickness

Metabolic Causes

Metabolic causes of vomiting include the following:
Pregnancy
Uremia
Alcohol
Chemoreceptor trigger areas responding to drugs absorbed by the body (Hope et
al 1993)

CONVENTIONAL APPROACHES TO TREATING VOMITING

There are seven basic categories of antiemetic agents used in conventional medicine: antihistamines, anticholinergics, corticosteroids, cannabinoids, benzodiazepines, dopamine antagonists, and serotonin antagonists.

Antihistamines (dramamine, diphenhydramine, hydroxyzine) affect the organ of balance as well as the vomiting center of the brain. These drugs also have an effect on the chemoreceptor trigger zone (CTZ), and they block the histamine and dopamine receptors. In addition, they inhibit acetylcholine. Antihistamines work by reducing the sensitivity of the vomiting center to input from the inner ear, although they do not directly affect the inner ear.

Because the vomiting center of the brain is stimulated by the neurotransmitter acetylcholine, one of the most direct ways of inhibiting vomiting is to use anticholinergic drugs (atropine, scopolamine, hyoscyamine). Transdermal scopolamine provides up to 72 hours of antiemetic treatment. However, long-term use of anticholinergic drugs can cause side effects such as poor digestion, dry mouth, blurred vision, and constipation. Corticosteroids (dexamethasone, prednisone) can help to reduce nausea associated with chemotherapy but can cause side effects such as mania, insomnia, and gastric irritation. Cannabinoids (dronabinol) have been used to treat nausea and vomiting in patients with end-stage illness, but they have limited effectiveness resulting from irregular absorption rates. Cannabinoids often take several days to weeks to reach therapeutic blood levels and have the side effect of uncomfortable dizziness or euphoria. Benzodiazepines such as lorazepam have been used to treat nausea. These drugs often cause dry mouth and drowsiness.

The neurochemical that stimulates the CTZ is dopamine. Dopamine agonists (e.g., prochlorperazine, chlorpromazine, haloperidol) work by blocking dopamine-mediated transmission, thereby relieving nausea. Dopamine agonists have common side effects of extrapyramidal symptoms, which limit their use.

The new serotonin agonists (e.g., ondansetron) are safe and effective in controlling nausea and are frequently considered first-line antiemetic agents. However, these drugs are often prohibitively expensive.

AROMATHERAPY APPROACHES

Although conventional approaches are often very effective in managing nausea and vomiting, some patients are intolerant of the drugs' side effects or are unable to afford them. In some cases, aromatherapy can be used both as adjunctive therapy and alternative therapy for the control of nausea. Alexander (2001) suggests that dopamine and serotonin can "cross talk," and believes that essential oils affect nausea in this manner.

Specific Essential Oils with Antiemetic Properties

Cardamom

Cardamom *(Elettaria cardamomum)* is listed in the *Indian Materia Medica* as checking vomiting and nausea (Nadkarni 1992); it is one of the oldest essential oils known (Arctander 1994). Tisserand (1989) also suggests it can relieve nausea. Cardamom contains 50% α-terpinyl acetate and 1,8-cineole, with small amounts of borneol, α-terpineol, and limonene. Borneol was shown to be an effective antagonist of acetylcholine in a study by Cabo et al (1986), and perhaps this compound imbues cardamom with its antiemetic property.

Peppermint

Peppermint *(Mentha piperita)* has been a classic choice for the treatment of nausea for hundreds of years. However, too much peppermint can cause nausea, so only a few drops are needed. Used primarily to treat nausea, rather than actual vomiting, peppermint has carminative effects both *in vitro* and *in vivo*. Peppermint also has recognized antispasmodic effects; in a study of endoscopy spasm, peppermint was found to relieve colonic spasm within 30 seconds (Leicester & Hunt 1982).

In another study, patients were given peppermint following colostomies. Among these patients, 18 of 20 individuals displayed reduced postoperative colic and nausea (McKensie & Gallacher 1989). Valnet (1980) states that peppermint is useful for the treatment of nervous vomiting. Franchomme (1980) also states that peppermint is an antiemetic. Peppermint floral water is one of the active ingredients of babies' gripe water, a traditional remedy recommended by hospitals in the United Kingdom.

The effect of peppermint was audited in a study with 10 patients at the oncology center of St. Luke's Hospital in New Bedford, Massachusetts, and found to be effective in reducing the nausea of patients undergoing chemotherapy when used instead of the drugs Zofran and Compazine (Figuenick 1998). Zofran is very expensive. Peppermint proved so effective that those in the control group demanded the peppermint, and the control part of the study collapsed! Of patients in this study, 84% stated that essential oil of peppermint relieved their nausea, and 71% found it enhanced their standard antiemetic medication. One patient found it enhanced the ability to eat. Aromatherapy is now routinely offered in many chemotherapy units in the United States and United Kingdom.

Tate (1997) carried out a controlled study of postoperative nausea on 18 patients who underwent major gynecologic surgery. Group 1 received no treatment, group 2 received peppermint essence, and group 3 received peppermint essential oil. Participants in group 3 were asked to inhale directly from the bottle when they were nauseated. Measurement was made on a five-point scale ranging from 0 (no nausea) to 4 (about to vomit). The amount of antiemetic drugs (metoclopramide [Maxolon], prochlorperazine [Stemetil], and ondansetron [Zofran]) used was measured. Participants in the experimental group needed 50% fewer antiemetics. The Kruskal-Wallis test was used to establish significance, $P = 0.0487$. The cost per treatment was approximately 75 cents (48 pence).

Spearmint is thought to also have an antiemetic effect and, according to Lawrence (2001), may prove effective for longer periods than peppermint. Several US hospitals are conducting clinical trials on peppermint and spearmint as this text is being written.

Ginger

Ginger *(Zingiber officinale)* was introduced in Europe during the Middle Ages. The essential oil, which does not smell anything like the dried root or candied ginger, contains zingiberene. In China, ginger root is classically given to new mothers following the birth of their children. Although it is often used topically in the treatment of chronic pain, inhaled essential oil of ginger is a very effective remedy for nausea and is particularly suitable for pregnancy. Vutyavanich et al (1997) studied 70 expectant mothers over a period of 5 months in a double-masked, placebo-controlled trial. They found baseline nausea and vomiting decreased significantly in the group using ginger. Ginger had no adverse effects on the mothers' pregnancy outcomes. However, ginger may not be as effective for nausea associated with CNS disturbances. Visalyaputra et al (1998) found that 2 gr ginger powder taken orally was ineffective at reducing the incidence of postoperative nausea and vomiting the day after gynecologic laparoscopy. This could be because many people find it difficult to take anything orally when nauseated.

Lavender

Everson (2000) carried out a small project with lavandin *(Lavandula intermedia* CT Super) to treat postoperative nausea. She became intrigued with the antiemetic properties of lavender while undergoing chemotherapy herself. During the 26 weeks Everson received chemotherapy, she never vomited and only used six of the prescribed antiemetic pills. All of the women in her cancer support group were nauseated, and all used most of their antiemetic pills. Ten patients were included in the exploratory postoperative study, which was not randomized or controlled. Consent was given by the hospital and each patient signed an informed consent. After inhaling lavender, only two patients required an antiemetic postoperatively, a much lower than usual incidence. Although no conclusions can be reached from this study, this chemotype of lavandin might be worth pursuing for treatment of postoperative nausea alongside spearmint, peppermint, cardamom, and ginger.

Clove *(Eugenia caryophyllata)* is listed in *Potter's New Cyclopaedia of Botanical Drugs and Preparations* as an antiemetic (Wren 1988). Pharmacognosy books suggest that cardamom, which has an antispasmodic action on the gastrointestinal tract, and peppermint are both suitable as carminatives (Evans 1994). Fennel *(Foeniculum vulgare)* and aniseed *(Anethum graveolens)* are also mentioned, but more as carminatives than as antinausea essential oils.

Other Anticholinergic Essential Oils

In a study investigating the activity of major components of various essential oils of aromatic plants from Granada, borneol and myrcene were found to be active against acetylcholine. In this instance, borneol and myrcene were from essential oils of thyme *(Thymus granatensis)* and Spanish sage *(Salvia lavendulaefolia).* The experiment was carried out with isolated duodenum. However, if borneol and myrcene do display anticholinergic activity, it would be logical to try other essential oils that contain these compounds to provide relief from nausea and to inhibit vomiting. Myrcene and borneol are found in many essential oils. Gas chromatography linked to mass spectrometry indicates how much myrcene or borneol is present in an essential oil.

Importance of Individual Preference in Choice of Essential Oil

Several of my students have completed case studies on nausea using ginger and peppermint and found that patients tended to prefer one essential oil over another. The essential oil patients preferred was more effective against their nausea than one they did not like. This highlights the importance of learned memory and of involving patients in choosing their oils. The method of choice is usually inhalation. However, a gentle abdominal rub can be very beneficial to a child or anxious patient who is sick with worry, rather than nauseated for physical reasons.

REFERENCES

Alexander M. 2001. How Aromatherapy Works, Vol 1. Odessa, FL: Whole Spectrum Books.

Arctander S. 1994. Perfume and Flavor Materials of Natural Origin. Carol Stream, IL: Allured Publishing.

Cabo J, Crespo M, Jimenez J et al. 1986. The spasmolytic activity of various aromatic plants from the province of Granada. The activity of the major components of their essential oils. Plantes Medicinales et Phytotherapie. 20(3) 213-218.

Evans W. 1994. Trease & Evan's Pharmacognosy, 13th ed. London: Bailliere Tindall.

Everson C. 2000. *Lavandula intermedia* (DT Super) as a post-operative anti-emetic. Unpublished dissertation. R J Buckle Associates, Hunter, NY.

Figuenick R. 1998. Essential oil of peppermint: A 3-part audit on nausea. Unpublished dissertation. R J Buckle Associates, Hunter, NY.

Franchomme P, Penoel D. 1980. L'aromatherapie Exactement. Jollois, Limoge, France.

Hope R, Longmore J, Hodgetts T et al. 1993. Oxford Handbook of Clinical Medicine, 3rd ed. Oxford, UK: Oxford University Press.

Leicester R, Hunt R. 1982. Peppermint oil to reduce colonic spasm during endoscopy. Lancet. 2(8305) 989-990.

Lawrence B•. 2001. Personal communication in September 2001.

McKenzie J, Gallacher M. 1989. A sweet-smelling success: Use of peppermint oil in helping patients accept their colostomies. Nursing Times. 85(27) 48-49.

Nadkarni K. 1992. Indian Materia Medica, Vol. 1. Prakashan, India: Bombay Popular.

Tate S. 1997. Peppermint oil: A treatment for postoperative nausea. Journal of Advanced Nursing. 26(3) 543-549.

Tisserand R. 1989. The Art of Aromatherapy. Saffron Walden, UK: CW Daniels.

Valnet J. 1990. The Practice of Aromatherapy. Saffron Walden, UK: CW Daniels.

Visalyaputra S, Petcchpaisit N, Somcharoen K et al. 1998. The efficacy of ginger root in the prevention of postoperative nausea and vomiting after outpatient gynaecological laparoscopy. Anaesthesia. 53(5) 506-510.

Vutyavanich T, Kraisarin T, Ruangsri R. 1997. Ginger for nausea and vomiting in pregnancy: randomized, double-masked, placebo controlled trial. Obstetrics and Gynecology. 97(4) 577-582.

Wren R. 1988. Potter's New Cyclopaedia of Botanical Drugs and Preparations. London: Churchill Livingstone.

12

PAIN AND INFLAMMATION

How did the rose ever open its heart and give to this world all its beauty?
It felt the encouragement of light against its being,
otherwise we all remain too frightened.

Hafiz
The Gift

PAIN

Pain is an unpleasant sensation localized to part of the body (Fields 1997). Although there are physical dimensions that reflect a commonality of pain in humans, the experience of pain is unique to the individual. People who live with pain on a daily basis have what is to them a clear way of describing what they feel. If the pain changes, they know it. However, describing pain to someone who does not experience it is very subjective and can be problematic. Descriptions of pain vary greatly. Apart from the site of the pain (for example, abdominal), one of the most important aspects to consider is the onset of pain. The onset clarifies which kind of pain is involved: acute or chronic.

Chronic pain costs the United States approximately $70 billion per year and affects approximately 80 million Americans (Berman & Swyers 1997). Pain is one of the most commonly addressed symptoms in a clinical setting.

Physiology of Pain

Pain is a complex neurophysiological phenomenon (Alavi et al 1997) and can be described as somatic, neuropathic, or visceral. Somatic pain is well localized, persistent, and is often described as sharp or stabbing. Neuropathic pain is usually described as burning, numbing, or shooting and originates from compression or stimulation of a nerve. Visceral pain tends to be poorly localized, dull, and aching and involves an A-C fiber ratio of 1:10 in visceral afferents. In normal adults the ability to detect pain is completely removed when A and C axons are blocked (Fields 1997). When pain triggers the nociceptors (pain receptors), it is translated or transduced into electrical activity. The electrical impulse is then transmitted to the spinal cord via the dorsal root and relayed to the thalamus via the afferent pathways.

Pain is often divided into acute and chronic. Acute pain is short lasting and has a well-defined pattern of onset. Chronic pain persists beyond the expected period of healing (Casey 2002) and is associated with a degenerative or chronic pathological process such as arthritis. However, sometimes the cause of the pain is elusive.

The thalamus is involved in pain perception and interpretation (Alavi et al 1997) and is, of course, part of the limbic system, which analyzes smell; therefore there is an implicit suggestion that smell may affect the perception of pain. Primary afferent nociceptors activate spinal pain-transmission cells through two neurotransmitters: glutamate (an amine) and substance P (a peptide) that are present in C fibers (Fields 1997). Greer (1995) noted substance P immunoreactive processes throughout the laminae of the olfactory bulb. A variety of chemical agents can activate the primary afferent nociceptors. These include serotonin and potassium. If the tissue is damaged or inflamed, the sensitivity of the nociceptors is heightened. The whole process results in a subjective, sensory, and emotional experience of pain.

Visceral pain is usually blocked by opioids (Sofaer & Foord 1993). Actually, the body itself produces enkephalin, an opioid-like peptide that occurs in two forms, Met-enkephalin and Leu-enkephalin.

Etiology of Pain

There are many possible causes of pain: a simple headache can have a dozen predisposing factors including low blood sugar, hormonal imbalance, or a brain tumor. Pain is an emotional issue because it is so intensely personal. Pain is closely linked to feelings. Pain sufferers frequently feel guilty or that somehow they should be able to bear their pain better, and many patients with chronic pain talk of feeling helpless or vulnerable. Goleman (1996) writes "humanity is most evident in our feelings." Feelings such as despair and anxiety are known to heighten pain, and pleasure and relaxation appear to decrease pain. It is difficult to relax and feel pleasure unaided when in pain, and it is all too easy to feel despair and anxiety. Changing perception of pain can be difficult when tackled alone.

Orthodox Approach to Pain

In January 2001, the Joint Commission on Accreditation of Healthcare Organizations (JCAHO), which accredits the majority of the United States' medical facilities, developed a new mandatory standard for the assessment and treatment of pain. It was the first time JCAHO, or any other accrediting body, had issued standards focusing on pain. Institutions began to scramble to work out how they were going to meet the new standards and what they needed to do to deal properly with a patient in pain. As part of the standards, medical institutions are required to inform patients of their right to appropriate pain assessment and treatment. The assessment includes documenting the level and characteristics of each person's pain using a numeric scale of 0-10 or pictures of expressive faces (www.JCAHO.org). No patient should score his or her pain above a four. Institutions are required to develop protocols for pain management and to educate their staff on pain management.

Orthodox Pain Relief

Analgesics (pain relievers) are divided into opioids (narcotics) and nonopioids. The use of opioids is strictly controlled. Originally narcotics were opioid derivatives and came from the plant *Papaver somniferum*. Recent advances in pharmacology have resulted in the development of several synthetic analgesics that work on the opioid receptors in the brain.

Narcotic/Opioid Drugs

Morphine is possibly the most common analgesic in this category. Derived from the opium poppy, morphine works by depressing the cerebral cortex, resulting in reduced powers of concentration as well as reduced pain. However, the respiratory and cough centers are also depressed by morphine, as is the neurotransmitter acetylcholine. *Cananga odorata* var. *genuina* (ylang ylang) has mild, opioid-like properties and can sometimes enhance the effect of opioid drugs. Codeine is a common but milder narcotic also derived from the opium poppy (Martin 1994). Codeine is used to suppress dry coughs as well as for the relief of general pain. Morphine, codeine, and opioid-like drugs are addictive, although they are less likely to be addictive for someone in severe or chronic pain. Such a patient's chances of addiction then fall to 1 in 3000 (Carter 1996). Another side effect of opioids is constipation. Narcotics have an extremely important role to play in health care.

Common Nonopioid/Nonnarcotic Drugs

The two most important drugs in this category are aspirin and acetaminophen. Aspirin (acetylsalicylic acid), as well as having antiinflammatory effects, is a well-recognized analgesic. Originally this analgesic was derived from salacin, a glycoside found in willow tree bark. Aspirin blocks prostaglandin synthesis in the central nervous system (CNS) and peripheral nervous system. Acetaminophen (Tylenol) is a painkiller that has no antiinflammatory effects because it blocks prostaglandin synthesis only in the CNS (Parish 1991). A list of undesirable side effects of antiinflammatory drugs can be found in many textbooks (Goodman-Gilma et al 1985). They are outlined in the following sections and are divided into the two main categories: nonsteroidal and steroidal.

Nonsteroidal Antiinflammatory Drugs

Aspirin is the most common nonsteroidal antiinflammatory drug (NSAID) and has a long history of use. Yin et al (1998) found aspirin inhibited transcription factors that coded the production of prostaglandin sythase enzymes. Lyss et al (1997) discovered helenalin, a lactone found in arnica, also inhibits the same transcription factor but in a different way. However, blocking prostaglandin synthesis can give rise to specific side effects. All NSAIDs, including aspirin (salicylic acid)-based antiinflammatories, can increase gastric bleeding in patients with gastric ulcers due to the inhibition of prostaglandin PGE2, which suppresses gastric acid secretion. NSAIDs can also prolong bleeding as they inhibit production of thromboxane (Ward 1993), upset the fluid balance by decreasing excretion due to inhibition of renal blood flow, cause bronchospasm and nasal polyposis in susceptible individuals, and delay the onset of labor due to loss of contractile effects of prostaglandins on the uterine muscles (Kvam 1994). Indomethacin is often used when salicylates are not tolerated. However, in arthritic patients, indomethacin can lead to a high incidence of CNS effects if the dose is high.

Phenylbutazone-like drugs can also cause gastrointestinal irritation, hepatitis, vertigo, and headaches. With prolonged usage, they can also depress the bone marrow, leading to leukemia and aplastic anemia (Craig & Stitzel 1994).

Steroid-Based Antiinflammatory Drugs

Despite being superior in effect to NSAIDs (and affecting the inflammatory process at each level), steroidal antiinflammatory drugs have many side effects. These include hyperglycemia leading to diabetes, myopathy, increased intraocular pressure with the potential for glaucoma, electrolyte imbalance leading to hypertension, thinning of the skin with an increased tendency for poor healing and skin breakdown, hirsutism, insomnia, depression, and psychosis (Craig & Stitzel 1994). These drugs are usually avoided in long-term treatment. However, steroidal antiinflammatory drugs have provided relief for chronic inflammatory conditions and will continue to be used until other drugs with fewer side effects are found.

Disadvantages of Orthodox Treatments

Despite advances in pain medication, many patients suffer chronic, and sometimes severe, pain before they die. Articles published in the *New England Journal of Medicine* and the *Journal of the American Medical Association* disclosed that children as well as adults suffered unnecessarily from pain. Carter (1996) suggests the poor pain-control in the studies could be because narcotics are often so tightly controlled in hospitals that staff cannot get them when their patients most need them. He suggests patient-controlled analgesia as the answer.

The barriers to pain management are patients' fear of addiction and their reluctance to report pain, plus their concerns about the side effects of medication and their fear their pain will not be controlled. These barriers have been compounded by inadequate reimbursement, poor administrative support, the high cost of technology, lack of continuity of care, and the lack of accountability for poor pain management. Muddying the whole issue of pain control are drug controversies such as that surrounding Oxycontin: a drug as potent as morphine that was heavily marketed to physicians without warning them of its addictive potential, which has had devastating consequences (Meier & Petersen 2001). However, things are changing for the better. As of January 2, 2002, pain management was recognized and reimbursed by Medicare, along with nutrition therapy (Pear 2002), and it is hoped that many health-insurance companies will follow suit.

Chronic Pain Syndrome

Chronic pain syndrome has been described as a complex dysfunction and is extremely difficult to treat successfully. Allopathic medicine treats CPS with a mixture of opioid and nonopioid drugs backed with tricyclic or Valium-type drugs that are not antidepressants, although they are used for that purpose in this instance.

Aromatherapy in Chronic Pain Management

Touch, relaxation, and pleasure each play an important part in how individuals perceives the world around them, and how they feel about themselves. This includes the perception of pain (Beck & Beck 1987). Aromatherapy works on the sensory system and appears to enhance the parasympathetic response, which is closely linked with endorphins (Weil 1996). The intensity and depth of pain is influenced by external factors such as previous experience, attitude, and culture. Pain can be "put on hold" by strong emotions such as anger, fear, or elation. Conversely, fear can make pain feel worse. Pain is a warning system. By deadening it, the warning system is dulled. A headache pill does not make the cause of the headache go away; it just allows the person to carry on functioning.

Aromatherapy using touch is very gentle and can be helpful in alleviating chronic pain. An application of diluted essential oils with either massage or sequenced movements (the "m" technique) is very relaxing. The odor of the essential oils is pleasurable. Even ignoring the possibility that essential oils might have pharmacologically active components or the possible pharmacokinetic enhancement of orthodox drugs by essential oils, there is still a potential role for aromatherapy as part of an integrated, multidisciplinary approach to pain management.

Aromatherapy enhances the parasympathetic response through the effects of touch and smell, encouraging relaxation at a deep level. Relaxation has been shown to alter perceptions of pain. Aromatherapy also enables patients to get "in touch with" feelings of relaxation and pleasure through smell and touch. These allow patients to "let go," often for the first time. A compress or gentle massage can draw attention either to the site of the pain, or away from it, depending on what will most meet the patient's psychological needs. Diffusing a relaxing essential oil can alter perceptions of pain (Buckle 1999).

The analgesic effects of aromatherapy can be traced to several factors:
1. A complex mixture of volatile chemicals reaching the pleasure memory sites within the brain;

2. Certain analgesic components within the essential oil, which may or may not be known, affecting the neurotransmitters dopamine, serotonin, and noradrenaline at receptor sites in the brain;
3 The interaction of touch with sensory fibers in the skin, which could possibly affect the transmission of referred pain;
4. The rubefacient effect of baths or friction on the skin.

Two thousand years ago, man used the plants Salix (willow) and Populus (poplar) to alleviate pain (Lewis & Elvin-Lewis 1977). Gattefosse (1937) states "almost all essential oils have analgesic properties," but some are more effective than others. Tables 12-1 and 12-2 list essential oils that are particularly suited to the treatment of chronic pain.

Table 12-1 ❧ Essential Oils Suitable for Chronic Pain

Common Name	**Botanical Name**	**Application**
Black pepper	*Piper nigrum*	Topical
Clove bud [a,b]	*Syzygium aromaticum*	Topical
Frankincense	*Boswellia carteri*	Inhaled, topical
Ginger [c]	*Zingiber officinale*	Topical
Juniper	*Juniperus communis*	Topical
Lavender (Spike) [d]	*Lavandula latifolia*	Topical
Lavender (True)	*Lavandula angustifolia*	Inhaled, topical
Lemongrass [e]	*Cymbopogon citrates*	Inhaled, topical
Marjoram (Sweet)	*Origanum majorana*	Inhaled, topical
Myrrh	*Commiphora molmol*	Topical
Peppermint	*Mentha piperita*	Topical
Rose	*Rosa damascene*	Topical
Rosemary [f]	*Rosmarinus officinalis*	Inhaled, topical
Verbena	*Aloysia triphylla*	Inhaled, topical
Ylang ylang	*Cananga odorata*	Inhaled

a = Clove bud is safer than clove leaf. Phenols can be harsh on the skin.
b = Best avoid regular use of clove with patients on anticoagulant therapy.
c = The CO_2 extraction contains gingerol thought to have analgesic action.
d = Spike lavender can be a stimulant; best avoid regular use in hypertension.
e = Lemongrass contains aldehydes; avoid in high concentrations on sensitive skin.
f = Rosemary is a stimulant; best avoid regular use in hypertension or epilepsy.

Table 12-2   🌿   *Essential Oils Particularly Suitable for Children*

Common Name	Botanical Name	Application
Chamomile (Roman)	*Chamaemelum nobile*	Inhaled, topical
Geranium	*Pelargonium graveolens*	Inhaled, topical
Mandarin	*Citrus reticulate*	Inhaled, topical
Neroli	*Citrus aurantium*	Inhaled, topical
Palma rosa	*Cymbopogon martini* var. *motia*	Inhaled, topical
Sandalwood	*Santalum album*	Inhaled, topical

Inhaled: 2 drops on cotton ball inhaled for 5-10 minutes

Topical: 2-5 drops diluted in a compress or in a vegetable cream/gel/oil

Animal Studies

Lorenzetti et al (1991) found myrcene, a terpene found in up to 20% in lemongrass (*Cymbopogon citratus*), had a direct analgesic effect on rats. The effect lasted 3 hours and was similar to that of peripheral-acting opioids, but did not affect the CNS, which was remarkable as the essential oil was administered orally. The analgesic effects did not lead to tolerance during a period of 5 days (which would have occurred with a narcotic). This is interesting as Seth et al (1976) had previously investigated the effect of lemongrass on pain and found it enhanced the effect of morphine in rats. However, Seth also investigated *Cymbopogon nardus* (East Indian lemongrass) and found it to be less effective as an analgesic. *Cymbopogon nardus* contains considerably less myrcene than *Cymbopogon citratus* (Boelens 1994). Lorenzetti et al (1991) conclude their paper with the suggestion that terpenes should be investigated with the "possibility of developing a new class of analgesic with myrcene as the prototype." Myrcene is found in small amounts in a number of essential oils, including rosemary, frankincense, juniper, rose, ginger, and verbena (Sheppard-Hangar 1995), all of which have traditional analgesic qualities. The analgesic effects of lemongrass in mice was the subject of another paper by Viana et al (2000) who concluded the essential oil worked at both central and peripheral levels when given by oral and intraperitoneal routes.

Artemisia caerulescens was found to have an analgesic effect on rats in a study by Moran et al (1989). Nepetalactone, a lactone found in *Nepeta caesarea*, was found to have analgesic properties in a controlled, comparative study with morphine on mice and hailed the "new opioid" (Aydin et al 1998). The essential oil was given by intraperitoneal injection. The lactone appeared to affect mechanical, not thermal, algesic receptors, which "suggests specificity for specific opioid receptor subtypes excluding mu-opioid receptors." Because the lactone is the main component of *Nepeta caesarea* (92%-95%) it was thought to have specific, opioid-receptor-subtype agonistic activity. The essential oil also had marked sedative effects. Aydin et al (1996) had previously studied *Origanum onites* and found it too had analgesic activity.

Lavandula angustifolia was found to have a local anesthetic effect in rabbits by Ghelardini et al (1999).

Human Studies

The analgesic effect of essential oils also occurred in human studies as reported by Woolfson and Hewitt (1992) who found a 50% pain reduction in 100 patients nursed in a critical care unit. Thirty-six patients were randomly allocated into three groups of 12: one group received massage plus lavender, one group received massage without lavender, and a control group received no massage but were left to "rest curtained off" from the remainder of the unit. Treatment consisted of 20 minutes of foot massage twice a week for 5 weeks. This was an interesting study as 50% of the patients were artificially ventilated, and therefore the effects of the essential oil could not be from inhalation. The most striking difference between the group receiving massage with lavender (Group A) and without lavender (Group B) was in the effect upon heart rate. Ninety percent of Group A showed a reduction of between 11 and 15 beats per minute whereas only 58% of Group B showed any reduction, and it was consistently less. Only 41% of the control group showed any reduction. The study gives no formal statistics or analysis.

Wilkinson (1995) investigated the effects of 1% Roman chamomile (*Chamomelum nobile*) on 51 patients with cancer in a randomized study. The participants ranged in age from 26 to 84 years. Ninety-four percent of the participants were female, and 6% were male. Forty-one percent had been referred for pain control. During the study, 45% of the participants were receiving morphine, with the remainder on weak opioids, nonopioids, or nothing. Seventy-six percent of the participants had metastases. Mann-Whitney U tests on all independent variables revealed no significant differences between conditions in the pretest scores for the Rotterdam Symptom Checklist on physical or psychological symptoms, activities, and top 10 symptoms. The data were analyzed using the Statistical Package for the Social Sciences (Nie et al 1975) and nonparametric tests were employed for all statistical analysis. State Trait Anxiety Inventory (STAI) scores fell by an average of 16 points in the aromatherapy massage group but only 10 points in the plain massage or standard group ($p = 0.005$), and pain was reduced statistically ($p = 0.003$). One patient is quoted as saying "I know now, almost definitely, that it (aromatherapy) has helped me in my quest for pain relief. I have told Dr. R at the pain clinic how pain free I was while having regular (aromatherapy) treatment" (Wilkinson 1995).

Gobel et al (1991) studied the effect of peppermint on headaches. Pain was induced in healthy humans using pressure, thermal, and ischemic stimuli. The intensity of the pain, neurophysiology, performance-related activity, and mood states were monitored. Peppermint diluted in ethanol and applied topically produced a significant analgesic effect. Perez-Raya et al (1990) found *Mentha rotundifolia* and *Mentha longifolia* (both types of peppermint) had analgesic properties in mice and rats. Peana et al (1999) found essential oil of clary sage to have an antiinflammatory and analgesic action at a local level. Extracts of myrrh (*Com-*

miphora momol) were found to have a strong local anesthetic effect in a study by Dolara et al (2000). The anesthetic action blocked the sodium current of excitable mammalian membranes. Local anesthetic activity on nerve cells was measured by incubating hippocampal brain slices, freshly dissected with a tissue chopper, from the brain of one of the experimental male rats. The slices were stimulated with a positive electrical current applied though electrodes.

Krall and Krause (1993) conducted an open, randomized study of 100 patients to evaluate the effects of a topically applied gel containing peppermint oil (30%) on periarticular pain. Effects of the peppermint gel were measured in acute (n = 49) and subacute (n = 51) conditions compared to the standard treatment of 10% hydroxyethyl salicylate gel. Different aspects of pain (intensity on pressure and spontaneous and movement pain) were examined using visual analog scales (0 = no symptom to 100 = severe symptom) for a period of 20 days. No statistical details were given. In 78% of cases both the physician and patient considered the results with the mint therapy to be highly effective, as opposed to 50% and 34 % respectively with the standard gel. There were 10 instances of side effects from the hydroxyethyl salicylate gel (three of erythema and seven of itching) and only one (smell of peppermint in the nose) from the mint oil. At the end of the study, 19% of the mint-oil patients were still suffering from pain, as were 36% of the aspirin gel group. The results of this comparative study were dependent on the severity of the symptoms.

Hot-pepper cream containing capsaicin has been found useful for arthritis and shingles and also appears to relieve postsurgical pain in cancer patients. Patients who used a cream containing 0.075% capsaicin around the incision site for 8 weeks following surgery experienced a 53% reduction in pain, compared with a 17% reduction for those using a placebo cream. Side effects included redness and burning of the skin, but those effects diminished with time. Capsaicin also appears to inhibit substance P.

Ginger (*Zingiber officinale*) can also have an analgesic and deeply warming action, but the topical analgesic gingerol (a phenol) only occurs in the CO_2 extract, not in the essential oil (Wren 1988). *Oleum spica* was traditionally used as a topical analgesic. *Oleum spica* contains one part spike lavender to four parts turpentine. It is thought the analgesic effect of turpentine is enhanced by the presence of spike lavender (Von Frohilche 1968).

Benzoin, camphor, clove, coriander, ginger, hops, lemongrass, marjoram, black pepper, pine, savory, and ylang ylang have analgesic properties (Rose 1992). Other suggestions include white birch, chamomile, frankincense, wintergreen, clove, lavender, and mint. Lawless (1994) writes that during the pre-Christian era, myrrh was added to wine to provide pain relief to those about to be crucified. Myrrh contains terpenes, esters, and a phenol called eugenol, all of which are reputed to be analgesics (Franchomme & Penoel 1991). Eugenol (and myrcene) are found in West Indian Bay (*Pimenta racemosa*) and in clove (*Syzygium aromaticum*). Use clove-bud oil (which also contains esters) not the leaf or stem oil that is higher in phenols. Diluted clove oil is useful to use prior to venipuncture as it make the veins more prominent and gives some local-anesthetic effect. Borneol (an alcohol) and myrcene (a terpene) were found to be effective antagonists of acetylcholine in a study by Cabo et al (1986). This study was conducted on isolated duodenum to counter contractile tissue. Acetylcholine is a central and peripheral nervous system transmitter (Craig 1994).

Muscle Spasm and Pain

Some pain is caused by muscle spasm. Several essential oils have antispasmodic effects, particularly those high in esters. The greater the number of different esters in an essential oil, the greater is thought to be the antispasmodic effect. Roman chamomile has more esters than any other essential oil and is also a recognized analgesic (Wren 1988). Lis-Balchin (1997) found clary sage, dill, fennel, frankincense, nutmeg, and lavender reduced the "twitch response to nerve stimulation; in isolated rat tissue." Historically the essential oils listed in Table 12-3 have been used for their antispasmodic effect.

Enteric-coated peppermint-oil capsules were used in the treatment of irritable bowel syndrome symptoms (Kline et al 2001). Fifty children took part in the controlled, multicentered study. The gelatin capsules did not release the oil until they were in the small intestine (an environment of pH 6.8 or higher). Between one capsule (187 mg) and two capsules were given three times a day. During the study eight children withdrew for various reasons. However, 76% of the peppermint group showed significant reduction in symptoms compared to the placebo group (43%). No side effects were reported and no change in stool consistency.

INFLAMMATION

Sometimes pain is caused by inflammation. Inflammation is a fundamentally protective mechanism (Betts 1993) and has been called "the most important of the

Table 12-3 ✖ *Some Antispasmodic Essential Oils*

Common Name	Botanical Name	Reference
Roman chamomile	*Chamaemelum nobile*	Franchomme & Penoel 1991
Petitgrain	*Citrus amara*	Reiter & Brandt 1985
Dill	*Anethum graveolens*	Lis-Balchin 1997
Clary sage	*Salvia sclarea*	Lis-Balchin 1997
Fennel	*Foeniculum vulgare*	Lis-Balchin 1997
Frankincense	*Boswellia carteri*	Lis-Balchin 1997
Lavender	*Lavandula angustifolia*	Lis-Balchin 1997
Sage	*Salvia officinalis*	Taddei et al 1988; Giachetti et al 1988

body's defense mechanisms" (MacSween & Whaley 1992). Derived from the Latin *inflammare*, meaning "to burn," the function of inflammation is to restore the body to normal functioning as quickly as possible. The symptoms of inflammation are redness, swelling, heat, and pain—through history listed as rubor, tumor, calor, and dolor (Mills 1991)— and a loss of function (Craig & Stitzel 1994).

Antiinflammatory Essential Oils

Essential oils have some of their most poignant antiinflammatory effects on the dermis and epidermis (Bowles 2000). Mascolo et al (1987) screened 75 species of plants (chosen from medicinal folklore) and their extracts for antiinflammatory activity. The experiments were performed on rats with carrageenan-induced foot edema. The control drug was indomethacin. Herbal extracts (not essential oils) from the plants were administered orally. However, many of the plants selected also produce essential oils used for antiinflammatory purposes in aromatherapy. *Coriandrum sativum* (coriander), *Foeniculum vulgare* (fennel), and *Juniperus communis* (juniper) all produced 45% reduction of inflammation, comparable with the control. However, if the essential oils had been applied topically, the response might have been greater. Essential oils are absorbed through the skin, with 70% of the oil being absorbed within 24 hours (Bronaugh et al 1990).

Rossi et al (1988) investigated Roman chamomile (*Anthemis nobilis*) in a comparative, controlled study on rats with carrageenan-induced edema. The control was indomethacin. Three essential oils of chamomile were used. White-headed, double-flowered chamomile flowers showed a greater antiinflammatory action than the yellow-flowered variety. Nevertheless, all three essential oils of Roman chamomile produced significant antiinflammatory effects. In this study the chamomile was given subcutaneously into the peritoneal cavity. Jakovlev et al (1979) demonstrated the antiinflammatory effect of German chamomile and suggested the antiphlogistic effects were due to bisabolol and bisabolol oxides. Tubaro et al (1984) found when German chamomile (*Matricaria recutita*) was applied topically to mouse ears, with hydrocortisone as the control, the chamomile showed an antiinflammatory action, although the effect was only half as strong as that of the steroid.

Nutmeg (*Myristica fragrans*) may have been the inspiration for Nostradamus' prophecies, but it also has antiinflammatory activities. Benet et al (1988), attributed nutmeg's antiinflammatory action to eugenol. They found the greatest effect was observed after 4 hours and was comparable to the effects of phenylbutazone and indomethacin. However, most essential oils of nutmeg contain very small amounts of eugenol (Lawrence 1995).

Wagner et al (1986) screened various essential oils traditionally used for their antiinflammatory action. They concluded eugenol, eugenyl acetate, thymol, capsaicin, curcumin, and carvacrol were present in most of the essential oils screened, and the antiphlogistic effects were closely linked to the vascular reaction of early inflammation. In herbal medicine this is called the counterirritant effect. Clove and cinnamon had the strongest effect, Dwarf pine (*Pinus mugo* var. *pumilo*) and eucalyptus (*Eucalyptus globulus*) had a mild effect and *Chamomelum nobile* had a weak antiinflammatory effect.

Where there is topical inflammation, essential oils should be applied topically. Essential oils are absorbed into and through the skin, and they can enhance the penetration of other medication. Godwin and Michniak (1999) found terpenen-4-ol and a-terpineol enhanced the penetration of a hydrocortisome cream on mouse skin by between three and five times. Sesquiterpenenes and sesquiterpenoids (found in many antiinflammatory essential oils) caused a 20% increase in penetration of 5-fluorouracil, and this effect lasts for 4 days (Cornwall & Barry 1994).

Sometimes, in cases of arthritic pain, heat can help. If this is the case, essential oils that have rubefacient effects, such as *Piper nigrum* (black pepper), *Syzygium aromaticum* (clove), or *Zingiber officinale* (ginger) can be useful, as CO_2 extracts. Sometimes cooling will help and an essential oil like *Mentha piperita* (peppermint) can be added to the topical-application mix.

It is important patients be allowed to smell the mixture before it is applied; they will have to live with it, after all! Be gentle and slow. Allowing someone to touch a painful area takes courage, and that courage needs to be rewarded with respect. All the essential oils mentioned are safe to use for relief of pain. While a 1-5% solution is usually adequate, much higher concentrations can be used. In some circumstances, and depending on the essential oils selected, 100% solutions can be used. Lavender and tea tree are good examples of oils that can be used at full strength.

Plant flavonoids have measurable effects on the CNS (Paladini et al 1999). Some semisynthetic derivatives of plant favonoids were found to have an anxiolytic effect 30 times that of diazepam. Both natural and synthetic flavonoids are a part of Western living and are ingested by millions of people on a daily basis.

Finally, the pain experienced by patients with sickle cell anemia, an inherited disease, may be helped with herbal medicine. Fakim and Sewaj (1992) found an aqueous extract of *Pelargonium graveolens* (geranium) successfully reverted sickled cells in vitro. Fennel has also been shown to reverse sickling (Fakim et al 1990). The extract used was aqueous, and therefore not found in the essential oil, but there could be a similar response using the CO_2 extract.

There is no suggestion that essential oils should replace conventional analgesia. However, topical or inhaled, applications of essential oils appears to enhance orthodox analgesia either through the placebo response, the effect of touch and smell on the parasympathetic nervous system, or because of pharmacologically active ingredients within the essential oils that may have an analgesic effect. There have been few published clinical trials, but there is growing anecdotal evidence to suggest essential oils could have an important role in augmenting conventional analgesia. Finally, anethole, methyl salicilate, and camphor are all analgesic components found in essential oils, and they are all found in root beer!

REFERENCES

Alavi A, LaRiccia P, Sadek A et al. 1997. Neuroimaging of acupuncture in patients with chronic pain. Journal of Alternative & Complementary Medicine. 3(Suppl 1) S47-S53.

Aydin S, Beis R, Ozturk Y et al. 1998. Nepetalactone: a new opioid analgesic from *Nepeta casesarea* Boiss, Journal of Pharmacy & Pharmacology. 50(7) 813-817.

Aydin S, Ozturk Y, Beis R et al. 1996. Investigation of *Origanum onites, Sideritis congesta* and *Saturega cuneifolia* essential oils for analgesic activity. Phytotherapy Research. 10:342-344.

Beck D, Beck J. 1987. The Pleasure Connection: How Endorphins Affect our Health and Happiness. Anaheim, CA: Synthesis Press.

Benett A, Stamford F, Tavares I. 1988. The biological activity of eugenol, a major constituent of nutmeg: studies on prostaglandins, the intestine and other tissues. Phytotherapy Research. 2(3) 125-129.

Berman B, Swyers J. 1997. Establishing a research agenda for investigating alternative medical interventions for chronic pain. Primary Care. 24(4) 743-758.

Betts A. 1993. An overview of pathology. In Hinchcliff S, Norman S, Schrober J (eds.), Nursing Practice and Health Care. London: Edward Arnold, 148-149.

Boelens M. 1994. Sensory and chemical evaluation of tropical grass oils. Perfumer & Flavorist. 19:29-45.

Bowles J. 2000. The Basic Chemistry of Aromatherapeutic Essential Oils. Sydney, Australia: Pirie Publishing.

Bronaugh R, Wester R, Bucks D. 1990. In vivo percutaneous absorption of fragrance ingredients in Rhesus monkeys and humans. Food and Chemical Toxicology. 28(5) 369-373.

Buckle J. 1999. Use of aromatherapy as a complementary therapy of chronic pain. Alternative Therapies in Health & Medicine. 5(5) 42-51.

Cabo J, Crespo M, Jimenez J et al. 1986. The spasmolytic activity of various aromatic plants from the province of Granada. The activity of the major components of their essential oils. Plantes Medicinales et Phytotherapy. 20(5) 213-218.

Carter R. 1996. Give a drug a bad name. New Scientist. 150(2024)27-29.

Casey M. 2002. Aromatherapy: Pain management. Aromatherapy Today. 21:26-29.

Cornwall P, Barry B. 1994. Sesquiterpene components of volatile oils as skin penetration enhancers for the hydrophilic permeant 5 fluorouracil. Journal of Pharmacy & Pharmacology. 46(4) 261-269.

Craig C. 1994. Introduction to CNS pharmacology. In Craig C, Stitzel R (eds.), Modern Pharmacology, 4th ed. Boston: Little, Brown & Co., 329-336.

Brestel E, Van Dyke K. 1994. Lipid mediators of homeostasis and inflammation. In Craig C, Stitzel R (eds.), Modern Pharmacology, 4th ed. Boston: Little, Brown & Co., 477-485.

Dolara P, Corte B, Ghelardini C et al. 2000. Local anesthetic, antibacterial and antifungal properties of sesquiterpenes from myrrh. Planta Medica. 66(4) 356-358.

Fakim G, Sofowora E, Sewaj M. 1990. Reversal of sickling and crenation in erythrocytes by aqueous extracts of *Pelargonium x asperum, Foeniculum vulgare* and *Sideroxylon puberulum.* Revue Agricole et Sucriere de l'Ile Maurice. 69, 91-93.

Fakim G, Sewaj M. 1992. Studies on the antisickling properties of extracts of *Sideroxylon puberulum, Faujariopsis flexuosa, Cardispermum halicacabum* and *Pelargonium graveoleus.* Planta Medica. 58 (Suppl.) A648-A649.

Fields H. 1997. Pain: Anatomy and physiology. Journal of Alternative & Complementary Medicine. 3(Suppl 1) S41-S46.

Franchomme P, Penoel D. 1991. L'aromatherapie Exactement. Limoges, France: Jollois.

Gattefosse R. 1937. (Translated in 1993 by R. Tisserand.) Aromatherapie: Les Huile Essentielles-Hormones Vegetales (Gattefosse's Aromatherapy.) Saffron Walden, UK: CW Daniels, 89.

Ghelardini C, Galeotti N, Salvatore G et al. 1999. Local anesthetic activity of essential oil of *Lavandula angustifolia.* Planta Medica. 65(8) 700-703.

Gobel H, Schmidt G, Soyka, D. 1991. Effect of peppermint and eucalyptus oil preparations on neurophysiological and experimental algesimetric headache parameters. Cephalalgia. 14:228-234.

Godwin D, Michniak B. 1999. Influence of drug lipophilicity on terpenes as transdermal penetration enhancers. Drug Development and Industrial Pharmacy. 25(8) 905-915.

Goleman D. 1996. Emotional Intelligence. New York: Bantam.

Goodman-Gilma A, Goodman L, Murad F (eds.). 1985. The Pharmacological Basis of Therapeutics. New York: Macmillan.

Greer C. 1995. Anatomical organization of the human olfactory system. In Gilbert A (ed.), Compendium of Olfactory Research 1982-1994, 3-7.

Jakovlev V, Isaac O, Thiemer K et al. 1979. Pharmacological investigations with compounds of chamomile. II. New investigations on the antiphlogistic effects of a bisabolol and bisabolol oxide. Planta Medica. 35:125-140.

Kline R, Kline J, Di Palma J et al. 2001. Enteric coated pH dependent peppermint oil capsules for the treatment of irritable bowel syndrome in children. Journal of Pediatrics. 138(1) 125-128.

Krall B, Krause W. 1993. Efficacy and tolerance of *Mentha arvensis aethoeroleum.* Paper presented July 21-24 at 24th International Symposium on Essential Oils. Berlin, Germany.

Kvam D. 1994. Anti-inflammatory and anti-rheumatic drugs. In Craig C, Stitzel R (eds.), Modern Pharmacology, 4th ed. Boston: Little, Brown & Co., 485-500.

Lawless J. 1994. Aromatherapy and the Mind. London: Thorsons.

Lawrence B. 1995. Essential Oils 1992-1994. Carol Stream, IL: Allured Publishing.

Lewis W, Elvin-Lewis M. 1977. Medical Botany. New York: Wiley Interscience.

Lis-Balchin M. 1997. A preliminary study of the effect of essential oils on skeletal and smooth muscle in vitro. Journal of Ethnopharmacology. 58(3) 183-187.

Lorenzetti B, Souza G, Sarti S et al. 1991. Myrcene mimics the peripheral analgesic activity of lemongrass tea. Journal of Ethnopharmacology. 34(1) 43-48.

Lyss G, Schmidt T, Merfort I et al. 1997. Helenalin, an anti-inflammatory sesquiterpene lactone from arnica, selectively inhibits transcription factor NF-kappaB. Biological Chemistry. 378(9) 951-961.

MacSween R, Whaley K (eds.). 1992. Muir's Textbook of Pathology, 13th ed. London: Edward Arnold.

Mascolo N, Autore G, Capasso F. 1987. Biological screening of Italian medicinal plants for anti-inflammatory activity. Phytotherapy Research. 1:28-31.

Martin B. 1994. Opioid and nonopioid analgesics. In Craig C, Stitzel R (eds.), Modern Pharmacology, 4th ed. Boston: Little, Brown & Co., 431-450.

Meier B, Petersen M. 2001. Sales of painkiller grew rapidly but success brought a high cost. New York Times. CL(51,683) A15.

Mills S. 1991. Out of the Earth. London: Viking Arkana.

Moran A, Martin N, Montero M. 1989. Analgesic, antipyretic and anti-inflammatory activity of essential oil of *Artemisia caerulescens* subsp. *gallica.* Journal of Ethnopharmacology. 27(3) 307-317.

Nie N, Hull C, Jenkins J et al. 1975. Statistical Package for the Social Sciences. New York: McGraw-Hill.

Paladini A, Marder M, Viola H et al. 1999. Flavonoids and the central nervous system: from forgotten factors to potent anxiolytic compounds. Journal of Pharmacy & Pharmacology. 51(5) 519-526.

Peana A, Moretti M, Juliano C. 1999. Chemical composition and antimicrobial action of the essential oils of *Salvia desoleana* and *Salvia sclarea.* Planta Medica. 65(8) 752-754.

Pear R. 2002. Nutrition therapy to fall under Medicare umbrella. New York Times. CLI(51,985) A16.

Perez-Raya M, Utrilla M, Navarro M et al. 1990. CNS activity of *Mentha rotundifolia* and *Mentha longifolia* essential oil in mice and rats. Phytotherapy Research. 4:232-234.

Rose J. 1992. The Aromatherapy Book. San Francisco: North Atlantic Books.

Rossi T, Melegari M, Bianchi A et al. 1988. Sedative, anti-inflammatory and anti-diuretic effects induced in rats by essential oils of varieties of *Anthemis nobilis:* a comparative study. Pharmacological Research Communications. 20(Suppl.) 71-74.

Seth G, Kokate C, Varma K. 1976. The effect of essential oil of *Cymbopogon citratus* on central nervous system. Indian Journal of Experimental Biology. 14(3) 370-371.

Sheppard-Hangar S. 1995. Aromatherapy Practitioner Reference Manual, Vol. II. Tampa, FL: Atlantic School of Aromatherapy.

Sofaer B, Foord J. 1993. Care of the person in pain. In Hinchcliff S, Norman S, Schrober J (eds.), Nursing Practice and Health Care. London: Edward Arnold, 374-401.

Tubaro A, Zillia,C, Redaeli C et al. 1984. Evaluation of anti-inflammatory activity of chamomile extract topical application. Planta Medica. 50(4) 359-360.

Von Frohilche A. 1968. A review of clinical, pharmacological and bacteriological research into *Oleum spicae.* Wiener Medizinische Wochenschrift. 15:345-350.

Wagner H, Wierer M, Bauer R. 1986. In vitro inhibition of prostaglandin biosynthesis by essential oils and phenolic compounds. Planta Medica. 52 (3)184-187.

Ward K. 1993. Care of the person with an infection. In Hinchcliff S, Norman S, Schrober J (eds.), Nursing Practice and Health Care. London: Edward Arnold, 402-434.

Weil A. 1996. Spontaneous Healing. New York: Fawcett.

Wilkinson S. 1995. Aromatherapy and massage in palliative care. International Journal of Palliative Nursing. 1(1) 21-30.

Woolfson A, Hewitt D. 1992. Intensive aromacare. International Journal of Aromatherapy. 4(2) 12-14.

Wren R. 1988. Potter's New Cyclopaedia of Botanical Drugs and Preparations. London: Churchill Livingstone.

Yin M, Yamamoto Y, Gaynor R. 1998. The anti-inflammatory agent aspirin and salicylate inhibit the activity of I(kappa)Bkinase-beta. Nature. 396(6706) 77-80.

13

STRESS MANAGEMENT

History is filled with examples that demonstrate how human contact acts as one of nature's most powerful antidotes to stress.

James Lynch (1979)

Patients' stress levels will directly impact the rate of their recovery. However, it is sometimes easy for health professionals to forget patients (and those who care for them) are under stress as all attention is fixed on their symptoms or their disease. The reliability of previously used tools to measure stress is now questioned, and there are moves to create different tools more sensitive to psychological stress. Frazier et al (2002) found reliance on the top recognized anxiety indicators in health care: agitation, increased blood pressure, increased heart rate, patients' verbalization of anxiety, and restlessness, produced an inaccurate and incomplete anxiety evaluation of vulnerable patients. Frazier et al (2002) wrote that reliance on these indicators could lead to "serious underestimation of the extent of anxiety because anxiety is an uncomfortable, subjective phenomenon that precedes the development of the most objectively detectable signs and behaviors." O'Brien et al (2001) found no correlation of rating of stress between coronary care patients and their attending health-care professionals. Van der Does (1989) found a similar mismatch between patients and their caregivers in a burn unit.

Despite these problems, health professionals now recognize stress has serious consequences, and procedures are in place to help reduce stress when possible. Redd and Manne (1995) investigated the effect of using aroma to reduce distress during magnetic resonance imaging and found that a pleasant smell reduced the stress and enhanced the coping ability of patients who had undergone traumatic experiences. Fifty-seven participants received either heliotropin (a vanilla-like scent) or plain air via a small tube inserted into their nostrils. Patients who received the heliotropin reported 64% less anxiety than patients who had plain air. However, their respiration and heart rate were not affected. Aromatherapy appears to be a quick, economical, and effective way of relieving, avoiding, and removing stress, not just for patients, but also for staff and relatives.

DEFINITIONS OF STRESS

There are many definitions and types of stress, but it is generally agreed that Hans Selye of McGill University conceived of the idea of stress in 1935. He was carrying out research on rats and discovered those that had been injected with various hormonal extracts developed enlarged adrenal glands, shrunken lymphatic glands, and bleeding gastrointestinal ulcers. He called this "the stress syndrome" (Anthony & Thibodeau 1983).

Rahe (1975), a psychiatrist at the University of Washington School of Medicine, found the more stress a person experienced, the more likely he or she would fall ill. He interviewed more than 5000 people and devised what was to become a classic, systematized method for correlating the events in people's lives with their illnesses (Pelletier 1992). Until that time it had been assumed only adverse stress would have a significant effect. However the survey indicated any change in the normal pattern of life, even good stress, was found to produce symptoms.

Today, the word *stress* is used to describe the cause of all ills that cannot be explained in any other way, even though the meaning of the word is unclear. A 1991 article in the *British Medical Journal* called stress a "chimera – an unreliable word to be used sparingly" (Wilkinson 1991). However, there is such a thing as good stress, which everyone feels occasionally and which galvanizes action.

A major conference held in Arizona in the 1980s brought together leading psychologists, immunologists, and physicians to discuss stress and try to define it. After heated debate, it was agreed there was no absolute definition of stress but that "things" outside people caused stress. These "things" were labeled *stressors*. It was suggested that people react and adapt to stressors differently. Some individuals seem to be able to cope, while others do not, and there is no way of telling who will cope and who will not.

The conference delegates agreed that stressors had measurable psychological and physiological effects. This was borne out by Cohen et al's later research on stress and human susceptibility to the common cold (Cohen et al 1991), which showed an individual under stress was more likely to "catch" a cold than someone not under stress.

Anthony and Thibodeau (1983) wrote of the ancient Chinese custom using anticipated physiological effects of stress. Individuals suspected of lying were forced to chew rice powder and then spit it out. The Chinese believed the stress of lying would render a person incapable of salivation. Indeed, perhaps this is the origin of the saying "the dry mouth of fear."

INDICATORS OF STRESS

Selye's List of Common Stressors (Anthony & Thibodeau 1983)

Extreme stimuli includes too much of almost anything. Consider a patient in a hospital, perhaps in a high-dependency unit. It is obvious the patient is receiving continuous extreme stimuli in the form of bright lights and loud or sudden noises.

Extreme deficiency including social deficiency incurred during solitary confinement, blindness, deafness, etc. This is called *sensory deprivation,* but some patients are physically isolated for either their own protection or that of others. Others can be made to feel outsiders to society because of their illness, such as those with AIDS, HIV, hepatitis, or the physically handicapped. Perhaps a semiconscious patient would also fit into this category.

Stressors are often injurious, unpleasant, or painful. Hospital personnel do not set out to injure their patients in the accepted sense of the word. However, many medical procedures are unpleasant or painful.

Stressors are things an individual perceives to be a threat, whether real or imaginary. Many hospital and nursing procedures are perceived to be threatening, such as injections or lumbar punctures.

Stress is an intangible phenomenon. It cannot be tasted, heard, smelled, or measured directly.

Stressors are individual. What is stressful today may not be tomorrow, and what is stressful to one patient may not be to another.

Some indicators of stress can be easily measured, such as blood pressure rise, tachycardia, pupil dilation, etc. But often stress cannot be measured in this way and a psychological tool such as the stress and self-esteem questionaire developed by Dr. Edward O'Brien (www.marywood.edu) needs to be used. Stress can be divided into that which is necessary for survival and that which will eventually lead to break down. Selye divided the physiological response to stressors into three stages: alarm, resistance, and exhaustion. The alarm response can be life-saving—the fight or flight phenomenon. During the alarm response, physiological changes produced by receptors in the brain increase heartbeat and respiration rates. Unnecessary metabolism, such as digestion, is curbed, while blood and oxygen are swiftly redirected to the more vital centers of the body. When the danger is over, the body quickly returns to its original state. Sweaty, clammy hands and cold feet become warm and dry again. Respiration and pulse slow down to a normal level, and digestion recommences.

Nixon (1976), a British cardiologist, found that when stress continued, a person reached a point of no return. Fig. 13-1 indicates the point at which a person under chronic stress would break down. Nixon thought if that person was isolated and encouraged to rest, the mind, body, and spirit would be able to mend. Many cardiac patients were treated successfully in this way when working with Nixon in the 1970s.

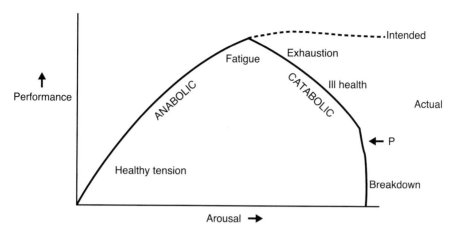

FIGURE 13-1   The human function curve: a performance arousal curve used as a model for a systems or biopsychosocial approach to a clinical problem.   Reproduced from: Nixon P. 1976. The human function curve. Practitioner. 217(76) 769, 935-944, with kind permission of the author.

In chronic stress, the "arousal state" of a person is never completely amelio- rated. The measurable levels of stress in the body do not return to normal, and cor- tisol levels remain above average. Throughout a period of time, small but damag- ing physiological changes occur: blood sugar and pressure are raised, hormonal functions change, and digestion and elimination are affected. Psychological stres- sors are the most common cause of chronic stress. Pitts (1969) found lactate con- centrations in the blood increased in patients with high levels of psychological stress, producing anxiety neurosis. Barasch (1993) wrote prolonged stress could create "fibrin cocoons" that prevented T cells from attacking cancerous metastases.

Stress is now recognized as one of the most serious health issues of the 20th century. In 2002, the workforce still continues to push itself to the limit. It is al- most as though being stressed is the acceptable face of modern life. No one seems to consider changing his or her lifestyle. However if stress remains relentless, change is often forced through breakdown.

If a person is unable to "switch off," either physically or mentally, he or she will eventually break down. It may be slow in coming, but break down they will because the body cannot maintain that level of stress. Wilde McCormick (1992), a British psychologist, wrote in her book on breakdown, "if we start to break down in our bodies with symptoms that don't seem to have an organic cause, it is a mes- sage to us from the unconscious that we need to be taken into areas we have not yet explored or made conscious."

Occasionally, some individuals who have undergone stringent training in the handling of potentially stressful situations (such as army personnel, firefighters, or paramedics) will only show signs of stress when the situation is over, almost as if their body is allowing them to "let go" when it is safe. Only then do they experience the palpitations and interrupted sleep patterns their colleagues experienced while in the stress situation. Survivors of the 9/11 terrorist attacks in the United States have written and spoken of this phenomenon.

Pelletier (1992a) quotes Sir William Osler: "the care of tuberculosis depends more on what the patient has in his head than what he has in his chest." In other words how a patient feels will affect how he recovers. This is very relevant to the way a patient is cared for in the hospital. Perhaps the word *treat* should be reassessed.

Stressors can be divided into several categories: physical, emotional, behavioral, environmental, cultural, and political. A patient in the hospital could be experiencing physical, emotional, behavioral, and environmental stress simultaneously. Physiological stress is usually accompanied by some psychological stress. Psychological stress produces measurable physical changes. Even though psychophysiology has found a wide range of physiological responses to psychological stress, very little is done to address the psychological stress of patients in hospitals (Anthony & Thibodeau 1983).

Physical responses to stress are governed by the hypothalamus, which is positioned next to the pituitary gland for easy hormone control (Clark & Montague 1993). The hypothalamus controls the autonomic nervous system and forms part of the limbic system, so it is immediately apparent that stress will have a direct effect on almost all bodily functions, from temperature to hormone balance. Anything that affects the sensory systems, like an odor, has a direct pathway to the limbic system, in particular to the amygdala. LeDoux (1996) suggests this pathway "does not allow for cortical processing and may be responsible for emotional responses a person does not understand."

The secretion of almost every hormone is altered in response to stress, and the altered chemical signals immediately affect the immune system. The immune system governs the ability to repair and heal (Linn et al 1988). Therefore the suggestion that aromas might affect a response to stress is a very important one.

Common Measurable Physical Responses

Measurable physical responses to stress include the following:
Increased concentrations of adrenaline/noradrenaline in the blood and urine;
Increase in the rate and force of the heartbeat;
Rise in systolic blood pressure;
Dilation of the pupils;
Decrease in the number of white blood cells;
Increase in the level of blood adrenocorticoids;
Increase in the level of lactate in the blood;
Increase in the level of urinary adrenocorticoids.
An increase in eosinophils and lymphocytes during times of stress will lead to immunosuppression and decreased resistance to infection. An increase in aldosterone,

thyroxine, and glucagon will increase the level of blood glucocorticoids. An increase in cortisol levels will affect carbohydrate, lipid, and protein metabolism. This can lead to muscle wasting, thinning of the skin, and depression of immune responses, as well as raised blood-cholesterol levels and a reduction in vitamin D levels and calcium absorption resulting in osteoporosis.

The effect of stress is determined by whether a person becomes angry or frightened. Proportions of adrenaline and noradrenaline are directly related to the emotion displayed (Clark & Montague 1993). Predatory animals produce more noradrenaline, while domestic animals produce more adrenaline. Patients in the hospital tend to become frightened rather than angry. It would be interesting to measure the levels of adrenaline and noradrenaline in patients to determine which is higher and therefore what their stress response might be.

Psychological stress negatively impacts the skin and blocks the cutaneous permeability barrier function. Coadministration of tranquilizers blocks this stress-induced deterioration in barrier function (Garg et al 2001). This is why so many skin diseases appear to be precipitated and exacerbated by stress. Walsh (1996) reports on the case study of a 57-year-old mother of four who had experienced psoriasis for 30 years. Severe plaque psoriasis affected both her knees and elbows. She had tried many orthodox treatments unsuccessfully. Bergamot, jasmine, sandalwood, and lavender in sweet almond oil were applied (2%) and improvement "beyond the normal" for prescribed medication was experienced. The dry, flaky skin and red "scabs" disappeared, and she was able to wear a short-sleeved blouse and knee-length skirt for the first time in years without embarrassment. While the psoriasis did not clear up completely, there was a great improvement. It is unclear whether the essential oils reduced her stress thus impacting her psoriasis, or if the essential oils directly impacted the psoriasis.

Rimmer (1998) wrote about using aromatherapy to reduce stress in a patient with terminal cancer. By using pleasant-smelling essential oils to reduce stress, the patient was able to relax deeply, began to sleep better, and was better able to cope with her pain.

Symptoms of Stress (Wilson-Barnett & Carrigy 1978)

Physical

Clenched jaw, leading to bruxism and referred neck pain

Hostility, depression, introspection, overemotionalism, nervous twitches, nail-biting

Sweating for no obvious reason

Inability to sit still

Frequent crying or wish to cry

Lack of appetite or unnatural craving for food

Dyspepsia, indigestion/heartburn, constipation, diarrhea

Constant tiredness

Insomnia, vivid dreams, sleep disturbances

Headaches, migraines

Breathlessness without exertion, palpitations, tachycardia
Dry mouth, dysphagia
Hypertension
Infertility, impotence

Mental

Constant irritability
Loss of sense of humor
Difficulty in concentrating
Lack of interest in life
Feeling unable to cope
Depression, being unable to show feelings
Dreading the future
Fear of being alone

Illnesses

Eczema, psoriasis, acne, skin disorders
Asthma
Dysmenorrea, premenstrual syndrome, hormonal imbalance, alopecia
Pruritus
Diabetes mellitus
Overactive thyroid
Colitis, irritable bowel syndrome

Pitt (1969), in *Scientific American,* made a list of 26 symptoms that are a result of prolonged stress. The list is as follows:

1. Tires easily	14. Insomnia
2. Breathlessness	15. Unhappiness
3. Nervousness	16. Shakiness
4. Chest pain	17. Fatigued all the time
5. Sighing	18. Sweating
6. Dizziness	19. Fear of death
7. Faintness	20. Smothering
8. Apprehensiveness	21. Syncope
9. Headache	22. Nervous chill
10. Paresis	23. Urinary frequency
11. Weakness	24. Vomiting and diarrhea
12. Trembling	25. Anorexia
13. Breath unsatisfactory	26. Palpitations

Stress and Immunology

The immunological effects of stress are not always clear because each person deals with them in his or her own way and because the effects are cumulative. However, there is a growing body of published evidence (both scientific and anecdotal) to show that specific stressors are linked to depressed immune function. A decrease in immunoglobulin A was measured in a study of dental students during their first year (Ng et al 2002; Klecolt-Glaser & Glaser 1993). A similar study of medical students prior to and during the first day of their final examinations repeated those findings; the students' ability to produce interferon was drastically reduced. Pelletier (1992a) discussed Bartrop's study on bereavement, which showed a lower lymphocyte function during the first 8 weeks following bereavement. Quinn (1993) used this knowledge for her research on bereavement, which looked at lowered immunological function and the effects of therapeutic touch.

Pert (1997), a molecular biologist and research scientist, described immunology as a network of information with the mind flowing along it. Karl Pibram (1976), who carried out neurophysiological research at Stanford University for many years, describes the brain as a hologram storing information available to all its different parts. In this case, could it be that when a person becomes stressed, this hologram is affected and communication between neuropeptides (the network of information) becomes blocked? Certain types of people appear to be protected from feelings of chronic stress. Jeanne Achterberg, an American psychologist, noted that at two institutions for the criminally insane, inmates who had carried out horrendous crimes had been unusually protected from life-threatening diseases such as cancer, despite poor health habits such as heavy smoking. Further studies showed mentally handicapped people were less likely to die from cancer. On the basis of these studies it was suggested that a higher level of intelligence could be linked to a higher incidence of chronic diseases such as cancer (Barasch 1993). Do intelligent people tend to suppress their feelings, which then suppress their immunological systems?

STRESS AND PATIENTS

Arguably, one of the most stressful situations in anyone's life is to be institutionalized. To many people a hospital can seem like a prison. This attitude is well documented (Jamison et al 1987). In a hospital is it all too easy for patients to lose their sense of identity. Patients often feel anonymous. This feeling of anonymity is compounded by Western medicine, which treats the medical condition rather than the patient. An appendix is removed or a cancer is irradiated with little regard for the gender, age, or weight of the person. Yet human beings are all unique, so how can such a blanket treatment be right?

Patients in hospital are encouraged to conform. Questioning procedures often labels a patient as "difficult". The medical profession is trained to diagnose, not to discuss. Responsibility and choice of treatment are often removed from the patient in the current medical model. Patients are rarely asked how they feel about their treatment, or given a choice in it.

One of the most stressful things in life is to feel a loss of control. Being a hospital patient means exactly that. This is not just the loss of control produced by an alien environment (being unable to choose when to sleep or eat) but also the loss of control of intimate bodily functions. The more seriously ill the patient, the more severe the loss of control and the ensuing stress. Compounding this sense of loss is the feeling of invasion. Privacy, personal space, and the body itself are invaded.

Of all surgery, perhaps heart surgery is the most feared, and a high percentage of patients experience psychological disturbances following open-heart surgery (Layne & Yudofsky 1971). This may be due to the bypass machinery, but it may have a closer connection to being in an intensive care unit and the relentless stressors found there: total loss of privacy, loss of sleep, bright lights, and continuous noise (Roberts 1991). It is ironic that the stress induced by a high-dependency unit may impact the psyche of a patient to such an extent that he or she may not survive the miracle of modern medicine.

AROMATHERAPY AND STRESS

Familiar smells associated with happy memories can help reestablish feelings of happiness. To be happy is to be unstressed. Most essential oils from plants and flowers have the potential to reduce stress. Certain essential oils, such as lavender, rose, neroli, and petitgrain, are well known for this ability.

Each hospital department, whether oncology or dermatology, carries its own particular brand of stress and fear. One of the most common, but least life-threatening, stresses in oncology is a patient's fear of hair loss. For women especially, this may produce profound anxiety. The simple act of a gentle head massage with a diluted essential oil such as lavender (*Lavandula angustifolia*) can do a tremendous amount to "touch the spot" and help reassure the patient that their hair *will* grow back. In a randomized, controlled study, hair loss due to alopecia responded well to topically applied essential oils (Hay et al 1998).

Organ transplant brings with it intense relief but also feelings of guilt and anger. Sometimes these two emotions are not fully addressed, despite counseling. For the patient receiving the transplant, it may not be the fact that another human being has had to suffer, or die, but that a part of their own body has been "thrown away" (Sylvia & Novak 1997). In the case of heart transplants, when patients have literally "lost their hearts," aromatherapy can introduce smell and touch to help release these feelings of grief and pain. Essential oils such as frankincense, ylang ylang, angelica, and neroli can be useful tools in the healing process.

Outpatient departments are associated with long waits, dark corridors, fraught staff, and physicians who rarely have time to look up from their notes. Aromatherapy can help reduce the stress of waiting. Lehrner et al (2000) conducted a randomized, controlled study with 72 participants and found *Citrus sinensis* (sweet orange) had a calming and relaxing effect on patients waiting in a dentist's office.

Schulz et al (1998) conducted two multiple-crossover studies, each involving 12 female subjects and electroencephalograms to screen for acute sedating effect of eight different plant extracts. *Lavandula angustifolia* (1200 mg) was given in capsule form (orally), and 140 minutes later 100 mg of caffeine was given orally in tablet form. Conventional medications decreased theta frequency but increased beta in these studies. However, several plant extracts increased theta but had no effect on beta. Theta and beta are brain waves generated by the thalamus (http://brain.web-us.com/brainwavesfunction.htm).

Tasev et al (1969) and Sugano and Sato (1991) found rose was gently uplifting. Muruzzella and Sicurella (1960) found eucalyptus was antibacterial. So, a vaporizer containing rose (*Rosa damascena*) or eucalyptus (*Eucalyptus globulus*) could gently uplift patients and staff and reduce the possibility of cross-infection.

Stress and Hospital Staff

Stress in hospitals is not confined to patients. The nursing staff is under tremendous stress; their numbers have been cut even though their workload has remained just as heavy, and morale is very low. Hospital managers show signs of stress as they attempt to keep hospitals functioning. Physicians, too, are often depressed and stressed. They have been forced into the "role of God" by the public, and are then pilloried if they get it wrong. Healthcare is not healthy.

From the interns, many of whom still work 80-hour weeks, to consultant surgeons who dash between operating rooms, there is no way these people could avoid stress. Few physicians find it easy to linger over a meal or to resist answering the telephone by the second ring. Stress is something accepted as part of the job in medicine. Alcoholism, drug abuse, and suicide were the downsides of working in medicine in the 1980s (Bennett 1987), and little has changed.

Health professionals find it hard to look after themselves. Since September 11, 2001, it has become more acceptable to acknowledge a sense of vulnerability but it is still not OK for a health professional to admit being overwhelmed. The pressure may be more manageable if some aromatherapy is used. Mandarin (*Citrus reticulata*), lavender (*Lavandula angustifolia*), or chamomile (*Chamaemelum nobile*) inhaled for 5 minutes to help relaxation, or a few drops of peppermint (*Mentha piperita*), black pepper (*Piper nigrum*), or rosemary (*Rosmarinus officinalis*) oil on a tissue, to revive and stimulate, might make long nights more tolerable.

Health professionals experience many emotional and disturbing scenes. This is always distressing. Often there is no way of ameliorating emotions until the next break, and frequently there are no breaks. However, a 2-minute hand "m" technique with some neroli (*Citrus aurantium* var. *amara*) could be a quick, effective, and therapeutic pick-me-up (Penson 1991). Just inhaling angelica, petitgrain, or rose could also be helpful. Touch and smell may be as old as the hills, but they can be deeply comforting.

Stress and Visitors

Visiting a sick relative is stressful. What to say? What to do? Where to sit? Frequently, the patient has insufficient energy to carry on a conversation, and the silences become longer and longer. The sicker the patient, the more stressed the visitors, and yet they come, sometimes long distances, if only for a few moments, to show that they care. Learning a simple hand or face "m" technique and using familiar smells can empower a visitor and make the patient feel wanted and cared for. No words are necessary; touch can say it all.

It does not matter how ill patients are, they still need this kind of compassion, especially from their loved ones. Research indicates the sicker the patients, the less likely they are to be touched by their relatives, who are frequently afraid to upset the complicated equipment around the patients. Research has also shown patients with the poorest prognosis, or who are the most acutely ill, are often touched least by the hospital staff (Ashworth 1984), although one of the most basic human, emotional needs is to feel physical contact (Weiss 1979).

Nurses, physicians, physical therapists, and others represent a large reservoir of professionals who touch other people throughout life—from pediatrics to the care of the elderly. For nurses in particular, aromatherapy offers a simple and acceptable way of care. Children can learn how to give a gentle aromatherapy "m" technique to elderly relatives, such as grandparents, in long-term care. Often a child visitor is restless and awkward. This kind of structured touch is easy for a child to learn. It is a simple and loving thing to do and costs little in terms of money, time, or energy, but it communicates a great deal. Learning the "m" technique can be empowering. It is the little things in life that are important, and in sickness the little things become more significant, including fresh air, natural light, plants, peace and quiet, kindly touch, and pleasant smells. Few of these occur in a hospital. Perhaps this is what Florence Nightingale meant when she said the "least fortunate were those who found themselves nearest to a hospital" (Landsdown 1994).

RELAXATION

Relaxation is not just the opposite of stress, it is the answer to stress, and is important to our quality of life and to our survival. However, sometimes it is difficult to "switch off," especially in a strange environment. The harder a person tries, the more elusive relaxation seems to become. Modern life is geared to doing, not being. What do you do? What do you want to do? These are the questions we use, not Who are you? or Who do you want to be? When people become sick, the ability to do is replaced with an enforced "being." This alone is stressful to people who have spent most of their lives in a doing mode. Dossey (1993) writes, "The most effective way to reverse illness is sometimes to focus primarily on being."

Health professionals frequently ask the impossible. "Just relax," nurses murmur before plunging hypodermic needles deep into the upper, outer quadrant. "Just relax," physicians suggest before probing the rectum with a finger. "Just breathe naturally," the voice murmurs as a gowned, masked man inserts a cardiac catheter into the femoral artery, aimed at the heart. What do health professionals actually do to help patients relax?

Relaxation brings with it manifold benefits both for patients and health professionals. Benson (1975) suggested many years ago that a relaxation break should replace a coffee break. Despite this, stress management is not emphasized enough in nurses' or physicians' training. However, there are programs developing to address this issue.

In a discussion of massage and aromatherapy as supportive therapies in health care, Sheena Hildebrand (1994) quotes from Wang Wei, who wrote in the 8th century, "Look in the perfumes of flowers and of nature for peace of mind and joy of life." Drury (1989) also wrote:

> Caring, loving, touching,
>
> Absence of connection to stress factors,
>
> Being a part of reality but
>
> Being centered in caring
>
> for the whole person, Functioning with a positive
>
> confident, loving presence.

Touch and relaxation

Many people find it pleasant and soothing to be stroked gently with something that smells pleasant. In *The Caring Touch* (1981), reference is made to Sidney Simon, who wrote of "skin hunger" and said "every human being comes into the world needing to be touched, and the need for skin contact persists until death, despite society's efforts to make us believe otherwise"(Pratt & Mason 1981). He also pointed out that "touch is quite distinct from sexual contact" and called for "touch nourishment strategies."

Touch presents a large body of reference that indicates a relaxation response. In *Palliative Care for Patients with Cancer*, Victor Brewer, a patient with advanced cancer, is quoted as describing the effects of touch as follows: "You unwind with the gentleness of the human touch. It would be marvelous if nurses could do it in hospital. . . . With touch, as soon as the hands go on, you know she's there, she's calm, she has time for you" (Penson 1991). The type of touch used in the "m" technique is different from regular massage. It is much lighter and slower and is not intended to address muscle tone, but to address soul tone. Please see the section in Chapter 8 on the "m" technique.

Relaxation and Pain Relief

Touch aids the release of endorphins. Some endorphins can block the release of substance P, one of the neurotransmitters involved in the sensation of pain. Some pain can also be alleviated by rubbing the skin. In the gate theory, rubbing the skin stimulates large-diameter afferent sensory fibers that excite interneurons, causing enkephalin release (Turk & Nash 1993). Enkephalin release inhibits the release of substance P from activated unmyelinated C fibers. This prevents T cell activation and closes the pain gate (Fields 1997). The pain most often relieved by massage is chronic pain that is poorly localized (Sofaer & Foord 1993). This type of pain can be associated with many chronic conditions and with postoperative recovery, although not with immediate postoperative care. Although deep massage is contraindicated following recent surgery, the gentleness of the "m" technique around the affected area is highly appropriate and is a very useful adjunct to pain control.

Some fragrances have deeply relaxing effects. Japanese research has shown contingent negative variation (CNV), namely the upward shift in the brain waves recorded by electrodes attached to the scalp, occurs in situations in which subjects are expecting something to happen. CNV alters in response to odor. Following experiments with diazepam and caffeine that produced central nervous system (CNS) depression or stimulation, Torii et al (1988) found lavender had a depressing effect and jasmine had a stimulating effect on the CNS. Further investigation revealed that although odor had an effect on the brain, it did not appear to affect physiological functions. Even in individuals who have no sense of smell (anosmia), a chemical reaction to odors occurs in the brain if the olfactory nerve is intact.

In conclusion, touch and smell are two powerful relaxation tools available to health professionals. It would be a shame not to use them.

Stress, Relaxation, and Psychoneuroimmunology

The American physicians Bernie Siegal and Larry Dossey have done much to raise awareness of the importance of psychoneuroimmunology (PNI). The term first became popular in 1986 with the publication of Siegal's book, *Love, Medicine and Miracles* (1986). In the book he wrote of patients who had survived cancer. He calls them "exceptional cancer patients." In one famous address to eminent, orthodox physicians (many of whom were openly hostile to his views), he read aloud from the novel *Lady Chatterley's Lover*. He read for some time, until the conservatively dressed men in front of him were fidgeting and red-faced. Then he paused, closed the book, and said quietly "Now then, gentlemen, don't tell me that your mind has not affected your body!"

PNI is a medical subspeciality that involves the study of the connection between the mind (*psycho*), the brain (*neuro*), and the body's ability to defend itself against disease (*immune*). Humans do have the ability to affect their wellness or disease-susceptibility through the power of thought. This finding has not been accepted readily within orthodox medicine. Indeed, Siegal quotes from Dostoevsky at the beginning of his book: "A new philosophy, a way of life, is not given for nothing. It has to be paid for dearly and is only acquired with much patience and great effort." Perhaps this quote is as relevant to aromatherapy as it is to PNI.

Norman Cousins, a patient, decided to apply the principle of PNI to himself. Diagnosed with ankylosing spondylitis, he was told his spinal connective tissue was dissolving (Cousins 1979). A regimen of medication consisting of 26 aspirin and 12 phenylbutazone tablets daily resulted in hives all over his body but no pain relief. Appalled by his hospital treatment (one day he had to give four separate samples of blood for the same test because the pathology laboratory was in chaos), he checked out of the hospital and into a hotel. Cousins knew pain could be affected by attitude, and he instinctively chose to try laughter instead of medication.

It was a brave and desperate move, but one that showed him 10 minutes of genuine belly laughter had an anesthetic effect and gave him 2 hours of pain-free sleep. Wanting "real" proof, Cousins took blood tests that confirmed his erythrocyte sedimentation rate fell by at least five points following laughter therapy. Better still, the effect was cumulative. It seems laughter was stimulating the production of endorphins, which resulted in a profound reduction of his joint inflammation. Bolstered by this discovery, he refused to let his friends see him unless they could bring a new joke, cartoon, or film to make him laugh. Cousins understood how he felt affected how he was, and that included his illness.

It would be interesting to see if laughter could become a commodity provided by hospitals. True, some get-well cards can be slightly amusing, but laughter therapy, although effective, is not an approach easily incorporated into either a Western medical model or the Western temperament. Illness is serious business, and in the private sector, serious illness means serious money and long faces. No one wants to be seen laughing! However Wilde McCormick (1990), in her book on changing one's life through self-help psychotherapy, advises "Make sure you laugh every day."

The relationship between an emotional reaction brought on by an illness and the survival rate of a patient is highlighted by Fiore (1979), a patient with cancer. Health professionals are in a unique position to encourage PNI, because "care givers have the power to be dispiriting or inspiring to their patients" (Young 1990). Yet how many health professionals actually use this power to encourage patients to draw on their own self-healing abilities?

Aromatherapy and PNI

Aromatherapy is a perfect way of utilizing PNI. Many patients find themselves lulled by repeated stroking movements, which encourage a series of endorphins into play. The pleasant smell of an essential oil will enhance this effect. Together, smell and touch can produce a synergy of social, physical, psychological, and neurological interactions in the patient. The most common comment made by patients is how relaxing they find the treatment and how the feeling of relaxation remains for several days. This may be highly relevant. Although it is recognized that smell is instant, the effect of smell wears off very quickly as olfactory neurons become inured to the odor. Perhaps by administering the "smell" transdermally, a slow-release smell that produces a longer-lasting effect could be achieved.

Antoni et al (1990) wrote relaxation "may influence the immune function of those patients with HIV, and retard disease progression among early HIV-1 seropositive individuals." Supportive personal relationships improved the immune function of women with breast cancer (Kiecolt-Glaser & Glaser 1993). Dean Ornish's study on reversing heart disease was based on diet, exercise, and stress management. He wrote he was "increasingly convinced that the root of chronic stress is a sense of isolation—from oneself, from others, and from something spiritual" (Ornish 1991).

Farrow (1990) used massage in an acute medical ward. She found it reduced anxiety in patients receiving morphine-pump therapy for pain during the period when the pump was being changed, and it enabled a teenager to cope better with her disfiguring postoperative ileostomy tubes and drains. Tisserand and Balacs (1988) wrote about the "emotionally uplifting and comforting oils" that can be used with cancer patients. King (1993) wrote about the ability of odor impressions to "produce effects partly through mood changes" and concludes "fragrance provides a useful adjunct for relaxation and has considerable potential for future development."

Birchall (1990), writing for the *New Scientist,* asked whether aromatherapy matches the potency of Valium and Librium, two drugs often used for stress, stating many of aromatherapy's claims are now being validated by research. In fact, as early as May 1988, the *International Journal of Aromatherapy* bore the headline "Lavender beats benzodiazepines"(Tisserand 1988).

Reed and Norfolk (1993) found 36 of 38 patients experienced a feeling of relaxation following aromatherapy. This British study was carried out by two midwives who were investigating whether lavender might reduce pain during childbirth. Patients took baths with five drops of lavender during labor. There was no control to this study. However, the results suggested aromatherapy did alter pain perception in 30 women, and 36 women felt their ability to relax during labor was enhanced. Stevenson (1992) concluded 100% of patients found the effects of a foot massage with essential oil relaxing. She was investigating the effects of neroli (*Citrus aurantium flos*) on 100 patients in London's Middlesex Hospital cardiac intensive-care unit following open-heart surgery. This was a controlled, randomized study using a modified Spielberger State Trait Anxiety Inventory for Adults State Evaluation Questionnaire to measure pain, anxiety, tension, calmness, rest, and relaxation. Physiological measurement showed a decrease in respiration, suggesting an increased parasympathetic response. This conclusion was supported by the psychological measurements. Stevenson showed patients who received a neroli foot massage felt their anxiety decreased more than the patients who received a foot massage without neroli essential oil.

Woolfson and Hewitt (1992) found 91% of patients experienced a reduction in their heart rate of between 11 and 15 beats per minute following aromatherapy massage. This study was carried out in the intensive-care unit of Royal Sussex County Hospital in the United Kingdom. A total of 36 patients were allocated to one of three groups: those massaged with essential oils, those massaged without essential oils, and a control group who just rested. The results of this study appear to agree with Stevenson's findings that massage with an essential oil, in this case lavender, was more effective in reducing stress than massage without an essential oil.

Dunn et al (1995) found 122 patients felt anxiety reduction following aromatherapy massage with lavender in an intensive-care unit. Dunn led one of the first formal trials to be conducted in a hospital, which paved the way for further trials. Burns and Blamey (1994) studied 585 women in labor to determine whether aromatherapy with any of 10 essential oils could reduce anxiety, increase contractions, and reduce pain. The oils used were lavender, clary sage, peppermint, eucalyptus, mandarin, chamomile, jasmine, rose, frankincense, and lemon. The study was set up when the two investigators discovered aromatherapy was part of the curriculum and examination syllabus for all student midwives in Germany. Their results showed much satisfaction expressed by the mothers and the delivery team concerning the reduction of stress with all of the essential oils used. The study was not randomized or controlled but was an important investigation and has led the way for the use of aromatherapy in other maternity units. A further analysis of 8058 mothers who had received aromatherapy between 1990 and 1998 indicated more than 50% of mothers found it helpful for relaxation (Burns et al 2000).

More than 10 years ago Wise (1989) wrote, "Aromatherapy helps to take the anxiety out of being in hospital and quickens the patient's return to self-care." Whether patients choose drops of essential oil on a pillow or an aromatic "m" technique, there is no doubt that aromatherapy as a method of stress therapy is a valid and important part of health care.

Spontaneous Remission

Finally, no chapter that refers to PNI would be complete without a mention of spontaneous remission. The Institute of Noetic Sciences was founded in 1973 by astronaut Edgar D. Mitchell, following his experience of walking on the moon. It is a research foundation and educational institution and has 30,000 members worldwide. The word *noetic* comes from the Greek word *nous,* meaning mind, intelligence, and transcendental knowing.

In 1993, the Institute of Noetic Sciences and the Fetzer Institute published a book documenting the results of a 10-year research program on the healing response. Their program was "based on the belief that the ability of the physician to promote health and to heal the sick in the future may be as dependent on the deeper understanding of the mind-body relationship as on the development of new technologies."

Their study revealed a large body of evidence of extraordinary healing, including regression of normally fatal tumors, with no currently available scientific explanation (O'Regan & Hirschberg 1993). This discovery was not new to medicine. Nearly a century earlier Handley (1909) wrote in the *British Medical Journal* that "the recorded cases of natural repair of cancer, far from being anomalous and exceptional, merely illustrate more strikingly than usual the natural laws which govern every case of the disease." The study carried out by the Institute of Noetic Sciences was the largest investigation of spontaneous remission to date. It concluded, "The evidence suggests this kind of healing can be triggered by a variety of stimuli, diverse in nature, including signals, suggestions and guidance from the physical, mental and/or spiritual realm of every individual."

Sadly, Brendan O'Regan, the visionary responsible for the program, died in 1992 before the study was completed. Although a great portion of the study was completed in 1990, more than 300 additional references to spontaneous remission from cancer and other diseases (which were published in medical journals between 1990 and 1992) have been collated subsequently.

There is no suggestion that aromatherapy could result in spontaneous remission, but aromatherapy does have a profound impact on the mind-body link. It would be interesting to measure immune levels before and after an aromatherapy treatment. To quote the Institute of Noetic Sciences, "We are at the threshold of a new field of inquiry." Ralph Waldo Emerson wrote that "thought is the blossom, language the bud, action the fruit behind it." I hope this chapter will serve as the bud to encourage a little fruit!

REFERENCES

Anthony G, Thibodeau G. 1983. Textbook of Anatomy and Physiology. London: CV Mosby.

Antoni M, Fletcher M, Goldstein D et al. 1990. Psychoneuroimmunology and HIV-1. Journal of Consulting and Clinical Psychology. 58(1) 38-49.

Ashworth P. 1984. Staff-patient communication in coronary care units. Journal of Advanced Nursing. 9(1) 35-41.

Barasch M. 1993. The Healing Path. New York: Putnam.

Bennett G. 1987. The Wound and the Physician. London: Secker & Warburg.

Benson H. 1975. The Relaxation Response. New York: Avon.

Birchall A. 1990. A whiff of happiness. New Scientist. 127(1731) 44-47.

Burns E, Blamey C. 1994. Soothing scents in childbirth. International Journal of Aromatherapy. 6(1) 24-28.

Burns E, Blamey C, Ersser S et al. 2000. An investigation into the use of aromatherapy in intrapartum midwifery practice. Journal of Alternative & Complementary Medicine. 6(2) 141-147.

Clark E, Montague S. 1993. The nature of stress and its implications for nursing practice. In Hinchcliff S, Norman S, Schober J (eds.), Nursing Practice and Health Care. London: Edward Arnold, 214-247.

Cohen S, Tyrrell D, Smith A. 1991. Psychological stress and susceptibility to the common cold. New England Journal of Medicine. 325(9) 606-612.

Cousins N. 1979. Anatomy of an Illness as Perceived by a Patient. New York: WW Norton.

Dossey L. 1993. Healing Words. San Francisco: Harper.

Drury M. 1989. Caring. In McGuire C (ed.), Visions of Nursing. Sedona, AZ: Light Technology, 44.

Dunn C, Sleep J, Collett D. 1995. Sensing an improvement: an experimental study to evaluate the use of aromatherapy, massage and periods of rest in an intensive-care unit. Journal of Advanced Nursing. 21(1) 34-40.

Farrow J. 1990. Massage therapy and nursing care. Nursing Standard. 4(17) 26-28.

Fields H. 1997. Pain: Anatomy and Physiology. Journal of Alternative and Complementary Medicine 3 (suppl. 1). 541-546.

Fiore N. 1979. Fighting cancer: one patient's perspective. New England Journal of Medicine. 300(21) 284-289.

Frazier S, Moser D, Riegel B et al. 2002. Critical care nurses' assessment of patients' anxiety: reliance on physiological and behavioral parameters. American Journal of Critical Care. 11(1) 57-64.

Garg A, Chren M, Sands L et al. 2001. Psychological stress perturbs epidermal permeability barrier homeostasis. Archives of Dermatology. 137(1) 53-59.

Handley W. 1909. The natural cure of cancer. British Medical Journal. 582-589.

Hay L, Jamieson M, Ormerod D. 1998. Randomized trial of aromatherapy: successful treatment for alopecia areata. Archives of Dermatology 134(11) 1349-1352.

Hildebrand S. 1994. Massage and aromatherapy. In Wells R (ed.), Wells' Supportive Therapies in Health Care. London: Bailliere Tindall, 110-111.

Jamison R, Parris W, Maxson W. 1987. Psychological factors influencing recovery from outpatient surgery. Behavioural Research Therapies. 25(1) 31-37.

Kiecolt-Glaser J, Glaser R. 1993. Mind and immunity. In Goleman D, Curin J (eds.), Mind-Body Medicine. New York: Consumer Reports Books, 39-65.

King J. 1993. Have the scent to relax. World Medicine. 29-31.

Landsdown R. 1994. Living longer? Qualitative survival. Journal of the Royal Society of Medicine. 87:636.

Layne O, Yudofsky S. 1971. Postoperative psychosis in cardiotomy patients. New England Journal of Medicine. 284(10) 518-520.

LeDouz J. 1996. The Emotional Brain. New York: Simon & Schuster.

Lehrner J, Eckersberger C, Walla P et al. 2000. Ambient odor of orange in a dental office reduces anxiety and improves mood in female patients. Physiology & Behavior. 71(1-2) 83-86.

Linn B, Linn M, Klimas N. 1988. Effects of psychophysical stress on surgical outcomes. Psychosomatic Medicine. 50(3) 230-244.

Lynch J. 1979. The broken heart—the medical consequences of loneliness. San Francisco: Harper-Row.

Muruzzella J, Sicurella N. 1960. Antibacterial activity of essential oil vapors. Journal of the American Pharmaceutical Association (Scientific Edition). 49(11) 692-695.

Ng V, Koh D, Mok B et al. 2002. Stressful life events of dental students and salivary diomarker (abstract). International Journal of Immunopathology and Pharmacology 15(2) 5.

Nixon P. 1976. The human function curve. Practitioner. 217(76) 769, 935-944.

O'Brien J, Moser D, Riegel B et al. 2001. Comparison of anxiety assessments between clinicians and patients with acute myocardial infarction in cardiac critical care units. American Journal of Critical Care. 10(2) 97-103.

O'Regan B, Hirshberg C. 1993. Spontaneous Remission. Sausalito, CA: Institute of Noetic Sciences.

Ornish D. 1991. Reversing heart disease through diet, exercise and stress management. Journal of the American Dietetic Association. 91(2) 162-165.

Pelletier K. 1992. Mind-body health: research, clinical and policy implications. American Journal of Health Promotion. 6(5) 345-348.

Pelletier K. 1992a. Mind as Healer, Mind as Slayer. New York: Delta.

Penson J. 1991. Complementary therapies. In Penson J, Fisher R (eds.), Palliative Care for People with Cancer. London: Edward Arnold, 233-246.

Pert C. 1997. Molecules of emotion. New York: Scribner.

Pibran K. 1976. Consciousness and the brain. New York: Plenum Press.

Pitts F. 1969. The biochemistry of anxiety. Scientific American. 220(2) 69-75.

Pratt J, Mason A. 1981. The Caring Touch. London: Heyden.

Quinn J. 1993. Psychoimmunologic effects of therapeutic touch on practitioners and recently bereaved recipients. Advanced Nursing Science. 15(5) 13-26.

Rahe R. 1975. Epidemiological studies of life change and illness. International Journal of Psychiatry in Medicine. 6(2) 133-146.

Redd W, Manne S. 1995. Using aroma to reduce distress during magnetic resonance imaging. In Gilbert A (ed.), Compendium of Olfactory Research 1982-1994. New York: Olfactory Research Fund Ltd., 47-52.

Reed L, Norfolk L. 1993. Aromatherapy in midwifery. International Journal of Alternative and Complementary Medicine. 11:15-17.

Rimmer L. 1998. The clinical use of aromatherapy in the reduction of stress. Home Healthcare Nurse. 16(2) 123-126.

Roberts R. 1991. Preventing PDD (post-pump delirium) after surgery. Nursing. 4(27) 28-31.

Schulz H, Jobert M, Hubner W. 1998. The quantitative EEG as a screening instrument to identify sedative effects of single doses of plant extracts in comparison to diazepam. Phytomedicine. 5(6) 449-458.

Siegal B. 1986. Love, Medicine and Miracles. New York: Arrow.

Sofaer B, Foord J. 1993. Care of the person in pain. In Hinchcliff S, Norman S, Schrober J. (eds.), Nursing Practice and Health Care. London: Edward Arnold, 374–401.

Stevenson C. 1992. Orange blossom evaluation. International Journal of Aromatherapy. 4(3) 22-24.

Sugano H, Sato N. 1991. Psychophysiological studies of fragrance. Chemical Senses. 16:183-184.

Sylvia C, Novak W. 1997. A Change of Heart. Boston: Little, Brown & Co.

Tasev T, Toleva P, Balabanova V. 1969. The neuro-psychic effect of Bulgarian rose, lavender and geranium. Folia Medica. 11(5) 307-317.

Tisserand R. 1988. Lavender beats benzodiazepines. International Journal of Aromatherapy. 1(1) 1-2.

Tisserand R, Balacs T. 1988. Essential oil therapy for cancer. International Journal of Aromatherapy. 1(4) 20-25.

Torii S, Fukuda H, Kanemoto H et al. 1988. Contingent negative variation (CNV) and the psychological effects of odor in perfumery. In Van Toller S, Dodd G (eds.), Perfumery: The Psychology and Biology of Fragrance. London: Chapman & Hall, 107-120.

Turk D, Nash J. 1993. Chronic pain: New ways to cope. In Goleman D and Gurin J (eds.). Mind/Body Medicine. New York: Consumer Reports. 111-131.

Van der Does A. 1989. Patients' and nurses' rating of pain and anxiety during burn wound care. Pain. 39(1) 95-101.

Walsh D. 1996. Using aromatherapy in the management of psoriasis. Nursing Standard. 11(13-15) 53-56.

Weiss S. 1979. The language of touch. Nursing Research. 28(2) 76-80.

Wilde McCormick E. 1990. Change for the Better. London: Unwin-Hyman Ltd.

Wilde McCormick E. 1992. Healing the Heart. London: Optima Books.

Wilkinson G. 1991. Stress: another chimera? British Medical Journal. 302(3) 191-192.

Wilson-Barnett J, Carrigy A. 1978. Factors influencing patients' emotional reactions to hospitalization. Journal of Advanced Nursing. 3(3) 221-229.

Wise R. 1989. Alternative therapies: Flower power. Nursing Times. 85(22) 45-47.

Woolfson A, Hewitt D. 1992. Intensive aromacare. International Journal of Aromatherapy. 4(2) 12-13.

Young S. 1990. The exceptional cancer patient support group: coping with cancer. In Clements S, Martin E (eds.), Nursing and Holistic Wellness. Dubuque, IA: Kendall/Hunt Publishing, 233-247.

14

CARDIOLOGY

Whatever the physiological problem with the heart, its function is affected by what each individual asks of their heart in terms of effort. This is determined by the person we are, by the way we live within our own body and by the relationship we do or do not make with it.

Elizabeth McCormick (1997)

Alterations in mental status are common among patients in a cardiac intensive-care unit. These changes can be due to medication, brain trauma, or metabolic function (Beauchamp et al 2000). However, continuous stress, insomnia, sensory deprivation, and loss of privacy can also cause changes in mental state. These all occur in an intensive-care unit. The heart is often described as the seat of emotion, and aromatherapy can play an important role in assisting patients as they come to terms with feelings that may have been blocked. Aromatherapy can also help them cope with a highly stressful situation. While aromatherapy cannot replace a damaged valve or repair an atrial septal defect, it can be useful for reducing the stress that surrounds a heart attack and may reduce the period of recovery following a heart attack or surgery. Aromatherapy is used in some medical and surgical cardiac units, and many of the essential oils have a history of being supportive to the heart, as well as being generally relaxing.

Several cardiac conditions can benefit from aromatherapy: borderline hypertension, anxiety associated with myocardial infarction, and postpump depression or delirium (PPD).

BORDERLINE HYPERTENSION

Hypertension and its complications affect an estimated 50 million Americans, 30% of whom are unaware they have hypertension. Only 70% of those who are aware of their condition receive treatment (Manger & Gifford 2001). Approximately 35,000 Americans die each year from conditions directly associated with hypertension. Hypertension, an abnormal rise in blood pressure, occurs when the arterioles become constricted, reducing the ability of the blood to flow and making the heart work harder. Ninety percent of all cases of hypertension are essential hypertension, which means there is no apparent reason. However, there are some associated risk factors: obesity, smoking, alcohol consumption, a diet high in fat or salt, gender (men are more likely to have hypertension than women), race (African Americans are more likely to develop hypertension than any other group), and genetics. Secondary hypertension is defined as an elevation in blood pressure caused by a preexisting condition such as coarctation of the aorta, kidney disease, or thyroid malfunction. However, Samuel Mann, a professor of clinical medicine at Cornell University, believes emotion may play a major role in hypertension (Mann 1997).

An elevated blood-pressure reading is above 140/90. Antihypertensive drugs appear to be effective at reducing mortality and morbidity in the elderly (Mulrow et al 1997). However, the British National Health Service Center for Reviews and Dissemination at the University of York (1999) reported all the main classes of antihypertensive drugs are associated with adverse side effects, although the majority of symptoms were mild, such as dizziness, headache, or rash. In addition, the report continued, the older the patient, the more severe the side effects become, including arrhythmias or renal dysfunction. Both the older types of beta-blocker and diuretic drugs and the newer angiotensin-converting enzyme (ACE) inhibitors and calcium-channel blockers had side effects. Instead, light exercise, change in diet, relaxation, and meditation are often encouraged to reduce borderline blood pressure.

Aromatherapy can help as an adjunctive relaxing therapy, and some essential oils are thought to help reduce borderline hypertension. Thymol isolated from essential oil of *Trachyspermum ammi* reduced the blood pressure of anesthetized rats (Aftab et al 1995). This herb has a history of being used in Pakistan to reduce hypertension. However, in this study quite large amounts of thymol were given (1-10 mg/kg) by intraperitoneal injection. The authors postulate the hypotensive effect of thymol was due to its calcium-channel-blocking ability. Thymol is also found in *Thymus vulgaris* (common thyme), an inexpensive essential oil. Thymol is a phenol and as such is not something that immediately comes to mind for hypertension, as phenols are generally thought to be stimulating.

Tisserand and Balacs (1995) state "it is extremely unlikely that an essential oil could exacerbate hypertension or hypotension." Guba (2000), an Australian clinical aromatherapist, completed an extensive search of the available literature and concluded that an essential oil was unlikely to elevate high blood pressure and many aromatherapy cautions regarding essential oils and hypertension were based on myth.

A recent study carried out on human subjects did show inhaled rosemary increased systolic and diastolic measurements, but the effects were transient, lasting only a few minutes (Saeki & Shihora 2001). The same study found lavender reduced systolic pressure, again for a short period of time. Other essential oils such as geranium and clary sage have shown measurable hypotensive effect in animal studies. Essential oils, like herbs, appear to be adaptogenic; they balance the body when it is out of balance. Adaptogens constitute a novel class of metabolic regulators that can have different psychological and physiological effects depending on the requirement of the host (Panossian et al 1999).

Despite a lack of evidence, many schools of aromatherapy suggest avoiding stimulant essential oils such as *Rosmarinus officinalis* (rosemary), *Mentha piperita* (peppermint), or spike lavender(*Lavandula latifolia*) with any patient who has hypertension. These essential oils will be discussed individually.

O'Brien (1997) reported on her experiences with the hypertensive effects of rosemary in elderly, long-term-care patients suffering transient hypotension as a side effect of antidepressants. Patients inhaled two drops of rosemary for 5 minutes before getting up from a seated position. Blood pressure was measured before and after getting up. A control group was given carrier oil with no known pharmacological properties to smell. Blood pressures of all patients had been recorded since their admission to the hospital, prior to beginning the antidepressant medication. The number of instances in which a subject fell down immediately after rising from a sitting position (presumably as a result of hypotension) was compared with falls within the same timeframe the previous year. The number of falls dropped by more than 50%. Rosemary did not appear to have any hypertensive effect on normal blood pressure.

Rosemary was also found to have pharmacological stimulatory effects in animals by Kovar et al (1987). However, rosemary was shown to have slight anxiety-reducing effects in a study at the University of Wolverhampton. Unfortunately, the botanical name and chemotype of the rosemary used were not stated (Morris et al 1995).

Peppermint is traditionally considered to have stimulating properties. Menthol-flavored cigarettes and peppermint confections have both been responsible for atrial fibrillation in cardiac patients prone to that condition who were previously stabilized on quinidine (Thomas 1962). l-menthol was found to dilate systemic blood vessels when given intravenously (Agshikar & Abraham 1957). It is extremely unlikely that inhaled peppermint would have any negative effect on patients with high blood pressure, and peppermint is very useful for nausea. However, peppermint has a pervasive smell and is difficult to tolerate for several hours. Perez-Raya et al (1990) found two other mints, *Mentha rotundifolia* and *Mentha longifolia*, which grow wild in Spain, enhanced sodium barbitone-induced sleep in rats.

Spike lavender (*Lavandula latifolia*) has a history of being an expectorant and mycolytic and was found useful in upper respiratory-tract infection (Charron 1997). It is also thought to be a stimulant. Certainly a few drops of this camphorous-smelling lavender is more likely to clear the sinuses than induce sleep; however, there is no record of spike lavender increasing blood pressure.

Freund (1999) conducted a small pilot study on 13 patients with borderline hypertension. The age range was 21-71 years, and the group included five males and eight females. Eleven patients were more than 15 pounds overweight. Baseline blood pressure was taken with each patient in a supine position. Patients rated their stress level based on a visual analog. Subjects were asked to inhale five drops of ylang ylang essential oil for 15 minutes. Blood pressure was remeasured, and the stress level recording was reassessed. The same group received a control aroma (carrier oil with no pharmacological effect) at a different time. The ylang ylang (*Cananga odorata*) group experienced a 50% greater drop in systolic and diastolic pressure than did the control group. The stress visual analog also indicated the ylang ylang group felt a 50% greater reduction in stress. Ylang ylang has an anecdotal history of being used to reduce blood pressure and is used by British midwives to help reduce hypertension in pregnancy.

Essential oils that could help reduce hypertension are ylang ylang, Roman chamomile, true lavender, and clary sage. Neroli, sandalwood, spikenard, and sweet marjoram might also have advantageous effects. Whatever the choice of essential oil, it is important to ask patients which aromas remind them of pleasant memories and use those. Gentle touch is one of the most soothing actions that can be offered another human being in distress. Holism is about being present for the patient. Aromatherapy can put the heart back into health care.

ANXIETY AND MYOCARDIAL INFARCTION

Acute myocardial infarction (known more commonly as a heart attack) is the leading cause of death in the Western world with one million deaths each year (Rogers et al 1994). It is also a leading reason for hospitalization in the United States (Hill et al 1992). Approximately 90% of those who reach a hospital survive (Hill et al 1992). Twenty to 30% of the cost associated with acute myocardial infarction is related to the length of time a patient stays in the coronary-care unit (Sgura et al 2001). The main symptom of acute myocardial infarction is defined by the World Health Organization as intense, prolonged, or intolerable chest pain necessitating hospitalization. Fifty percents of deaths caused by myocardial infarction occur within 2 hours of the onset of symptoms (Hope et al 1993). In the United Kingdom, the number of deaths from heart attacks each year is equal to the number of babies born (McCormick 1993). Standard treatment is primary reperfusion therapy and the judicious use of aspirin, beta blockers, angiotensin-converting enzyme (ACE) inhibitors, and glyoprotein antagonists. These have reduced the length of time patients spend in a high-dependency unit (Sgura et al 2001).

Despite analgesics and sedatives, many patients are anxious when they arrive in a coronary-care unit. Their arrival at the hospital is usually unexpected, so they come unprepared. Unattended business meetings and unanswered e-mail are difficult to forget, and patients find it a challenge to switch off their worries. Anxiety can extend infarction areas or precipitate further arrhythmias (Summers Dunnington et al 1988). Anxious patients are more likely to experience severe or chronic psychological distress. Rowe (1989) discovered patients' anxieties tend to be focused on their own illness. The severity of the infarction and how close to death patients perceive themselves to be will influence the level of psychological distress they experience. Vlay and Fricchione (1985) reported on heart-attack patients' emotional disturbances, which are often expressed as depression, anger, frustration, and fear. Mood has a powerful influence on prognosis after acute myocardial infarction (Petty 2000).

Aromatherapy attempts to alleviate these feelings and to reduce anxiety. Because these patients have constant monitoring and/or visitors, it is important to select essential oils that will be acceptable to all those who will smell them. Aromas of citrus and herbs are usually acceptable. Gould et al (1973) reported on the relaxing cardiac effects of chamomile tea on a group of 12 hospitalized patients who were undergoing cardiac catheterization. They found there was a small but significant rise in the group's mean brachial-artery pressure, so there was some hemodynamic change but essentially no cardiac effect. However, the scientists were more struck that 10 of the 12 patients fell into a deep sleep within 10 minutes of drinking the tea. Sleeping is a rarity during cardiac catheterization. Patients had not been premedicated and received no other sedation during the procedure.

Yamada et al (1996) found chamomile essential oil reduced stress-induced increases in plasma adrenocorticotropic-hormone levels in rats and concluded essential oil of Roman chamomile might be useful against stress in humans. Finally, Avollone et al (1996) studied an aqueous extract of German chamomile flowers and found it behaved as both central and peripheral benzodiazepine receptor ligands, with anxiolytic effects. Viola et al (1995) identified the anxiolytic compound as apigenin. German and Roman chamomile are different essential oils with different chemistries. Roman may be more conducive to use in a cardiac unit as it has a more pleasant aroma. Table 14-1 lists essential oils used following myocardial infarction along with the studies that have been done on their effects.

Table 14-1 ✿ *Anxiolytic Essential Oils for Use Following Myocardial Infarction*

Common Name	Botanical Name	Reference
Melissa	*Melissa officinalis*	Wagner & Sprinkmeyer 1973 Buchbauer et al 1993
Lavender	*Lavandula angustifolia*	Bauhbauer et al 1991, Woolfson & Hewitt 1991
Roman chamomile	*Chamaemelum nobile*	Rossi et al 1988
Neroli	*Citrus aurantium flos*	Jager et al 1992
Rosewood	*Aniba rosaeodora*	Nacht & Ting 1921
Marjoram	*Origanum majorana*	Nacht & Ting 1921
German chamomile	*Matricaria recutita*	Viola et al 1995
Rose	*Rosa damascena*	Nacht & Ting 1921, Buchbauer et al 1994

POSTPUMP DEPRESSION/DELIRIUM

Alterations in mental status are common following bypass surgery (Beauchamp et al 2000). Up to 75% of patients have deterioration in performance on neuropsychiatric tests (Mahanna et al 1996), and up to 32% develop Postpump depression/delirium (PPD) (Roach et al 1996). Glick et al (1996) suggest PPD is often not recorded, so it is difficult to analyze how many patients are affected. A 2001 article in the *New York Times* suggested depression is more common after bypass surgery than other types of surgery (Epstein 2001) and occurs in 30%-75% of patients. The article quotes Dr. R. Scott Mitchell, a cardiovascular surgeon at Stanford, and Dr. Roy John, professor of psychiatry and director of the brain research laboratories at New York University Medical Center. Dr. John suggests atherosclerotic plaques in the aorta could become dislodged during surgery and bombard the brain, or that the anesthesia and cooling used during the operation could alter brain chemistry. A doctor at one British university suggests PPD (delirium) could be caused by sensory imbalance or disorientation (Lidster 2001).

Danilowicz and Gabriel (2001) compared two matched groups of patients from the National Heart Institute and found the incidence of PPD (delirium) was higher among men than women and higher in those who were not able to communicate in English. The study emphasizes the importance of communication. PPD is thought to play a major role in the development of sternal instability (Bimmel et al 2001), which has a major influence on postoperative recovery after bypass surgery.

Many patients arriving in a critical-care unit have undergone elective surgery, so they have been prepared for the ordeal that awaits them. British psychologist McCormick (1993) suggests "preparation by the feeling heart for the worker heart's surgery is essential." Many surgeons, including Mehmet Oz, MD, at Columbia Presbyterian Medical Center in New York, believe she is right. Patients who are prepared are better able to cope with their condition postoperatively (Roberts 1991), as fear of surgery is a factor that can strongly influence a patient's emotional response to hospitalization (Wilson-Barnett & Carrigy 1978). Of all the operations performed, open-heart surgery is possibly the most feared.

The symptoms of PPD are hyperventilation, tachycardia, auditory hallucinations, disorientation, and paranoid delusions (Layne & Yudofsky 1971). The symptoms are distressing for the patient, their relatives, and for those who care for them. The Rancho Los Amigos Cognitive Scale lists eight different states of consciousness (Herndon 1997). They range from no response, through confused-inappropriate, to purposeful appropriate and could be a very good tool to use in measuring PPD.

Although there are several theories concerning the pathogenesis of PPD, nothing is clear. It is thought that older patients, those undergoing aortic valve replacement, and male patients are more at risk. However, Layne and Yudofsky (1971) found a reduction in postoperative psychosis was achieved in 50% of patients by conducting a preoperative psychiatric interview. This interview allowed and encouraged patients to ask questions about their disease and surgery and to discuss openly any worries they had (Layne & Yudofsky 1971). Preoperative psychological preparation is now recognized as being important not just for the patient, but also for the relatives who will be supporting the patient postoperatively (Roberts 1991). Discussing current or potential marital or relationship problems can help indicate which patients are more likely to succumb to PPD (Egerton & Kay 1964). Any illness will force a relationship to change, and open-heart surgery will certainly test the strength of every relationship.

Utilizing the preparation time, aromatherapy can set a safe, gentle pattern which, when repeated postoperatively, could affect the patient positively through learned memory. If patients feel relaxation and pleasure when they receive a foot, hand, or face "m" technique with a favorite aroma preoperatively, chances are they will feel the same relaxation and pleasure when the aromatherapy is repeated postoperatively. Table 14-2 lists essential oils that have been used to prevent and/or treat PPD, along with the studies undertaken to determine the possible benefits.

Table 14-2 ✿ *Essential Oils for the Possible Reduction of PPD*

Common Name	Botanical Name	Reference
Neroli	*Citrus aurantium flos*	Jager et al 1992, Stevensen 1994
Angelica	*Angelica archangelica* (root)	Franchomme & Penoel 1991
Lavender	*Lavandula angustifolia*	Dunn et al 1995
Rosewood	*Aniba rosaeodora*	Nacht & Ting 1921
Marjoram	*Origanum majorana*	Nacht & Ting 1921
Rose	*Rosa damascena*	Nacht & Ting 1921, Rovesti & Columbo 1973
Lemon	*Citrus limon*	Komori et al 1995
Bergamot	*Citrus bergamia*	Komori et al 1995
Geranium	*Pelargonium graveolens*	Morris et al 1995
Roman chamomile	*Anthemis nobilis*	Rossi et al 1988, Moate 1995
Melissa	*Melissa officinalis*	Wagner & Sprinkmeyer 1973
Sandalwood	*Santalum album*	Kikuchi et al 1995

Komori et al (1995) demonstrated the positive effects of lemon oil (*Citrus limon*) mixed with bergamot, sweet orange, and cis-4-hexanol on depressed inpatients who were exposed to the fragrance for 4 to 11 weeks while their antidepressant medication was systematically reduced. By the end of the period, nine of the 12 patients no longer needed antidepressant medication. Their levels of urinary cortisol and dopamine became lower and were normalized with the citrus aroma. The authors posited that inappropriate use of antidepressants could weaken immune function.

Moate (1995) wrote of a patient suffering from depression who was treated with Largactil and Sertraline (a tricyclic) but found profound relief from aromatherapy massage using lavender and chamomile. In another study, Sano et al (1998) showed essence of cedarwood produced sedative effects on rats and reduced the time needed to achieve deeper stages of sleep in napping humans.

Templeton (2002) carried out a small study to investigate the effects of bergamot as an antidepressant. Ten volunteers from a natural-health clinic responded to an advertisement to take part in a study on depression. Each agreed to take six aromatic baths and six baths with no aroma. Subjects were to remain in the bath for 20 minutes. While the study was self-monitoring, several subjects commented on how this simple technique had empowered them. One wrote, "I experienced an overwhelming feeling of tranquility."

Vogley (2002) used bergamot in her study on anxiety in a psychiatric unit for the elderly. A psychiatric nurse assessed each patient each morning for 10 days and scored their level of anxiety on a scale of zero to 10. Then, bergamot was diffused and the patients were reassessed. There was a notable difference in many of the patients, which presented as enhanced communication and the ability to sit still. One participant was hospitalized for depression and had been taking Librium for 20 years. It was decided to withdraw her from the drug. She was having great difficulty sleeping and was feeling generally anxious. Several drops of bergamot were placed on a cotton ball and put inside her pillowcase. The following morning she reported it was the first good night's sleep since she had stopped taking Librium. She continued to use bergamot throughout her stay, and at discharge she asked for and was given bergamot essential oil to take home with her, along with instructions on how to use it.

A patient's "pleasure memory" could have an effect even when the patient is not fully conscious. Patients who have their chosen music played via headphones during an operation need less medication postoperatively (Good et al 1999). Patients receiving aromatherapy using the "m" technique in a critical-care unit postoperatively have experienced a decrease in their pain perception. Some patients remember receiving the "m" technique when they recover consciousness. What the patients probably remember is they received *care* in a manner they could recognize, even when they were not conscious. In today's "managed care," care seems to be in danger of becoming marginalized simply because it is not on the reimbursement form. Ten years ago, when I was carrying out a pilot study on post–open-heart surgery patients in an intensive-care unit in England, a patient said, "You were the first person who didn't hurt me." That made a deep impression on me that has remained to this day. Health professionals do not want to hurt their patients, but much of the time they do.

Talk with patients about the smells they enjoyed in their childhood and about the smells they did not like. Were they brought up in the country, near a wood? Have they traveled to far-away places? What kind of perfumes do they enjoy? The answers to all of these questions will provide guidelines as to which essential oils to use. This is a situation where, apart from trying to reduce the patient's anxiety, the focus is also on giving pleasure in circumstances in which pleasure is not often experienced.

Patients frequently experience a "high" of survival immediately after open-heart surgery. This is often followed by a "low" of exhaustion. Touch and smell can help a patient accept this rite of passage. Post-open-heart surgery patients need to feel celebrated, whole, and held. They have survived one of the greatest miracles orthodox medicine has to offer. Now it is time to help them to heal, through the comforts of gentle touch and familiar smell.

OTHER CARDIAC USES FOR AROMATHERAPY

Claudia Ogden, RN, (2001) used aromatherapy on a 19-year-old girl with an insufficient aortic valve as a result of a *Streptococcus* virus at the University of Michigan's Motts Children's Hospital. The girl had had an initial repair at age 13. During open-heart surgery for this subsequent repair, she developed compartment syndrome, which required fasciotomy. She was then required to be on bedrest, flat on her back, while the skin grafts had an opportunity to take hold. During this time she experienced considerable amounts of pain, anxiety, and depression. Compounding her discomfort was constipation, and she was experiencing considerable pain, anxiety, and profuse perspiration while attempting to have a bowel movement.

Ogden was called in to see if clinical aromatherapy could help. She used neroli floral water as a spray to immediately ease anxiety and then a 1% mixture of frankincense and rose on the patient's abdomen in a clockwise movement using the "m" technique. The same 1% mixture was also used on the patient's hands using the "m" technique. The patient calmed down a great deal. She was able to cooperate better with the staff and required less pain medication. She managed a bowel movement. The nurse showed the patient's mother how to apply the aromatherapy mixture to her daughter's foot or hand using the "m" technique whenever her daughter felt anxious. The mother reported being able to use aromatherapy, and stated that the "m" technique had both comforted her daughter and empowered her. The skin on the patient's feet had become red and sore from pushing against the sheets. After only two days, the dilute essential oils had softened and smoothed the girl's heels, and all redness disappeared.

COUMARINS IN AROMATHERAPY

There is some confusion over the possible anticoagulant effects of coumarins. A synthetic chemical called dicoumarol forms the basis of warfarin, an anticoagulant drug (Seth et al 1976). Dicoumarol is created naturally by the breakdown of sweet clover plant but is created synthetically for the drug companies (Budavari 1996). However, a careful look at the chemical drawing of warfarin will uncover a coumarin group within it (Bowles 2000). This does *not* mean an essential oil containing coumarin could or would cause bleeding. Coumarins are present in small amounts, less than 6%, in a few essential oils used in aromatherapy, and it is extremely unlikely they would affect anticoagulant therapy, especially using 1-5% dilutions on the skin. To put things into perspective, wintergreen, a common flavoring in chewing gum and toothpaste, is also used in proprietary topical applications for sprains and strains. Wintergreen is almost all methyl salicylate and as such much more likely to increase the effect of anticoagulant therapy. Despite this, there are no warnings on chewing gum, so the risk must be extremely small!

Unlike the commonly prescribed tranquilizer, droperidol, which caused fatal, irregular heartbeats at far lower doses than expected (prompting the manufacturer to enact a global withdrawal of the product), aromatherapy is a safe, gentle therapy to use in cardiology that may well help a patient's anxiety.

REFERENCES

Aftab K, Ur-Rahman A, Usmanghani K. 1995. Blood pressure lowering action of active principle from *Trachyspermum ammi*. Phytomedicine. 2(1) 35-40.

Agshikar N, Abraham G. 1957. The effect of l-menthol on the systemic blood pressure. Journal of the American Pharmaceutical Association. 46:82-84.

Akorm's injectable droperidol gets FDA black box warning on Label. Jan. 2002. http://www.mosbydrugconsult.com/drugconsult/newsaf2001.html −37.

Avollone R, Zanoli P, Corsi L et al. 1996. Benzodiazepine-like compounds and GABA in flower heads of *Matricaria chamomilla*. Physiotherapy Research. 10:S177-S179.

Beauchamp K, Baker S, McDaniel C et al. 2000. Reliability of nurses' neurological assessments in the cardiothoracic surgical intensive care unit. American Journal of Critical Care. 10(5) 298-305.

Bimmel D, Mellert F, Ashraff O et al. Dec. 20, 2001. Does postoperative delirium syndrome promote sternal instability? Thoracic Cardioavascular Surgery. Thema: Permanent Poster. www.theime.de/thoracic.abstracts2001/daten/pp6.html.

Bowles J. 2000. The Basic Chemistry of Aromatherapeutic Essential Oils. Sydney, Australia: Pirie Publishing.

Budavari S (ed.). 1996. The Merck Index, 12th ed. Whitehouse Station, NJ: Merck.

Charron J. 1997. Use of *Lavandula latifolia* as an expectorant. The Journal of Alternative & Complementary Medicine. 3(3) 211.

Danilowicz A, Gabriel H. 1971. Post cardiotomy psychosis in non-English-speaking patients. The International Journal of Psychiatry in Medicine. 2(4) 314-320.

Dunn C, Sleep J, Collett D. 1995. Sensing an improvement: an experimental study to evaluate the use of aromatherapy, massage and period of rest in an intensive care unit. Journal of Advanced Nursing. 21(1) 34-41.

Dunnington C, Johnson M, Finkelmeier B et al. 1988. Patients with heart rhythm disturbances: variables associated with increased psychologic distress. Heart and Lung. 17:381-389.

Egerton N, Kay J. 1964. PPD and relationship problems. British Journal of Psychiatry. 110(RSM) 433-439.

Epstein R. Nov. 27, 2001. Facing up to depression after a bypass. New York Times. F8.

Franchomme P, Penoel D. 1991. Aromatherapie Exactement. Limoges, France: Jollois.

Freund D. 1999. Does ylang ylang inhalation have a hypotensive effect on unmedicated resting blood pressure in individuals with borderline hypertension? Unpublished dissertation, Hunter, NY: R J Buckle Associates.

Gattefosse R. 1937. (Translated in 1993 by R. Tisserand.) Aromatherapie: Les Huile Essentielles-Hormones Vegetales (Gattefosse's Aromatherapy.) Saffron Walden, UK: CW Daniels, 89.

Good M, Stanton-Hicks M, Grass J et al. 1999. Relief of postoperative pain with jaw relaxation, music and their combination. Pain. 81(1-2) 163-172.

Gould L, Reddy R, Gomprecht R. 1973. Cardiac effects of chamomile tea. Journal of Clinical Pharmacology. 13(11-12) 475-479.

Guba R. 2000. Toxicity myths. International Journal of Aromatherapy. 10(1/2) 37-50.

Herndon R (ed.). 1997. Handbook of Neurologic Rating Scales. New York: Demost Medical Publishing.

Hill J, Brown R, Chu D et al. 1992. The Impact of Medicare Risk Program on the Use of Services and Cost to Medicare. Princeton, NJ: Mathematica Policy Research, Inc., 31-98.

Hope R, Longmore J, Hodgetts T et al. 1993. Oxford Handbook of Clinical Medicine, 3rd ed. Oxford, UK: Oxford University Press.

Jager W, Buchbauer G, Jirovetz L. 1992. Evidence of the sedative effect of neroli oil, citronella and phenylethyl acetate on mice. Journal of Essential Oil Research. 4(4) 387-394.

Kikuchi A, Shoj K, Nakamura S et al. 1995. Effect of fragrance on insomniac tendency in healthy human subjects. In published conference proceedings, Vol. 1: Flavors, Fragrances, & Essential Oils. Istanbul. 15-19 October.

Komori T, Fujiwara R, Tanida M et al. 1995. Effects of citrus fragrance of immune function and depressive states. Neuroimmunomodulation. 2(3) 174-180.

Kovar K, Gropper D, Friess D et al. 1987. Blood levels of 1,8 cineole and locomotor activity of mice after inhalation and oral administration of rosemary oil. Planta Medica. 53(4) 315-318.

Layne O, Yudofsky S. 1971. Postoperative psychosis in cardiotomy patients. New England Journal of Medicine. 284(10) 518-520.

Lidster G. 2001. Retrieved Dec. 20, 2001, from www.leeds.ac.uk/students/ugmodules/done3033.htm.

Lowe R. 1989. Anxiety in a coronary care unit. Nursing Times. 85(45) 61-63.

Macht D, Ting G. 1921. Experimental inquiry into the sedative properties of some aromatic drugs and fumes. Journal of Pharmacology and Experimental Therapeutics. 18(5) 361-372.

Mahanna E, Blumenthal J, White W et al. 1996. Defining neuropsychological dysfunction after coronary artery bypass grafting. Annals of Thoracic Surgery. 61(5) 1342-1347.

Manger W, Gifford R. 2001. 100 Questions and Answers About Hypertension. New York: Blackwell Science Inc.

Mann S. 1997. Healing Hypertension: Uncovering the Secret Power of Your Hidden Emotions. New York: Wiley.

McCormick E. 1997. Psychological interventions for patients with heart disease. The British Journal of Cardiology. 4(7) 268-271.

McCormick E. 1993. Healing the Heart. London: Optima.

McCormick E. 1997. Psychological interventions for patients with heart disease. British Journal of Cardiology. 4(7) 268-271.

Moate S. 1995. Anxiety and depression. International Journal of Aromatherapy. 7(7) 18-21.

Morris N, Birtwistle S, Toms M. 1995. Anxiety reduction. International Journal of Aromatherapy. 7(2) 33-39.

Mulrow C, Lau J, Cornell J et al. 1997. Pharmacotherapy for hypertension in the elderly. Cochrane Database Syst Rev. 2000(2):CD000028.

National Health Service Center for Reviews and Dissemination. 1999. The University of York. 4(2) 1-8. Retrieved Dec. 20, 2001, from www.york.ac.uk/inst/crd/em42.htm.

O'Brien B. 1997. Experience with aromatherapy in the elderly. Journal of Alternative & Complementary Medicine. 3(3) 211.

Ogden C. 2001. Personal communication.

Panossian A, Wikman G, Wagner H. 1999. Plant adaptogens III: Earlier and more recent aspects and concepts of their mode of action. Phytomedicine. 6(4) 287-300.

Perez-Raya M, Utrilla M, Navarro M. 1990. CNS activity of *Mentha rotundifolia* and *Mentha longifolia* essential oils in mice and rats. Phytotherapy Research. 4(6) 232-235.

Petty J. 2000. Surgery and complementary therapies: a review. Alternative Therapies in Health and Medicine. 6(5) 64-74.

Roach G, Kanchuger M, Mangano C et al. 1996. Adverse cerebral outcomes after coronary bypass surgery. New England Journal of Medicine. 335(25) 1857-1863.

Roberts R. 1991. Preventing PPD after surgery. Nursing. 4(6) 28.

Rogers W, Bowlby L, Chandra N et al. 1994. Treatment of myocardial infarction in the USA (1990-1993): observations from the National Registry of Myocardial Infarction. Circulation. 90(4) 2103-2114.

Rossi T, Melegari M, Blanchi A. 1988. Sedative, anti-inflammatory and anti-diuretic effects induced in rats by essential oils of varieties of *Anthemis nobilis:* a comparative study. Pharmacological Research Communications. 20(Suppl. V) 71-74.

Rovesti P, Columbo E. 1973. Aromatherapy and aerosols. Soap, Perfumery and Cosmetics. 46:475-477.

Saeki Y, Shihora M. 2001. Physiological effects of inhaling fragrances. International Journal of Aromatherapy. 11(3) 118-125.

Sanders K, Glick R, O'Gara H et al. 1991. Failure to record delirium as a complication of intra-aortic balloon pump treatment: a retrospective study. Paper presented at the Annual meeting of the Academy of Psychosomatic Medicine, Georgia. Spring.

Sano A, Sei H, Seno H et al. 1998. Influence of cedar essence on spontaneous activity and sleep of rats and human daytime naps. Psychiatry and Clinical Neuroscience. 8(6) 133-135.

Seth G, Kolate C, Varma K. 1976. Effect of essential oil of *Cymbopogon citratus* on central nervous system. Indian Journal of Experimental Biology. 14(3) 370-373.

Sgura F, Scott-Wright R, Kopecky S et al. 2001. Length of stay in myocardial infarction. Journal of Cost and Quality Association. 7(2) 1-17.

Stevensen C. 1994. The psychophysical effects of aromatherapy massage following cardiac surgery. Complementary Therapies in Medicine. 2(1) 27-35.

Templeton J. 2002. How effective is bergamot as an anti-depressant? Unpublished dissertation, Hunter, NY: R J Buckle Associates.

Thomas J. 1962. Peppermint fibrillation. Lancet. 222-223.

Tisserand R, Balacs, T. 1995. Essential Oil Safety. London: Churchill Livingstone.

Viola H, Wasowski C, Levi de Stein M et al. Jun. 1995. Apigenin, a component of *Matricaria recutita* flowers, is a central benzodiazepine receptors ligand with anxiolytic effects. Planta Med. 61(3):213-216.

Vlay S, Fricchione G. 1985. Psychological aspects of surviving sudden cardiac death. Clinical Cardiology. 8(4) 237-242.

Vogley G. 2002. Bergamot, anxiety and the elderly. Unpublished dissertation, Hunter, NY: R J Buckle Associates.

Wagner H, Sprinkmeyer L. 1973. Pharmacological effect of balm spirit. Deutsche Apotheker Zeitung. 113:1156-1166.

Wilson-Barnett J, Carrigy A. 1978. Factors influencing patients' emotional reactions to hospitalization. Journal of Advanced Nursing. 3(3) 221-229.

Yamada K, Miura T, Mimaki Y et al. 1996. Effect of inhalation of chamomile oil vapor on plasma ACTJ level in ovariectomized rat under restriction stress. Biological & Pharmaceutical Bulletin. 19(9) 1244-1246.

15

CARE OF THE ELDERLY

The body it crumbles. Grace and vigor depart.
There is now a stone where I once had a heart.
But inside this old carcass, a young girl still dwells,
And now and again my battered heart swells.
I remember the pain, and I remember the joys,
And I'm living and loving all over again.
And I think of the years, all too few, gone too fast,
And accept the stark fact that nothing will last.
So open your eyes, nurse, open and see, not a crabbed old woman.
Look closer. See me.

Anonymous—found in a nursing home after the author's death
(cited in Montagu 1986)

Improved diet and medical breakthroughs have allowed humans to survive longer and longer. The oldest woman thus far, Jeanne Calment, lived to the age of 121 years. Therefore it is hardly surprising that many older people will need care and, in some instances, supervision. It is a sad part of Western culture that age is not revered, and those who could impart so much information and life experience to younger members of society are frequently isolated in residential homes. This is not to denigrate such institutions, as they are obviously much needed, but to question why civilized society either cannot, or does not want to, look after its elderly own. Indian and Asian families who have moved to the United States often choose to maintain their cultural choice of extended family living.

However, for many Westerners, the world has become such a busy place there appears to be no time to nurture or just "be" with those whose sense of time has gone. Cases of dementia and Alzheimer's disease appear to be increasing. Whether this increase is because humans are living longer or because factors that may contribute to dementia are becoming more widespread is difficult to say. Nearly 20% of those over 80 suffer from dementia. Nearly half of those over 85 suffer from Alzheimer's disease. Some 4 million Americans are afflicted with Alzheimer's, and it is now the fourth leading cause of death among American adults. The average amount of time from onset of symptoms until death ranges from 3 to 20 years. Conventional treatment is with tacrine (Cognex) and donepezil (Aricept): drugs that can temporarily improve the cognitive capabilities but do not slow the progress of the disease (Weil 1997). Alzheimer's disease is a very difficult condition for relatives to accept. Several years ago, a family-practice physician in New Mexico who was investigating dementia among the Native American population commented that there was no record of Alzheimer's disease among the Navaho because "it just did not occur." She believed this was possibly because of genetic or environmental factors.

Until recently friends of mine ran a beautiful home for the elderly in the New Forest area of England. The average age of the residents was 88.4 years. However, the 82-year-old mother of one of the owners regularly came in to help on weekends. She was a sprightly, immaculately dressed lady, and she was older than many of the residents she cared for. This seems to indicate age often has little to do with aging. That residential home used aromatherapy regularly, and the immediate impression on walking into the lobby was of a beautiful, caring atmosphere.

Aromatherapy and the Elderly

There is no doubt the elderly become forgetful. Certain plants from the Labiatae and Asteracae family have long histories of use as restoratives of lost or declining cognitive functions (Wake et al 2000). Extracts from *Melissa* and three *Salvia* species were screened for contents able to displace $(3H)$-(N)-nicotine and $(3H0$-(N) scopolomine from nicotinic and muscarinic receptors of human cerebral-cell membranes. *Melissa officinalis* had the highest $(3H)$-(N)-nicotine displacement value, and *Salvia elegans* had the highest $(3H0$-(N) scopolomine deplacement value.

Helen Passant, a geriatric-nurse manager is recognized as one of the first nurses to use aromatherapy in care of the elderly (Passant 1990). Buckwalter (1992) a geriatric nurse researcher described Passant's work as "giving new meaning to the term holistic care. She and her staff were able to restore harmony, to bring body and mind together and to allow the spirit to shine through." Papadopoulos et al (1999) carried out a qualitative assessment of the use of aromatherapy for older patients in a hospital in Birmingham, England. Each of the 10 participants (six clients and four caregivers) were interviewed using a semistructured interview to explore which part of a session they liked best and what they perceived as benefits of essential oils of *Lavandula angustifolia* and *Chamaemelum nobile*.

There are classic problems that can occur among elderly patients. These include sleep-pattern alteration, dementia, constipation, skin ulcers and poor healing, and osteoarthritis. Each condition can often be treated and improved with aromatherapy.

Sleep Pattern Alteration and Insomnia

There have been a few published studies on aromatherapy and insomnia, and the *Lancet* published a letter explaining one of the studies (Hardy et al 1995). Hardy (1991) investigated the effects of lavender (*Lavandula angustifolia*) on four male residents over a 6-week period and found all four men slept approximately the same number of hours with lavender as they did with their previous conventional sleep medication. The worst sleeper of the four men, who also presented noisy, aggressive behavior during the day, appeared calmer. This could have been because of the lavender or the cessation of the sleep medication. Two of the other men in the study no longer required naps during the day, presumably because they were getting enough sleep at night. The lavender was cost effective: about $\frac{1}{3}$ the price of the sleep medication.

Hudson (1996) carried out a similar study on 51 patients using *Lavandula angustifolia* for 14 days. Sleep pattern and daytime alertness were monitored. During the first week, baseline measurements were taken. During the second week, two drops of lavender were put on the pillow of each participant; no other changes were made. Findings were an improved sleep pattern and increased alertness during the day with a 50% reduction in confusion.

Cannard (1994) investigated the effects of a "commercially pre-mixed blend of essential oils" on 10 patients in a nursing-development unit. Eight of the patients were aged over 70. In this study inhalation and hand massage were used. Baseline sleep patterns were established over 94 nights. Then inhaled lavender plus hand massage were introduced for two nights. On the third day, night sedation was discontinued and sleep patterns were recorded for a further 94 nights. Some patients required no sedation at all during the second 94-night period; only one person requested night sedation every night. Ninety-seven percent of patients felt they had a good night's sleep. Although the paper itself did not reveal what was in the mixture, another source reported it contained *Ocimum basilicum* CT linalool, *Lavandula angustifolia*, and *Origanum majorana* (Price & Price 1999).

Remember, the wrong lavender (*Lavandula latifolia* or *Lavandula stoechas*) will not produce a sedative effect and too much of even the right lavender (*Lavandula angustifolia*) can exacerbate a patient's insomnia. There could also be a problem with overdoing it if too much lavender is put in an electric nebulizer, and it is kept on incessantly. For some elderly people, lavender can be a disliked smell, associated with death.

The learned memory of lavender can trigger negative images of dying relatives or friends, as years ago lavender was used to protect linen from moths and mold and every linen cupboard was liberally stacked with lavender bags. In all cases, but especially with care of the elderly, it is important to allow patients to choose their own aromas when possible. Memories are very individual, and smell memories can be easily triggered (Ehrlichman & Halpern 1988).

Usha Rani & Naidu (1998) discuss the use of *Nardostachys jatamansi* (spikenard) to produce tranquility and sedation in conditions of insomnia and restlessness and cite Arora (1965) who suggests the sedative effect of spikenard is due to the sesquiterpene ketone, jatamansone. Gupta and Virmani's double-blind clinical study on children (1968) found isolated jatamansone caused significant improvement in restlessness and aggressiveness in 28 hyperkinetic children compared to amphetamine. This is interesting as jatamansone is identical in structure to valeranone, the ketone in *Valeriana officinalis* (Lawrence 1989) thought to produce valerian's sedative effect. Essential oil of spikenard also was found to produce marked relaxation of skeletal muscles and central nervous system depression by Bose et al (1957).

Sanderson and Ruddle (1992) found lavender and sweet marjoram were often offered as alternatives to Temazepan in an Oxford, UK, nursing-development unit. The comment was that although lavender was effective when inhaled, it was much more effective when given in a massage.

Studies are not limited to olfaction only. In two multiple-crossover studies, each involving 12 female subjects, Schulz et al (1998) demonstrated that extract of *Lavandula angustifolia* when taken orally produced a sedative effect only slightly less sedative than diazepam. Lavender drops have been taken orally for their digestive and relaxing properties for hundreds of years in Europe. Frankincense was found to enhance the effect of barbiturates in a study on rats by Menon and Kar (1971). Injected frankincense also appeared to have a sedative action on its own and in high doses (300 mg/kg) to have an action comparable to 7.5 mg/kg chlorpromazine. Suggested essential oils for insomnia are listed in Table 15-1.

Dementia

Dementia is present in 20% of individuals over 80 years of age (Jobst et al 1994). People who suffer dementia have been identified as a special-needs group (Kilstoff & Chenoweth 1998). Although there are more than 50 different causes of dementia, some of which are reversible, the majority are progressive and lead to premature death. The most common cause of dementia in the developed world is Alzheimer's disease. Although Alzheimer's can affect patients as young as 35 years of age, the most recent view is that this disturbing disease is part of a pathological cascade process linked with aging (Jobst et al 1994a). In total, 70% of patients older than 65 who have dementia will have Alzheimer's disease. Currently there is no cure.

Olfactory dysfunction is thought to be a marker for detecting early Alzheimer's disease (Burns 2000). While aromatherapy is not a cure for dementia, smell and touch are powerful messengers, often penetrating the fog of amnesia in a way words do not. Knasko and Gilbert (1990) suggest patients normally

Table 15-1 ✖ *Essential Oils for Insomnia*

Common Name	Botanical Name	Reference
Neroli	*Citrus aurantium flos*	Jager et al 1992
Mandarin	*Citrus reticulate*	Kilstoff & Chenoweth 1998
Melissa	*Melissa officinalis*	Mitchell 1993
Angelica	*Angelica archangelica*	Franchomme 1991
Spikenard	*Nardostachys jaamansi*	Usah Rani 1998
Lemongrass	*Cymbopogon citrates*	Seth et al 1976
Lavender	*Lavandula angustifolia*	Flanagan 1995
Geranium	*Pelargonium graveolens*	Flanagan 1995
Mandarin	*Citrus reticulate*	Flanagan 1995
Roman chamomile	*Chamaemelum nobile*	Rossi et al 1988
Sandalwood	*Santalum album*	Kikuchi et al 1995
Rose	*Rosa damascene*	Brud & Szydlowska 1991
Sweet marjoram	*Origanum majorana*	Price & Price 1999

unable to communicate would find it "refreshing to have a nonverbal interaction with their environment." Ho (1996) described the sensory-stimulation groups developed at Burton Hospital in Dudley, England. Odors were matched with colors, such as lavender with shades of mauve and purple. Music associated with the aroma was played, such as the nursery rhyme "Lavender Blue Dilly Dilly," and patients had access to herbs and photographs connected with the aroma. In many instances patients with dementia were able to make the correct connections.

Smith et al (1992) reported on ambient odor that elicited verbal memory in a study of 47 college students with a mean age of 20.5 years (age range was 17-25). The two odors used were jasmine incense and Lauren perfume. Superior memory for the 24 words chosen was found when the odor present during the relearning session was the same as the odor present at the time of the initial learning, thereby demonstrating a context-dependent memory.

Flanagan (1995) reported on the use of a variety of essential oils to improve atmosphere and behavior in institutionalized patients with Alzheimer's. One patient, who was so combative he required sedation injections, changed dramatically when a cotton ball with essential oil of lavender was pinned to his shirt lapel. Now, he no longer needs medication if the cotton ball can be pinned to his shirt in time. Kilstoff and Chenoweth (1998) reported on the effect of aromatherapy on patients in a multicultural dementia day-care center in Australia for a period of 18 months. They used a combination of lavender, mandarin, and geranium essential oils diluted in a hand massage. Patients were thought to have become more alert and less agitated, although it was unclear whether this was from the hand massage or the essential oils. The use of aromathreapy appeared to have had a positive effect on the staff and caregivers as well, possibly because of empowerment.

Smith (2000) studied the effects of inhaled lavender and sweet marjoram on 17 residents of the Northboro Senior Care Center in Northboro, Massachusetts. Subjects who had memory-impaired agitation were chosen for the study, and their relative or responsible party was approached for written consent. The most frequent time for agitation was between 6 pm and 7:30 pm, and behavior ranged from mild to severe agitation. The study took 9 weeks. During the first week, a baseline was taken, and it was noted how many times the alarm was set off. (This is a safety alarm set off when patients who cannot stand on their own attempt to get out of their seats unaided.) For the next 4 weeks, essential oil of *Lavandula angustifolia* was diffused into the meeting room 15 minutes prior to each session. As of the fifth week, *Origanum majorana* (sweet marjoram) was diffused into the meeting room 15 minutes prior each session. The whole residential-care team observed subjects during the study to avoid bias. The team discussed the effects and decided lavender had the best effect, as all subjects were able to remain engaged with a marked decrease in agitation. No alarms went off during the lavender, which was very unusual. Sweet marjoram appeared less effective.

MacMohan and Kermode (1998) found aromatherapy dramatically improved motivational behavior in a 2-month study (n=1). However, not all studies have shown improvement in dementia. Brooker et al (1997) investigated the effects of lavender inhalation and massage on four severely demented patients and found two patients became severely agitated. The lavender may have evoked distressing memories, or perhaps they did not like being massaged.

In cases where patients cannot or will not remain stationary, walking alongside them while simultaneously conducting a gentle, hand "m" technique can lead to some positive changes in the patient, such as renewed eye contact and speech coherence. In cases in which patients are confined to bed and incapable of walking or are violently resistant to any form of touch, vaporizers and nebulizers can be used. Even in instances such as these, when it seems the patient will be unable to help with the selection of an aroma, offering a choice of two different smells can elicit a response. Laraine Kyle, MSN, in Boulder, Colorado, has done much to introduce aromatherapy into the geriatric setting in the United States. She writes aromatherapy can help "transport Alzheimer patients to memories of their past. Seeing facial expressions change from mask-like to animated smiles is feedback enough to know that something is happening" (Kyle 1996).

Mitchell (1993) used melissa and lavender in a randomized, controlled crossover study of 12 patients with Alzheimer's aged between 64 and 91 at a residential and day-care unit. Six drops of lavender were added to the morning wash. A 3% solution of melissa was applied to the patients' chins at midday, and three drops of lavender were applied to their pillows at night. Mild behavioral and verbal improvements were observed.

Other suitable essential oils are those the patients might be familiar with either from their childhood or from positive life experiences. For example, Trumpers, possibly the oldest gentlemen's hairdressers in London, has used essential oil of geranium (Bourbon) in their pomade for more than 100 years (Freeman 1996).

Rosmarinus officinalis CT cineole or borneol (rosemary) will be remembered by most elderly patients as a common ingredient in cooking and from gardening. "There's rosemary—that's for remembrance" said Shakespeare's Ophelia, and it is a valid comment. Rosemary is traditionally thought to be helpful as a memory aid. Suggestions for other aromas to try are listed in Table 15-2. There are in no particular order. If a patient has lived in India or Asia, lemongrass, ginger, or ylang ylang might be appealing and soothing.

Dales Occupational Therapy Service in Derbyshire, United Kingdom, used aromatherapy to improve the quality of life of their Alzheimer's patients. Essential oils they found useful include pine, eucalyptus, and peppermint to trigger conversation and memory and lavender and geranium to trigger thoughts of cooking and plants (Henry 1993).

Table 15-2 ❧ *Essential Oils for Dementia*

Common Name	Botanical Name
Geranium	*Pelargonium graveolens*
Lavender	*Lavandula angustifolia*
Sandalwood	*Santalum album*
Patchouli	*Pogostemon patchouli*
Clary sage	*Slavia sclarea*
Rose	*Rosa damascene*
Lavender	*Lavandula angustifolia*
Mandarin	*Citrus reticulate*
Geranium	*Pelargonium graveolens*
Rosemary	*Rosmarinus officinalis*
Melissa	*Melissa officinalis*
Peppermint	*Mentha piperita*
Eucalyptus	*Eucalyptus globules*
Ginger	*Zingiber officinalis*
Ylang ylang	*Cananga odorata* var. *genuine*

Table 15-3 ✖ *Essential Oils for Constipation*

Common Name	Botanical Name
Black pepper	*Piper nigrum*
Ginger	*Zingiber officinale*
Fennel	*Foeniculum vulgare*
Marjoram	*Origanum marjorana*
Grapefruit	*Citrus paradisi*

Constipation

The slowed-down passage of food through the large intestine may be a result of reduced exercise or insufficient roughage in the diet. The latter could be due to poor appetite for various reasons ranging from ill-fitting dentures to boredom with institutional food. Another cause of constipation is regular use of night sedation.

One of the simplest and most gentle ways to ease constipation is through abdominal massage using essential oils. This is effective for mild constipation. A slight improvement was documented in a study by Klauser et al (1992), although in that instance no essential oils were used. In the residential home owned by my friends, this form of massage produced very good results and was used successfully for several years. See Table 15-3 for a list of essential oils Barker (1995) suggests for treating constipation.

Use a 3% solution (three drops of essential oil/s in 5ccs of cold-pressed vegetable oil). Let the patient choose which oil to use from the selection in Table 15-3. Work slowly and rhythmically up the ascending colon, along the transverse colon, and down the descending colon, paying attention to both hepatic and splenic flexures. This gentle massage only takes 5 minutes, but it can be really useful. It is best repeated up to five times a day or until relief is obtained.

Skin Ulcers and Slow Healing

Aging slows down the body's ability to heal. Skin becomes thinner and more fragile, and the slightest knock can cause a deep bruise, especially if the person is taking steroids. Very gentle massage with cold-pressed vegetable oils, such as oil of evening primrose, can aid the elasticity of aging skin, and certain essential oils can enhance aging skin's ability to heal. Alan Barker, a clinical aromatherapist employed by the British National Health Service, has used floral waters to irrigate wounds (Barker 1994). Table 15-4 lists some floral waters used for this purpose. Floral waters are the byproduct of steam distillation and can be obtained from many essential-oil suppliers. Slightly acidic, they are refreshing to use, smell lovely, and are excellent for skin care. (Floral waters are slightly acidic because they contain parts of the essential oil that are most soluble.) When using floral

Table 15-4 ❧ *Floral Waters Used to Irrigate Wounds*

Common Name	Botanical Name
Niaouli	*Melaleuca viridiflora*
Tea tree	*Melaleuca alternifolia*
German chamomile	*Matricaria recutitia*
Grapefruit	*Citrus paradisi*

water, make sure the distributor can supply an analysis to prove the floral water is not contaminated with bacteria or fungi.

After irrigating the wound, a compress soaked in diluted essential oils can be applied to aid healing. The essential oils will also reduce the chance of infection. Apply a fresh compress twice daily, or every 4 hours if the wound is infected. Areas immediately around the wound can be gently swabbed with oil of evening primrose or *Rosa rubiginosa.* Another excellent oil to use around the wound would be a macerated oil such as *Hypericum perforatum* (St John's wort) or calendula (*Calendula officinalis*).

Glowania et al (1987) found *Matricaria recutita* (German chamomile) effective in a controlled, double-blind study of slow-healing wounds in 14 patients. A further article, in the *Journal of Tissue Viability* in 1993, reported on two case studies using lavender and tea tree (Hitchin 1993). Thorne (1996) described the use of 3% oil of *Lavandula angustifolia* in a carrier oil of rosehip (*Rosa rubiginosa*) on a leg ulcer measuring 1.5 cm by 1 cm. After one month of applying the lavender solution to the area around the wound (not the wound itself), the wound was smaller (1cm by 1cm), and the whole area looked much healthier. It is not clear why the mixture was not applied to the wound itself. However, after tea tree was added to the dilution, the wound became inflamed, and a course of antibiotics was prescribed. This may have been due to an allergy to the tea tree. There is no indication a patch test was taken. Two months later the wound had healed, but there is no indication that this was due to the antibiotic rather than the essential oils.

Emeny (1994) reported on a 90-year-old woman with a diabetic foot ulcer that had become gangrenous: amputation was scheduled. Undiluted tea tree was applied to the ulcerated lesion between her toes in the form of soaks for 1 week. Her pain level decreased, and there was marked physical improvement. Tea tree was continued in a 10% solution, decreasing to 3% over the next 3 weeks. The foot gradually became warmer. Continuing tea tree at 3% for 9 weeks, the wound healed completely, and there was no evidence of gangrene. Belaiche (1985) a French physician, used undiluted tea tree daily on intertrigo under the breasts and in the groin and underarm with disappearance of all lesions within 2 months.

Ron Guba (1999) reported on the rapid healing of dermal wounds using his own essential oil-based cream (See Table 15-5 for details.) on selected patients in six nursing homes in Australia. Wounds were divided into two groups: skin tears received once-a-day treatment, while pressure-area and venous ulcers received treatment twice a day. Treatment consisted of putting the cream onto dry gauze and taping it over the wound. Detailed accounts of seven patients (aged 58-93) are given. All wounds healed, some within a week. This was remarkable as some of the wounds had been in stasis for several months. Guba also conducted a punch-biopsy, controlled study on five subjects who each sustained two wounds. The wounds treated with Guba's cream healed within an average of 12 weeks. The control wounds took an average of 26 weeks.

My own clinical experience confirms the excellence of Guba's wound-healing cream. I have also found frankincense very beneficial to superficial wounds and scars, and palma rosa is good for deeper wounds.

Finally, essential oils that contain high percentages of ketones are thought to be beneficial in wounds and may help reduce cheloid scars. This process may be accelerated if the carrier oil used is *Rosa rubiginosa* (rosehip).

Osteoarthritis

Degenerative joint pain is frequently part of the aging process, especially if there is a family history of rheumatism. As secondary changes occur in the underlying bone, pain and impaired function make life a misery for those who were once agile. This is particularly the case if one of the affected joints has been injured.

Table 15-5 ❧ *Guba's Wound-Healing Cream (reprinted with permission)*

Common Name	Botanical Name	Concentration
True lavender	*Lavandula angustifolia*	40 mg/g
Mugwort	*Artemesia vulgaris*	10 mg/g
Sage	*Salvia officinalis*	10 mg/g
Everlasting	*Helichrysum italicum*	18 mg/g
German chamomile	*Matricaria recutita*	12 mg/g
Calendula	*Calendula officinalis*	10 mg/g
Tamanu	*Calophyllum inophyllum* vegetable oil	62.5 mg/g
Borage	*Borago officinalis* vegetable oil	62.5 mg/g
Flaxseed	*Linum usitatissimum* vegetable oil	62.5 mg/g
Shea butter	*Butrospermum parkii* vegetable oil	62.5 mg/g
Grapefruit seed	*Citrus paradisi* (as preservative)	5.0 mg/g
Rosemary	*Rosmarinus officinalis* CT cineole CO_2 (antioxidant)	0.125 mg/g

Extract of ginger was found to be marginally effective in a randomized, controlled crossover study by Bliddel et al (2000). While in the crossover period no statistical difference could be demonstrated, during the first explorative period ginger was found to be better than the control. The extracts were taken orally, which may have contributed to the poor results. Ginger foot baths and compresses are very good for both feet and knees; use CO_2 extract that contains gingerol.

Cote (2002) investigated the effect of topically applied *Piper nigrum* (black pepper) on 11 self-selected subjects (10 women and one man) who were members of Panorama City Retirement Community in Lacy, Florida. Following baseline measurement of pain using a visual analog, a 4% dilution of black pepper in 5 ml of grapeseed oil was massaged into the painful joint of each subject (7 hands, one knee, one shoulder, one ankle, one foot). After the massage, the subjects were asked to rate their pain immediately, then again after 2 hours and after 4 hours. There was a slight reduction in perception of pain for most participants. It is difficult to assess whether the reduction was due to the massage or the essential oil.

Macdonald (1995) wrote about elderly patients and osteopathic pain. The following essential oils were used in her study: eucalyptus, juniper, marjoram, and rosemary. Unfortunately, no botanical names were given, so it is impossible to assess which essential oils were actually used (there are 400 different types of *Eucalyptus*). Traditional essential oils for osteoarthritic pain are rubefacient ones that will dilate the capillaries and give a peripheral warming effect. One such essential oil is black pepper. An antiinflammatory essential oil such as German chamomile or immortelle (*Helicrysum italicum*) can give relief, as can an analgesic essential oil such as lavender or peppermint. For more information on antiinflammatory essential oils, please see the section of Chapter 12 on inflammation. For more information on analgesic essential oils, please see the section of Chapter 12 on pain.

Franchomme and Penoel (1991) state that p-cymene has analgesic properties and is particularly suited to osteoarthritis. Paracymene is present in cajeput (6.8%), summer savory (7%), and *Thymus vulgaris* (21.9%) (Bowles 2000), although at these low percentages it is dubious that the cymeme will have much impact.

I have found *Cymbopogon citratus* (lemongrass) useful for alleviating osteoarthritic pain using a 5% compress. Lemongrass may be analgesic due to its myrcene content (Lorenzetti et al 1991). *Satureja hortensis* (summer savory) is also useful for pain, and it contains a small amount of myrcene.

Perhaps it would be pertinent to end this section with a mention of essential oils for aging. Deans (1991) conducted substantial research into the properties of polyunsaturated fatty acids (PUFAs) at Warwick University in England. PUFAs form part of plant oils and are used by the human body to make cellular components and steroid hormones. Aging is associated with a decline in PUFAs. In research on aging rats, essential oils were found to restore PUFA levels almost to the levels observed in young mice. Of the essential oils tested, red thyme and clove appeared to give the most impressive results (Deans 1991). This research involved feeding the rats essential oils by mouth. There is no suggestion we do the same for our patients or ourselves, but the antiaging properties of essential oils may turn out to be an exciting area. In the meantime, both West (1993) and Kyle (1999) suggest aromatherapy can be integrated into care of the elderly very simply, and many health professionals are following her lead.

REFERENCES

Arora R. 1965. *Nardostachys jatamansi:* a chemical, pharmacological and clinical appraisal. Special Report Series No 51. New Delhi, India: Indian Council of Medical Research.

Barker A. 1994. Pressure sores. Aromatherapy Quarterly. 41:5-7.

Belaiche P. 1985. Treatment of skin infections with the essential oil of *Melaleuca alternifolia*. Phytotherapy. 15:15-17.

Bliddel H, Rosetzsky A, Schlinchting P et al. 2000. A randomized placebo controlled cross-over study of ginger extracts and ibuprofen in osteoarthritis. Osteoarthritis and Cartilage. 8(1) 9-12.

Bose B, Gupta S, Bhatnagar J et al. 1957. *Nardostachys jatamansi* DC: its sedative and depressant action as estimated by Warburg technique. Indian Journal of Medical Science. 11:803-804.

Bowles E. 2000. The Basic Chemistry of Aromatherapeutic Essential Oils. Sydney, Australia: Pirie Printers.

Brooker D, Snape M, Johnson E et al. 1997. Single case evaluation of the effects of aromatherapy and massage on disturbed behavior in severe dementia. British Journal of Clinical Psychology. 36(Part 2) 287-296.

Brud W, Szydlowska I. 1991. Bulgarian rose otto. International Journal of Aromatherapy. 3(3) 17-19.

Buckwalter K. 1992. Geropsychiatry: confessions of a geriatric nurse researcher. Journal of Psychosocial Nursing. 30(6) 38-39.

Burns A. 2000. Might olfactory dysfunction be a marker for early Alzheimer's disease? Lancet. 355(9198) 84-85.

Cannard G. 1995. On the scent of a good night's sleep: trial project. Nursing Standard. 9(34) 21-22.

Cote S. 2002. The effects of essential oils of black pepper on arthritis. Unpublished dissertation, Hunter, NY: R J Buckle Associates.

Deans S. 1991. More life in your years. International Journal of Aromatherapy. 3(4) 20-22.

Ehrlichman H, Halpern J. 1988. Affect and memory: effects of pleasant and unpleasant odor on retrieval of happy and unhappy memories. Journal of Personality and Social Psychology. 55(5) 769-779.

Emeny P. 1994. Diabetic gangrene in case studies. International Journal of Aromatherapy. 6(4) 23.

Flanagan N. 1995. The clinical use of aromatherapy in Alzheimer's patients. Alternative & Complementary Therapies. 377-380.

Franchomme P, Penoel D. 1991. Aromatherapie Exactement. Limoges, France: Jollois.

Freeman G. 1996. Personal communication.

Glowania H, Raulin C, Svoboda M. 1987. Effect of chamomile on wound healing: a clinical double-blind study. Zeitschrift fur Hautkrankheiten (Berlin). 62(17) 1267-1271.

Guba R. 1999. Wound healing. International Journal of Aromatherapy. 9(2) 67-74.

Gupta B, Virmani V. 1968. Clinical trial of jatamansome in hyperkinetic behavior disorders. Neurology (India). 16(4) 168-173.

Hardy M. 1991. Sweet scented dreams. International Journal of Aromatherapy. 3(2) 12-13.

Hardy M, Kirk-Smith M, Stretch D. 1995. Replacement of drug treatment for insomnia by ambient odour (letter). Lancet. 346(8976) 701.

Henry J. 1993. Dementia. International Journal of Aromatherapy. 5(2) 27-29.

Hitchin D. 1993. Wound care and the aromatherapist. Journal of Tissue Viability. 3(1) 56-57.

Ho C. 1996. Stirring memories through all the senses. Journal of Dementia Care. 4(4) 15.

Hudson R. 1996. The value of lavender for rest and activity in the elderly patient. Complementary Therapies in Medicine. 4(1) 52-57.

Jager W, Buchbauer G, Jirovetz L. 1992. Evidence of the sedative effect of neroli oil, citronella and phenylethyl acetate on mice. Journal of Essential Oil Research. 4(4) 387-394.

Jobst K, Hindley N, Pearce M. 1994. Clinical investigation and therapeutic aspects of Alzheimer's disease. Continuing Medical Education. 12:401-412.

Jobst K, Smith A, Szatmari M. 1994a. Rapidly progressing atrophy of medial temporal lobe in Alzheimer's disease. Lancet. 343(8901) 829-830.

Kikuchi A, Shoji K, Nakamura S et al. 1995. Effects of fragrance on insomniac tendency in healthy human beings. In published conference proceedings, Vol. 1: Flavors, Fragrances & Essential Oils. Istanbul. 15-19 October.

Kilstoff K, Chenoweth L. 1998. New approaches to health and well-being for dementia day-care clients, family carers and day-care staff. International Journal of Nursing Practice. 4(2) 70-83.

Klauser A, Flaschentrager J, Gehrke A et al. 1992. Abdominal wall massage: effect of colonic function in healthy volunteers and in patients with chronic constipation. Zeitschrift fur Gastroenterologie. 30:247-251.

Knasko S, Gilbert A. 1990. Emotional state, physical well-being and performance in the presence of feigned ambient odor. Journal of Applied Social Psychology. 20(16) 1345-1357.

Kyle L. 1996. Clinical uses of aromatherapy. Aromatic Thymes. 4(1) 13-15.

Kyle L. 1999. Aromatherapy for elder care. International Journal of Aromatherapy. 9(4) 170-176.

Lawrence B. 1989. Essential Oils: 1981-1987. Carol Stream, IL: Allured Publishing, 116.

Lorenzetti B, Souza G, Sarti S, Gehrke A et al. 1991. Myrcene mimics the peripheral analgesic activity of lemongrass tea. Ethnopharmacology. 30(4) 43-48.

Macdonald E. 1995. Aromatherapy for the enhancement of the nursing care of elderly people suffering from arthritis. Aromatherapist. 2:26-31.

MacMohan S, Kermode S. 1998. A clinical trial of the effect of aromatherapy on motivational behavior in a dementia care setting using single subjects. Australian Journal of Holistic Nursing. 5(2) 47-49.

Menon M, Kar A. 1971. Analgesic and psychopharmacological effects of the gum resin of *Boswellia serrata*. Planta Medica. 19(4) 333-341.

Mitchell S. 1993. Dementia. International Journal of Aromatherapy. 5(2) 20-24.

Montagu A. 1986. Touching: The Human Significance of Skin. New York: Perennial.

Papadopoulos A, Wright S, Ensor J. 1999. Evaluation and attributional analysis of an aromatherapy service for older adults with physical health problems and carers using the service. Complementary Therapies in Medicine. 7(4) 239-245.

Passant H. 1990. A holistic approach in the ward. Nursing Times. 86(4) 26-28.

Price S, Price L. 1999. Aromatherapy for Health Professionals. London: Churchill Livingstone, 233.

Rossi T, Melegari M, Blanchi A. 1988. Sedative, anti-inflammatory and anti-diuretic effects induced in rats by essential oils of varieties of *Anthemis nobilis:* a comparative study. Pharmacological Research Communications. 20(Suppl. 5) 71-74.

Sanderson H, Ruddle J. 1992. Aromatherapy and occupational therapy. British Journal of Occupational Therapy. 55(8) 310-314.

Schulz H, Jobert M, Hubner W. 1998. The quantitative EEG as a screening instrument to identify sedative effects of single doses of plant extracts in comparison to Diazepam. Phytomedicine. 5(6) 449-458.

Seth G, Kolate C, Varma K. 1976. Effect of essential oils of *Cymbopogon citratus* on central nervous system. Indian Journal of Experimental Biology. 14(3) 370-373.

Smith D, Standing L, de Man A. 2002. Verbal memory elicited by ambient odor. Perceptual and Motor Skills. 74(2) 339-343.

Thorne D. 1996. Healing ulcers using essential oils. Journal of Community Nursing. 10(9) 14-16.

Usha Rani P, Naidu M. 1998. Subjective and polysomnographic evaluation of an herbal preparation in insomnia. Phytomedicine. 5(4) 253-257.

Wake G, Court J, Pickering A et al. 2000. CNS acetylcholine receptor activity in European medicinal plants traditionally used to improve failing memory. Journal of Ethnopharmacology. 69(2) 105-114.

Weil A. 1997. Preventing Alzheimer's. Dr. Andrew Weil's Self-Healing. 1, 6.

West B. 1993. The essence of aromatherapy. Elderly Care. 5(4) 24-25.

16

CRITICAL CARE

We may need to be cured by flowers.

Sharman Russell
Anatomy of a Rose

C ritical care encompasses patients with grave, long-term medical conditions, those with acute myocardial infarctions who will have shorter stays, and patients who have had major surgery. The one common factor will be the gravity of their condition. Patients in critical care experience one of the most stressful times in their lives (Dunn et al 1995). Often unable to breathe unaided, their survival depends on the experience and expertise of their professional caregivers. Communication and trust play a large role in the patient-caregiver relationship. Ingham (1989) suggests communication should be "written in to a patient's care-plan." Touch is a communication skill that can enhance trust. Ashworth (1984) wrote about the importance of teaching nonprocedural touch, commenting "it was more difficult to learn than defibrillation and cardiopulmonary resuscitation and at least as valuable."

A critical-care nurse who experienced being intubated as a patient in a critical-care unit described how "her worst nightmare came true." She felt "abandoned and longed for someone to reassure her." Following her experience she understood "why it was sometimes necessary to hold a patient's hand" (Urden 1997). It is greatly underestimated how important it is for intensive-care unit patients to feel trust and confidence in their caregivers. Nonprocedural touch and pleasant aromas can do much to relive anxiety and give comfort in what is perceived by patients to be a "hostile environment" (Welsh 1997). Essential oils can be used in many ways in a critical-care unit: from relieving the pain of intravenous insertions to alleviating bronchial spasm to reducing anxiety (Buckle 1998).

Most of the published research has focused on physical parameters that can be easily measured. These physical tools have not always conveyed what the patients have said if their perception of anxiety, pain, or stress have been relieved. This could be because a more accurate tool, such as measuring blood or saliva cortisol levels, has been too expensive for most nursing studies. However this would be an excellent area of study for the future.

AROMATHERAPY IN A CRITICAL-CARE SETTING

Dunn et al (1995) reported on the effects of reducing stress using a gentle massage with of 1% lavender (*Lavandula angustifolia*) on 122 patients in an intensive-care unit at Battle Hospital in Reading, United Kingdom. Patients were randomly assigned to three groups: one with plain massage, one with massage plus 1% lavender, and one with rest for 30 minutes. The areas of massage depended on the areas available and lasted between 15 and 30 minutes (mean time 16.5 minutes). The age of participants ranged from 2 years to 92 years. Physiological and psychological measurements were taken before and after the treatment. Although there appeared to be no difference between the group that received massage with and without an essential oil, this could be because the percentage used was very low. or it could be because when patients fell asleep during the aromatherapy massage they were not awakened! (Dunn 1996). However, the comments indicated all patients were very appreciative of the extra care they received. One patient who had received the aromatherapy massage commented, "Aromatherapy made me feel clean and like a whole person."

Woolfson and Hewitt (1992) used foot massage with 1% lavender in their study of 36 patients in a medical and surgery critical-care unit at the Royal Sussex County Hospital in the United Kingdom. Each patient was randomly assigned to three groups. The groups received either a 20-minute massage without oil, 20-minute massage with oil, or a 20-minute rest. Two treatments per week were given for 5 weeks. This means the majority of patients would have been medical (as surgical patients tend not to stay that long). The massage-with-lavender group showed the greatest benefits with a consistent decrease in blood pressure, heart rate, respiration, and anxiety. Patients in the lavender group perceived their stress as being less than patients in the control group.

Stevensen (1994) reported on the effects of a 2.5% neroli (*Citrus aurantium flos*) foot massage on 100 patients in the critical-care unit at Middlesex Hospital in London, England. In this study patients were randomly assigned to one of four groups: massage with neroli, massage with plain oil (apricot kernel), a rest period, or nothing. Results indicated the neroli group perceived they were less stressed, although there were only small differences in physical measurements.

In my study (Buckle 1993) *Lavandula* x *intermedia* (lavandin) was used as a control because at that time it was thought to have little therapeutic effect. The study was to find out if aromatherapy had an effect beyond that of massage. *Lavandula angustifolia* was chosen for the experimental group. Two-percent solutions of *Lavandula angustifolia* and *Lavandula* x *intermedia*, (called *Lavandula burnati* by Frachomme and Penoel 2000) were supplied by the Fragrant Earth Co. Ltd. The company labeled the solutions Lavender A and Lavender B.

At 2% dilution it was impossible to tell which lavender was which, so the investigator was blind to the intervention, and so were the patients. Each patient was randomly allocated to one of two groups. Following analysis, it did appear one of the lavenders was more effective at reducing respiration rate than the other one. When the identity of the experimental group lavender was revealed, it was lavandin, and it appeared to be twice as effective as *Lavandula angustifolia*. The results were rechecked as they appeared to contradict what was being taught about lavandin. This also indicated the relaxation was not simply due to massage as there was a difference between the two groups. One of the comments made was "You were the first person who didn't hurt me." Another was, "Why send flowers and cards if you can send this?" Others were, "I feel like you really cared about me," and "I felt like I was important, not just a number, and that you really would take care of me," and "Until you did that, I was really scared, but you made me feel it would be OK to relax."

Waldman et al (1993) suggested the following essential oils would be useful in a critical-care setting: lavender, clary sage, jasmine, peppermint, rose, rosemary, tea tree, and ylang ylang. The oils were used in a 2% massage solution and in electric burners. Others could include neroli, Roman chamomile, sandalwood, lemon, lemongrass, and palma rosa. Mitchell (2002), a critical-care nurse, has used aromatherapy in her unit for several years. She suggests frankincense, geranium, petitgrain, sweet marjoram, mandarin, juniper, and German chamomile.

Each patient is someone's child, no matter how old he or she is. Most patients in an intensive-care unit are frightened, no matter how brave they try to appear. Each patient belongs, in some capacity, to another, and the others are also in need of nurturing. Critical-care units can be very frightening for relatives, with so many tubes and complicated machinery around the motionless body of a loved one. Mitchell (2002) writes relatives are often stunned by the intensive-care unit, and they are very appreciative when their loved ones receive the loving care aromatherapy provides.

I remember seeing my father in a critical-care unit many years ago, and more recently my brother-in-law, and experiencing some of the feelings of helplessness many relatives and visitors feel even though I had trained and worked in critical care for many years. Often relatives feel there is nothing they can do except wait and pray. Aromatherapy presents a wonderful opportunity to give the family a sense of control and a simple way to contribute and promote comfort and quality of care for their loved one.

The gentle, stroking movements of the "m" technique, which can be used to apply dilute essential oils, are extremely simple both to teach and to learn. I taught them to a 5-year-old granddaughter who spent almost an hour lovingly stroking her grandfather's hands. Her sad, cross little face softened as she sang gently under her breath, moving her hands in time to her lullaby. Her parents watched her as she worked, amazed at the transformation. This little girl knew she had been given an important task, one that not only empowered her but was actually of therapeutic value.

Teaching relatives to touch in this way does not take very long—probably only 5 minutes. Everyone can find that amount of time. Talking with relatives about the aromas patients enjoyed before they came into hospital allows dialogue on a safe subject, but one still linked to the patient. Finding an aroma relatives feel could help their loved ones gives them something to think about and a way of becoming involved. It is best to offer just a few aromas known to have relaxing effects. The floral aromas are usually popular. The rose essential oil used on my brother-in-law in Papworth Hospital in Cambridge, England, produced a smile even though he was extremely ill and was appreciated by the staff who gravitated toward the lovely smell.

Clinical aromatherapy has much to offer critical care as it reveals the softer, more caring side of a hard, mechanistic world. In a place full of technical equipment, aromatherapy allows patient and health provider a chance to get in touch with their feelings, to trust, and to communicate. Human beings often forget how to "be" as they are programmed to "do." The transition from doing to being can be a hard one to learn, but in the learning, both patient and health provider can share in the healing process at a much deeper level. In critical care, patients have to *be*. Aromatherapy enables patients to feel better as well as get better. That is the essence of holistic care. Anxiety, pain, insomnia, and stress are major areas in which aromatherapy could help in a critical-care setting. These have been covered in-depth in other chapters of the book, so please refer to the index for more information. The remaining sections of this chapter address other specialized areas of critical care where aromatherapy could be of use.

Extubation

Extubation is an alarming procedure for a patient who needs to be awake enough to breathe without assistance, but sedated enough not to fight the endotracheal tube. Tremendous trust is needed. Aromatherapy using the "m" technique can help produce a deep level of trust in a very short period of time. Just because a patient is intubated does not mean aromatherapy will have no effect. Drugs such as fentanyl, scopolamine, and clonidine are absorbed through the skin. Some compound pharmacists for hospice care are even putting Ativan and other commonly used prescription drugs into a gel for topical delivery. Components within essential oils, such as linalyl acetate and linalool, are also absorbed through the skin.

During extubation, fear of oversedation can be a common cause of inadequate pain- and anxiety-relief. Aromatherapy has no side effects and can actually facilitate extubation by promoting relaxation, decreasing anxiety, relieving pain, and promoting trust between patient and caregiver. After extubation, clearance of secretions can be greatly aided by the skilled use of mucolytic essential oils, such as *Eucalyptus globulus* or *Lavandula latifolia*, which can be inhaled by the patient. Mitchell (2002) found it was possible to decrease the amount of opioid narcotics needed while enhancing pain relief with the use of the "m" technique and essential oils. She suggests applying essential oils to the skin with the "m" technique can alter the pain pathway by affecting the transduction, perception, and modulation of nociceptive (somatic and visceral) pain. For example, an application of an antispasmodic essential oil, such as Roman chamomile, clary sage, or lavender, can minimize the transduction phase of nociception by minimizing the effects of sensitizing substances, such as prostaglandin, bradykinin, serotonin, and substance P, which are released at the periphery. Mitchell (2002) has found aromatherapy in a critical-care unit reduces stress, anxiety, fear, and insomnia, improves mood, promotes relaxation, enhances coping, and increases a patient's sense of control, all without side effects.

Figure 6-1 in Chapter 6 shows the effect of 2% *Lavandula angustifolia* given in a hand "m" technique by Mitchell prior to extubation. There have been similar effects from Roman chamomile and rose essential oils with the "m" technique. Mitchell further explains the patient appeared much calmer and less anxious as she was carrying out the "m" technique procedure. The patient felt "able to trust" her, and extubation was achieved far more easily than normal.

Henneman et al (2002) suggest a collaborative weaning plan for patients requiring prolonged mechanical ventilation, which draws on a multidisciplinary team. One advantage of aromatherapy is it can be carried out by any member of that team.

Fear

Patients in a critical-care unit face more invasive and obnoxious procedures and diagnostics than in any other unit. Invasive procedures are those such as the insertion of hemodynamic monitoring lines, thoracentesis, paracentesis, and chest-tube placement and removal. Diagnostics include those such as computed tomography scans, magnetic resonance imaging, and angiograms. Inhaling a familiar aroma can do much to allay fears during these procedures and really helps the claustrophobia and hyperventilation that can ensue.

Carrying out a hand, foot, or face "m" technique prior to the scheduled procedure can minimize the fear of cardiac catheterization. This will take only 5-10 minutes and can have a dramatic effect on the need for anxiolytics during the procedure. It is also a great way to enhance trust between patient and caregiver. Essential oils to choose from are rose, neroli, mandarin, lavender, or Roman chamomile. Please see Chapter 14 on cardiology for more information.

Adding three or four drops of essential oils to bath water can greatly improve the mood of patients (and their caregivers!). Geranium is an excellent choice as it appears to lift mood and reduce anxiety and can cut through some unpleasant odors. Spritzing the room with a solution of *Eucalyptus citriadora* will do much to improve the ambience but will also help cut down cross-infection and the possibility of resistant organisms. Please see Chapter 9 on infection for a more in-depth discussion of specific pathogens and essential oils that would be effective.

Pressure Sores (Decubitus Ulcers)

Critically ill patients often cannot move by themselves and need to be turned every few hours to prevent skin breakdown. Despite good nursing care and alternating-pressure mattresses, decubitus ulcers (pressure sores) can occur. These lesions are notoriously difficult to heal. What is initially persistent erythema can develop into necrotic ulceration involving muscle, tendon, and bone.

Pressure sores can be caused by the following:

simple pressure exceeding that of the blood pressure at the venous or arterial end of capillaries (Pritchard & Mallett 1992);

shearing (when the patient is dragged up the bed) destroying the microcirculation in the underlying tissue; in serious cases, lymphatic vessels and muscle fibers can also become torn (Waterlow 1988);

friction causing stripping of the stratum corneum leading to superficial damage (Johnson 1989).

Specific areas of the body are at risk for the development of pressure sores. These include the sacral area when lying supine, the coccygeal area when lying supine, the ischial tuberosities when lying laterally, and the greater trochanters when lying laterally. Inactivity, immobility, malnutrition, altered sensation, and advanced age can contribute to the incidence of pressure sores, but they are also more common among patients with decreased levels of consciousness. Waterlow (1987) produced at-risk scales to show the type of patient found in a critical-care unit is more likely to be at risk for pressure sores than other type of patient.

Pressure sores can be graded according to their severity (stage I-stage IV) and need different treatments for each stage (David et al 1983). The degrees of severity range from unbroken skin with simple redness to destruction of skin and the underlying tissue. Once the skin has broken down, careful treatment of the ensuing wound is paramount to prevent infection. Gustafsson (1988) categorized wounds as dry and clean, wet and oozing but clean, or open and contaminated.

Turner et al (1985) described an appropriate material for wound dressing as "a material which, when applied to the surface of a wound, provides and maintains an environment in which healing can take place at the maximum rate". An essential oil diluted in a cold-pressed vegetable oil would fit this description.

When the skin is red and sore but still intact, floral waters can be used to bathe the skin and reduce surface heat. Chamomile (*Matricaria recutita*), helichrysum, rose, and lavender floral water are good choices. When the skin is broken, a compress using floral waters with added essential oils can be used. However, when the wound has deepened, it is kinder to dilute the essential oils in a carrier oil (or gel) to prevent the compress sticking to the sides of the wound and increasing the trauma when the compress is removed. *Calophyllum inophyllum* (palm kernel) carrier oil is an excellent medium in which to dilute the essential oil because of its antiinflammatory action and gentle analgesic effects. Rosehip (*Rosa rubiginosa*) carrier oil is also useful in the treatment of pressure sores. Aloe vera gel would be an another excellent choice, particularly as it is so effective in the treatment of burns, which show a similar healing pattern to pressure sores (Zawahry 1973).

See Table 16-1, 16-2, and 16-3 for some suggestions of suitable essential oils, phytols, and hydrolats. If the wound is grossly infected, a higher concentra-

Table 16-1 ✖ *Suitable Essential Oils for Treating Decubitus Ulcers*

Common Name	Botanical Name
Lavender	*Lavandula angustifolia*
Roman chamomile	*Chamaemelum nobile*
Frankincense	*Boswellia carteri*
Geranium	*Pelargonium graveolens*
Yarrow	*Achillea millefolium*
German chamomile	*Matricaria recutita*
Common thyme	*Thymus vulgaris* CT linalol and CT thujone
Rosemary	*Rosmarinus officinalis* CT verbenone
Myrrh	*Commiphora myrrha*
Bergamot	*Citrus bergamia*

Table 16-2 ✖ *Suitable Phytols (Infused Herbal Oils) for Treating Decubitus Ulcers*

Common Name	Botanical Name
Echinacea	*Echinacea purpurea*
St John's wort	*Hypericum perforatum*
Calendula	*Calendula officinalis*

Table 16-3 ✖ *Suitable Hydrolats (Floral Waters) for Treating Decubitus Ulcers*

Common Name	Botanical Name
Rosemary	*Rosmarinus officinalis* CT borneol
Myrtle	*Myrtus communis*
Elderflower	*Sambucus nigra*
Roman chamomile	*Chamaemelum nobile*
Lavender	*Lavandula angustifolia*
Rose	*Rosa damascena*

Table 16-4 ❧ *Some Examples of Antimicrobial Essential Oils*

Common Name	Botanical Name	Use Against	Reference(s)
German chamomile	*Matricaria recutita*	*Staphylococcus aureus, Proteus vulgaris*	Franchomme & Penoel 1991, Valnet 1993
Lemongrass	*Cymbopogon citratus*	*Shigella, E. coli, Bacillus subtilis*	Onawunmi & Ogunina 1986
Juniper	*Juniperus communis*	*Pseudomonas*	Janssen & Chin 1986
Sweet marjoram	*Origanum majorana*	*Clostrium, Salmonella*	Deans & Svoboda 1990

tion of essential oil will be needed to contain the infection; use up to 20% when necessary. However, if the wound is just slow in healing, 3%-10% will suffice. Hartman and Coetzee (2002) found 8% solution was effective in treating deep, slow-healing ulcers. solution in a carrier oil or phytol is necessary. Many stage II-III decubiti are now covered with hydrocolloidal dressings until healing has taken place. The suggestions in the tables are particularly relevant after initial healing has begun and the dressings are removed. The selection of essential oils, floral water, and infused herbal oils will decrease pain, promote ongoing healing, and can help prevent reoccurrence. Ensure that floral waters and infused herbal oils are purchased from a reputable supplier to avoid contaminated products.

In cases in which the ulcer is infected, please select essential oils that are effective against the relevant pathogen. See Table 16-4, as well as Chapter 9 on infection, for some suggestions.

REFERENCES

Ashworth P. 1984. Staff-patient communication in coronary care units. J Adv Nurs. 9(1) 35-42.

Buckle J. 1993. Aromatherapy: does it matter which lavender essential oil is used? Nursing Times. 89(20) 32-35.

Buckle J. 1998. Clinical aromatherapy and touch: complementary therapies for Nursing Practice. Critical Care Nurse. 18(5) 54-61.

David J, et al. 1983. Normal physiology from injury to repair. Nursing. 2(11) 296-297.

Deans S, Svoboda K. 1990. The antimicrobial properties of marjoram (*Origanum majorana*). Flavour and Fragrance Journal. 5(3) 187-190.

Dunn C. 1996. Personal communication.

Dunn C, Sleep J, Collett D. 1995. Sensing an improvement: an experimental study to evaluate the use of aromatherapy, massage and periods of rest in an intensive care unit. Journal of Advanced Nursing. 21(1) 34-40.

Franchomme P, Penoel D. 1990. Aromatherapie Exactement. Limoges, France: Jollois.

Gustafsson G. 1988. Guidelines for the application of disinfectant in wound care. Nursing RSA. 3(11-12) 8-9.

Hartman D, Coetzee J. 2002. Two US practitioners' experience of using essential oils for wound care. Journal Wound Care. 11(8) 317-320.

Henneman E, Dracup K, Ganz T, et al. 2002. Using a collaborative weaning plan to decrease duration of mechanical ventilation and length of stay in the intensive care unit for patients receiving long-term ventilation. American Journal of Critical Care. 11(2) 132-140.

Ingham A. 1989. A review of the literature relating to touch and its use in intensive care. Intensive Care Nurse. 5(2) 65-75.

Janssen A, Chin N. 1986. Screening for antimicrobial activity of some essential oils. Pharmaceutisch Weekblad Scientific Edition (Utrecht). 8(6) 289-292.

Johnson A. 1989. Granuflex wafers as a prophylactic pressure sore dressing. Care-Science and Practice. 7(2) 55-58.

Mitchell L. 2002. Personal communication.

Onawunmi G, Ogunina E. 1986. A study of the antibacterial activity of the EO of lemongrass. International Journal of Crude Drug Research. 24(2) 64-68.

Pritchard A, Mallett J (eds.). 1992. The Royal Marsden Hospital Manual of Clinical Nursing Procedures, 3rd ed. Oxford, UK: Blackwell Scientific Publications.

Redd W, Manne S, Peters B, et al. 1994. Fragrance Administration to reduce anxiety during MRI imaging. J Magnetic Resonance Imaging. 4(4) 623-626.

Sharman R. 2001. Anatomy of a rose. Cambridge, MA: Perseus.

Stevensen C. 1994. The psychophysical effects of aromatherapy massage following cardiac surgery. Complementary Therapies in Medicine. 2(1) 27-35.

Turner T. 1985. Semi-occlusive and occlusive dressing. In Royal Society of Medicine International Congress and Symposium Series No. 88. London: Royal Society of Medicine. 5-14.

Urden L. 1997. From the patient's eyes. Critical Care Nurse. 17(1) 104-105.

Valnet J. 1990. The Practice of Aromatherapy. Saffron Walden, UK: CW Daniels.

Woolfson A, Hewitt D. 1992. Intensive aromacare. International Journal of Aromatherapy. 4(2) 12-13.

Waldman C, Tseng P, Meulman P, et al. 1993. Aromatherapy in the intensive care unit. Care of the Critically Ill. 9(4) 170-174.

Waterlow J. 1987. Tissue viability. Calculating the risk. Nursing Times. 83(39) 58-60.

Waterlow J. 1988. Tissue viability. Prevention is cheaper than cure. Nursing Times. 84(25) 69-71.

Welsh C. 1997. Tissue viability. Touch with oils: a pertinent part of holistic hospice care. American Journal of Hospital Palliative Care. 14(1) 42-44.

Zawahry E. 1973. Leg ulcers, acne vulgaris, seborrhea and alopecea. International Journal of Dermatology. 12(1) 68-73.

17

DERMATOLOGY

I have seen cosmic beings and other worlds, yet without seeing a flower it is nothing.

William Elliott
Tying Rocks to Clouds

Increasingly, transdermal therapeutic systems (TTS) are used as an alternative to oral and parenteral pharmaceuticals. The skin, and therefore the care of skin (dermatology), has become an important part of new drug delivery. This is important to aromatherapy as many essential oils are applied to the skin. Fuchs et al (1997) reported on the ability of carvone to be absorbed systemically from a diluted massage. Carvone is a ketone that makes up 42.8% of spearmint (Bowles 2000).

However, many drugs are unsuitable for TTS because of their low permeability, and components within essential oils may improve their permeability. Almirall et al (1996) found that cineole, d-limonene, and pinene permeated the skin and affected topical application of conventional drugs such as haloperidol and chlorpromazine. Whereas cineole and d-limonene enhanced the transdermal permeability of haloperidol, d-limonene reduced the transdermal permiability of chlorpromazine. Cineole is an oxide found in rosemary, cardamon, spike lavender, sage, and eucalyptus (Bowles 2000). Limonene is found in many citrus-peel oils. Cornwall and Barry (1994) investigated the ability of 12 sesquiterpenes to enhance the drug 5 fluorouracil and concluded several showed promise as clinically acceptable penetration enhancers.

The skin is the largest organ of the body. It is also a stress barometer that provides the outside world with an indication of the serenity or confusion within. Much of dermatology is concerned with putting topical drugs onto the skin. However, skin problems may be linked to stress and diet. Possibly three of the most common skin conditions suitable for aromatherapy are eczema, herpes, and onychomycosis.

ECZEMA

Eczema is often used as a generic term to describe dermatitis although Ellis et al (2002) suggests the two are not synonomous. Eczema is described as a "common itching skin disease characterized by reddening (erythema) and vesicle formation which may lead to weeping and crusting" (McFerran 1996). Eczema can be divided into two definitive groups: specific, which includes atopic or allergic, and a broad generic term covering generalized dermatitis. Eczema becomes clearer if it is divided into four specific types: allergic, atopic, irritant, and seborrhoeic (Schultz 2002).

Allergic eczema is caused by an allergen, and the allergy is unique to each person. An example of this is latex allergy, one of the most common skin problems among health workers. Minute amounts of latex, sometimes only two molecules, can trigger a skin reaction. Other examples of allergens are wool, lanolin, nickel found in jewelry, and rubber. Atopic eczema is associated with hay fever and asthma and affects up to 20% of the population. Irritant dermatitis can affect anyone and is related to the use of irritants such as biological washing powders and detergent cleaning agents (Gascoigne 1993). The only difference is the amount of irritant needed to produce an eczematous reaction. Seborrhoeic dermatitis involves the nose, lips, eyes, and scalp and is associated with *Pityrosporum* yeast infections.

The traditional treatment for eczema involves corticosteroid creams, avoidance of foods such as dairy products, yeast, or food additives (in cases of allergic or atopic eczema), and reduction of topical irritants.

While aromatherapy may aid the treatment of eczema either by reducing stress or by acting at a topical, aniinflammatory level, if the underlying problems contributing to the condition are not removed, the condition will not improve greatly. Eczema could be made worse if an essential oil is chosen to which the patient is sensitive or, in the case of atopic eczema, if too high a concentration is used. For this reason, patch testing should be mandatory for all eczema patients (particularly atopic) who wish to try aromatherapy. Put double the concentration of essential oil you wish to use on an adhesive bandage and apply to the patient's inner forearm. Leave in situ for 12 hours. Look for redness and itching. In addition, a careful case history, including details of potential antagonists (especially herbal teas, flowers, and pollens in cases of atopic eczema) and cosmetics (for contact allergic eczema) should be tabulated.

Anderson et al (2000) carried out a study on atopic eczema that, at first glance, indicated massage with essential oils made the eczema worse. However, this was a very unusual study as mothers chose the essential oil for their children themselves from an offered selection of 36 "commonly used" essential oils. It was not clear whether the mothers had any previous knowledge of or experience with essential oils. Two of the oils they chose were spike lavender and *Litsea cubeba.* Spike lavender contains up to 30% oxide (1,8-cineole) a common skin irritant, especially among young children (Price & Price 1999). *Litsea cubeba* often called "May chang" is commonly used in natural perfumery and is 85% citral, a common skin (and mucous membrane) irritant (Bowles 2000). It might be interesting to revisit this study and analyze it without those two essential oils.

Kadir and Barry (1991) found that alpha-bisabolol (an ingredient in German chamomile) enhanced the penetration of triamcinolone acetonide (a weak steroid which was formerly used to treat severe eczema) by 73 times thereby suggesting German chamomile could be used successfully with conventional topical treatment. Another ingredient in German chamomile, chamazulene, was found to inhibit the production of leukotriene B4 in neutraphilic granulocytes in vitro (Safayhi et al 1994).

Listed in Table 17-1 are some essential oils considered to be beneficial in treating eczema, followed by a discussion of the reasons for their use.

Lavandula angustifolia (true lavender) is very useful because of its recognized healing properties for burns and wounds. Lavender appears to have a cell-regenerating action, is soothing and sedative, and has a topical analgesic action that will help the itching. It is also antibacterial and moderately antifungal. This was the essential oil that proved so effective for Gattefosse's burns (Tisserand 1993).

The almost antihistamine-like action of *Matricaria recutita* (German chamomile) essential oil is due to the strong antiinflammatory effect of its three sesquiterpenes: azulene, bisabolol, and farnesene (Mills 1991). This makes German chamomile invaluable in the treatment of eczema. Its antiinflammatory

Table 17-1 ✖ *Essential Oils for Eczema*

Common Name	Botanical Name	Reference
True lavender	*Lavandula angustifolia*	Tisserand 1994
German chamomile	*Matricaria recutita*	Carle & Gomaa 1992 Tubaro et al 1984
Frankincense	*Boswellia carteri*	Duwiejua et al 1992
Roman chamomile	*Chamamelum nobile*	Rossi et al 1988
Balsam	*Myroxylon balsamum*	Tisserand 1993
Nagar matha	*Cyperus scariosus*	Gupta et al 1972
Cedarwood	*Cedrus atlantica*	Tisserand 1993
Fennel	*Foeniculum vulgare*	Mascolo et al 1987
Everlasting	*Helicrysum italicum*	Buckle 2001
Juniper	*Juniperus communis*	Mascolo et al 1987

effects have been well researched, and it is used in several pharmaceutical preparations. Carle & Gomaa (1992) found the alpha-bisabolol chemotype was the most effective.

German chamomile was tested together with a steroid and a nonsteroid (hydrocortisone and benzydamine, respectively) preparation on mice. Although it was not as effective as hydrocortisone, it was as effective as benzydamine (Tubaro et al 1984). However, in another study on humans, Kamillosan Ointment, which contains German chamomile, was found to be as effective as hydrocortisone in 161 patients (Aertgeerts et al 1985). German chamomile was also found to be effective in wound healing of patients following dermabrasion of tattoos (Glowania et al 1987).

Roman chamomile, *Chamemelum nobile,* is also an antiinflammatory (Rossi et al 1988). Although not as antiinflammatory as German chamomile, Roman chamomile might be more acceptable. German chamomile is dark blue and very pungent. Roman chamomile is colorless to pale blue with a pleasant, apple-like aroma. The two chamomiles have very different chemistry.

A little-known essential oil, *Cyperus scariosus* (nagar matha in Sanskrit), which is a grass-like herb, showed antiinflammatory activity in rats within 3 hours of its application. The inhibition of granulous-tissue formation was thought to be comparable to that achieved with hydrocortisone (Gupta et al 1972). This essential oil is not readily available.

Resins such as *Boswellia carteri* (frankincense) have traditionally been used in India and Africa to treat inflammatory conditions (Duwiejua et al 1992). In a study of the antiinflammatory effects of 75 species of plants on artificially induced inflammation in rats, *Foeniculum vulgare dulce* (sweet fennel), *Juniperus communis* (juniper), and *Symphytum officinale* (comfrey) decreased inflammation by up to 50%. Comfrey (an infused oil) also has antiulcer properties (Mascolo et al 1987) and could form a useful base for the essential oil mix. Balsam and skin problems were the subject of a doctoral thesis by Descouleurs, written in 1896 (Tisserand 1993).

Gattefosse reported *Cedrus atlantica* (cedar) was used to treat skin disorders in an Algerian hospital in 1899 with great success (Tisserand 1992). Finally, my clinical experience and that of my students is that *Helicrysum italicum* diluted in aloe vera gel (3%) is very effective in reducing the heat and itchiness of eczema. It will work within a few hours if it is going to work at all and is definitely worth a try.

HERPES

Cases of herpes simplex I and II reached epidemic proportions in the 1980s, and currently statistics from the American Social Health Association show that up to 50 million Americans have genital herpes, and there are 1 million newly diagnosed infections each year (Susman 2001). Further, genital herpes affects one of every five teens and adults in the United States and has increased 30% during the past 10 years, according to ASHA, a private, nonprofit organization dedicated to stopping sexually transmitted diseases (ASHA 2003).

The painful clusters of blisters reappear, usually in the same area, with agonizing regularity—often monthly—and once the disease has been contracted, the patient is infected for life. Outbreaks can be triggered by sexual activity, stress, heat, hormonal changes, diet, and low immunity. Although the blisters often occur in the genital area (either internally or externally), they may also be found on the thighs and buttocks. Extremely contagious at the blister stage, herpes can remain dormant for months or years in the spinal cord, ready to migrate down the sensory nerves to the skin.

Orthodox treatment for herpes is with nucleoside analogues, such as Acyclovir, that introduce intracellular impediment to viral replication. These medications are taken orally and often leave a metal-like after taste. Essential oils that may be effective against herpes in tissue are shown in Table 17-2. The table was compiled with reference to various research studies carried out on human tissue using extracts from plants (Cohen et al 1964; Kucera & Herrmann 1967; May & Willuhn 1978).

A randomized, controlled, multicentered study on 115 patients by Wolbling and Leonhardt (1994) found the aqueous extract of *Melissa* effective in treating herpes. On the final day (fifth day) of treatment, 24 patients in the *Melissa* group were symptom free versus 15 symptom-free patients in the placebo control group. Scabbing and swelling were more reduced in the *Melissa* group, indicating reduced cell damage and accelerated healing. Method of treatment was a proprietary-brand cream (Lomaherpan) that contains 1% *Melissa* extract. The control was an identical cream base without *Melissa*. The site of the herpes treated was the lips in 34 in the *Melissa* group and 33 in the control group and on the genitals in four

Table 17-2 ❧ *Essential Oils for Treating Herpes Simplex I & II*

Common Name	Botanical Name	Reference
Cubeb	*Piper cubeba*	May & Willuhn 1978
Blue gum	*Eucalyptus globulus*	May & Willuhn 1978
Juniper	*Juniperus communis*	May & Willuhn 1978
Melissa	*Melissa officinalis*	Wolbling et al 1994
Tea tree	*Melaleuca alternifolia*	Buckle 2001
Palma rosa	*Cymbopogon martinii*	Buckle 2001
Rosemary	*Rosmarinus officinalis*	May & Willuhn 1978
Rose	*Rosa damascena*	Buckle 2001
Ravensara	*Ravensara aromatica*	Buckle 2001
Moroccan thyme	*Thymus satureioides*	Buckle 2001

in the *Melissa* group and six in the control group. A subgroup of 67 patients tested positive for herpes labialis (type II, on the lips). The decline of the lesions remained statistically faster in the *Melissa* group than the placebo group.

One-percent *Melissa* aqueous extract was tested for topical treatment of recurring herpes labialis (Koytchev et al 1999). This was a double-blind, placebo controlled, randomized trial on 66 patients who had a history of four episodes of herpes labialis per year. The *Melissa* cream was applied four times a day. There was significant reduction in size of affected area and blisters at day 2 in the *Melissa* group. There was a rapid ameliorating effect on typical symptoms, reduction in healing time, and prolonged periods between occurrences.

Both these studies used an aqueous extract. This is not the same as an essential oil. However, clinical experience of myself and my students indicates the essential oil of *Melissa* is also extremely effective against herpes simplex I and II.

Melissa is the most expensive of all essential oils, and therefore is the most often adulterated. Frequently it is mixed with synthetics, lemongrass, or citronella. These contaminants may have a worsening effect on irritated or abraded lesions in irritant dermatitis, or, indeed, herpes.

A certain amount of anecdotal evidence indicates essential oils, applied to the area when the tingling begins, can prevent herpes blisters from forming. There is also anecdotal evidence that, when such oils are applied to the blisters, the pain and itching are greatly relieved. The most commonly used essential oils have been isolated from the 75 plants found to have virustatic activity. Despite the age of the papers cited that investigated the first four essential oils listed for treating herpes (see Table 17-2), I have found these and the other essential oils in the table effective in 10 years of clinical experience. Severity, duration, and frequency of herpes outbreaks have decreased substantially with their use. A suggested protocol for application is shown in Table 17-3. Each patient will respond to one particular essential oil or mix of oils. The reason the essential oils work could be because they are lipophyllic and appear to dissolve the lipid capsule (or capsid) of the virus. The most successful essential oil I have used has been *Ravansara aromatica* (ravensara).

Table 17-3 & *Protocol for Using Essential Oils in Treating Herpes*

Symptom	Topical Application	Frequency
Tingling	Undiluted essential oil	Every 4 hours
Redness and swelling	Undiluted essential oil	Every 4 hours
Pustule formation	Undiluted essential oil	Every 4 hours
Broken pustule, raw skin	25% diluted essential oil*	Every 4 hours
Raw skin	5% diluted essential oil	Every 4 hours

*Dilute in cold-pressed vegetable oils, like sweet almond, or aloe vera gel.

In a study by Armaka et al (1999), isoborneol, a monoterpeneol found in several essential oils, demonstrated viricidal activity against herpes simplex virus I by inactivating the virus within 30 minutes of exposure. Further, a concentration of 0.06% isoborneol completely inhibited viral replication without affecting viral adsorption. Isoborneol did not show significant cytotoxicity when tested against human cell lines at 0.16%. Therefore essential oils containing a major proportion of isoborneol might be useful in treating herpes. A high amount of borneol (up to 70%.) is found in *Thymus satureoides* (Japanese thyme).

Geraniol, a monoterpenol found in many essential oils, was found to enhance the antiherpetic activity of conventional treatment in a study by Shoji et al (1998). Its action was thought to occur by changing the subcellular distribution of the oligonucleotides. Geraniol is found in palma rosa (80%) (Bowles 2000) and *Thymus vulgaris* CT gereniol.

Benencia and Courreges (2000) found eugenol was effective against herpes simplex type I and II in monkey kidney-cell cultures and in vivo (in rabbits). The monkey-cell cultures showed a dose-dependent sensitivity (higher doses increased treatment effectiveness), and at least 50% of the viral activity was lost after contact with the diluted eugenol (250ug/ml) for one hour. Eugenol also appeared to enhance the effect of Acyclovir. Eugenol appeared to prolong the resistance of rabbits to developing herpes by 7 days, but all experimental animals eventually became ill.

The antiherpetic activity of buds of *Syzygium aromatica* (clove) were alluded to by Takechi et al (1985). However as clove is very high in phenols (70%), and phenols are irritant to the skin and mucous membrane, clove bud (or leaf) is best avoided.

ATHLETE'S FOOT AND ONYCHOMYCOSIS

Athlete's foot (*Tinea pedis*) is the most common form of superficial dermatophyte infection in the developed world and infects approximately 10% of the population (Tong et al 1992).

Onychomycosis (sometimes called *Tinea ingium*) is a superficial fungal infection that destroys the entire nail unit. It is a cousin of *Tinea pedis,* which causes athlete's foot. It is less contagious than athlete's foot, but susceptibility increases after trauma to the nail bed. Once contracted, it is extremely difficult to remove completely. Symptoms are a thickened nail that becomes discolored, brittle, or chalky and ultimately disintegrates. Medical treatment includes debridement and topical or systemic antifungals. Oral antifungal agents began with Griseofulvin in 1959 (Buck et al 1994), which was given orally for 6 months or until the nail grew out. Side effects to Griseofulvin are nausea, vomiting, diarrhea, mental confusion, and headaches.

Headaches are the most common side effect and can be severe, especially at the commencement of treatment. The cure rate is 3%-38%. Ketoconazole is another option, with the added advantage that it also treats yeast. The cure rate is higher at 50%-94%, and the side effects are less common, although they are more serious and include idiosyncratic liver dysfuntion, requiring liver transplantation (Knight et al 1991). Unfortunately, 50% of toenail infections recur within 4 years of completion of treatment (Torok & Stechlich 1986). Itraconazole has cure rates of 4%-92% but has only been evaluated in small studies (Piepponen et al 1992). The previously mentioned conventional treatments are expensive and involve oral medication.

The incidence of onychomycosis is increasing with no real satisfactory cure. Buck et al (1994) carried out a multicentered, double-blind, randomized, controlled study on onychomycosis using tea tree or clotrimazole. One-hundred seventeen patients with distal subungual onychomycosis proven by culture took part in the study. Patients received either twice-daily applications of clotrimazole solution or 100% tea tree. Debridement took place at 0, 1, 3, and 6 months. Topical use of tea tree produced a similar result to oral doses of clotrimazole, with 55% of the clotrimazole group and 56% of the tea tree group reporting improvement or resolution after 3 months. The number of adverse reactions were similar; three out of 53 for the clotrimazole group and five out of 64 in the tea tree group.

Syed et al (1999) carried out a randomized, double-blind, placebo-controlled study to examine the clinical efficacy and tolerability of 5% *Melaleuca alternifolia* with 2% butenafine hydrochloride incorporated in a cream. Sixty patients took part in the study. There were 39 men and 21 women, and the average age was 29 years. Each participant had a history of onychomycosis for 6-36 months. After using the cream for 16 weeks, 80% of the participants in the experimental group were cured. No participant was cured in the placebo group. Four participants in the experimental group experienced mild inflammation but did not discontinue treatment. During follow-up no relapse occurred in the cured patients, and no improvement was seen in the medication-resistant and placebo participants.

Elsethager (2000) investigated the effect of two essential oils (lemongrass and tea tree) on 12 study participants who had onychomycosis for a minimum duration of 1 year. One participant had it for more than 10 years. Two dilutions, 2% tea tree and 3% lemongrass, were mixed together in grapeseed oil and given to each participant, who rubbed the mixture well into the affected nail bed twice a day for 2 months. It was thought there would be some visual improvement during this time, although participants would need to continue treatment until the whole nail had grown out. Only four people completed the treatment for 2 months. All stated their nails were less discolored, scaly, and cracked, and the discomfort was less. A visual analog on effectiveness was completed, with zero as not effective and 10 as extremely effective. One person rated the treatment a seven, and the other three rated it a seven. Two of the four had previously used over-the-counter medications (Tinactin and Dr. Scholl's) which were rated zero. One of the four participants had been offered an oral course of Griseofulvin, which she had declined because she was concerned about the side effects.

Garg and Dengre (1988) found *Cymbopogon citratus* (West Indian lemongrass) effective against *Trichophyton mentagrophytes*. The most active component of lemongrass was citral (70%-80%), which is thought to be responsible for the antifungal activity of this plant. *Lippia alba,* which grows widely in Central and South America, also has strong antifungal activity against *Trichophyton mentagrophyes* var. *interdigitale.* Several chemotypes of the plant exist, and the essential oil from the plant grown in Aruba is thought to be most suitable as it contains 64% citral (Fun & Svendsen 1990).

Even at the low concentrations, essential oils can show very significant antimycotic activity against *Trichophyton mentagrophytes* (Rai & Acharya 2001). Sahi et al (1999) compared the efficacy of *Eucalyptus citriadora* with commercial antifungal drugs and found minimal concentration of the oil inhibited all the tested pathogens, *Microsporum nanum, Trichophyton mentagrophytes,* and *T. rubrum,* completely with fungistatic activity. Romagna et al (1994) reported the antifungal effects of alpha-terthienyl from *Tagetes patula* on five dermatophytes. Rai and Acharya (2000) found *Tagetes erecta, T. patula,* and *Eupatorium triplinerve* to be effective topical antimycotics.

REFERENCES

Aertgeerts P, Albring M, Klaaschka F, et al. 1985. Comparative testing of Kamillosan cream and steroidal (0.25% hydrocortisone, 0.75% fluocortin butyl ester) and non-steroidal (5% bufexamac) dermatologic agents maintenance therapy for eczematous diseases. Zeitschrift fur Hautkrankheiten (Berlin). 60(3) 270-277.

Almirall M, Montana J, Escribano E, et al. 1996. Effect of d-limonene, a pinene and cineole on in vitro transdermal human skin penetration of chlorpromazine and haloperidol. Arzneim-Forsch/Drug Research. 46(7) 676-680.

American Social Health Association. January 2003. www.ashstd.org.

American Social Health Association. June 2001. www.ashstd.org.

Anderson C, Lis-Balchin M, Kirk-Smith M. 2000. Evaluation of massage with essential oils on childhood atopic eczema. Phytotherapy Research. 14(6) 452-456.

Armaka M, Papanikolaou E, Sivropoulou A, et al. 1999. Antiviral properties of isoborneol, a potent inhibitor of herpes simplex virus type 1. Antiviral Research. 43(2) 79-92.

Benencia F, Courreges M. 2000. In vitro and in vivo activity of eugenol on human herpes virus. Phytotherapy Research. 14:495-500.

Bowles J. 2002. The basic chemistry of aromatherapeutic essenial oils. Sydney: Good Scents Aromapleasure.

Buck D, Nidorf D, Addino J. 1994. Comparison of two topical preparations for the treatment of onychomycosis: *Melaleuca alternifolia* (teatree) oil and clotrimazole. Journal of Family Practice. 38(6) 601-605.

Buckle J. 2001. Results of 200 case studies. Unpublished dissertation. Hunter, NY: R J Buckle Associates.

Cohen R, Kucera L, Herrmann C. 1964. Antiviral activity of *Melissa officinalis.* Proceedings of the Society of Experimental Biology and Medicine. 117: 431-434.

Cornwall P, Barry B. 1994. Sesquiterpene components of volatile oils as skin penetration enhancers for the hydrophilic permanent 5 fluorouracil. Journal of Pharmacy and Pharmacology. 46(4) 261-269.

Duwiejua M, Zeitlin I, Waterman P, et al. 1992. Anti-inflammatory activity of resins from some species of the plant family Burseraceae. *Planta Medica.* 59(1) 12-16.

Elliott W. 1995. Tying rocks to clouds. New York: Image Books/Doubleday.

Ellis C, Drake L, Prendelgast M, et al. 2002. Cost of atopic dermaitis and eczema in the USA. Dermatology. 46: 361-370.

Elsethager T. 2000. The use of lemongrass and teatree for fungal infections of feet and nails. Unpublished dissertation. Hunter, NY: R J Buckle Associates.

Fuchs N, Jager W, Lenhardt A, et al. 1997. Systemic absorption of topically applied carvone: influence of massage technique. Journal of Society of Cosmetic Chemists. 48: 277-282.

Fun C, Svendsen A. 1990. The essential oils of *Lippia alba.* Journal of Essential Oil Research. 2(5) 265-267.

Garg S, Dengre S. 1988. Antifungal activity of some essential oils. Pharmacie. 43(2) 141-142.

Gascoigne S. 1993. Manual of Conventional Medicine for Alternative Practitioners, Vol. 1. Richmond, VA: Jigme Press.

Gattefosse R. 1937. (Translated in 1993 by R. Tisserand.) Aromatherapie: Les Huile Essentielles-Hormones Vegetales (Gattefosse's Aromatherapy.) Saffron Walden, UK: CW Daniels, 89.

Glowania H, Raulin C, Svoboda M. 1987. Effect of chamomile on wound healing: a clinical double-blind study. Berlin: Zeitschrift fur Hautkrankheiten. 62(17) 1262, 1267-1271.

Gupta S, Sharma R, Aggarwal O. 1972. Anti-inflammatory activity of the oils isolated from *Cyperus scariosus.* Indian Journal of Experimental Biology. 10(1) 41.

Jandera V, Hudson S, de West P. 2000. Cooling the burn wound: evaluation of different modalities. Burns. 26(3) 265-270.

Kadir R, Barry B. 1991. A-bisabolol a possible safe penetration enhancer for dermal and transdermal therapeutics. International Journal of Pharmacology. 70: 87-94.

Knight T, Shikuma C, Knight J. 1991. Ketoconazole-induced fulminant hepatitis necessitating liver transplantation. Journal of the American Academy of Dermatology. 25(2 part 2) 398-400.

Koytchev R, Alken R, Dundarov S. 1999. Balm mint extract (Lo-701) for topical treatment for recurring herpes labialis. Phytomedicine. 6(4) 225-230.

Kucera L, Herrmann E. 1967. Antiviral substances in plants of the mint family. (Labiatae) Tannin of *Melissa officinalis.* Proceedings from the Society for Experimental Biology and Medicine. 124(3) 865-869.

Maiche A G, Grohn P, Maki-Hokkonen H. 1991. Effect of chamomile cream and almond ointment on acute radiation skin reaction. Acta Oncologica. 30(3) 395-396.

Mascolo N, Autore G, Capasso F 1987. Biological screening of Italian medicinal plants for anti-inflammatory activity. Phytotherapy Research. 1(1) 28-31.

May V, Willuhn G. 1978. Antivirale Wirkung waBriger Pflanzenextrakte in Gewebekulturen. Arzneim-Forsch/Drug Research. 28(1) 1-7.

McFerran T. 1996. A Dictionary of Nursing, 2nd ed. Oxford, UK: Oxford University Press.

Mills S. 1991. Out of the Earth. London:Viking Arkana.

Piepponen T, Blomqvist K, Brandt H, et al. 1992. Onychomycosis treated with itraconazole or griseofulvin alone with and without a topical antimycotic or keratolytic agent. International Journal of Dermatology. 30: 586-589.

Price S, Price L. 1999. Aromatherapy for Health Professionals. London: Churchill Livingstone.

Rai M, Mares M, editors. 2003. Plant Derived Antimycotics. Binghamton, NY: Haworth.

Romagna C, Mares D, Fasulo M, et al. 1994. Antifungal effects of alpha-terthienyl from *Tagetes patula* on five dermatophytes. Phytotherapy Research. 8(6) 332-336.

Rossi T, Melegari M, Blanchi A. 1988. Sedative, anti-inflammatory and anti-diuretic effects induced in rats by essential oils of varieties of *Anthemis nobilis:* a comparative study. Pharmacological Research Communications. 20(Suppl. V) 71-74.

Safayhi H, Sabieraj J, Sailer E et al. 1994. Chamazulene: an antioxidant-type inhibitor of leukotriene B4 formation. Planta Medica. 60(5) 410-413.

Sahi S, Shukla A, Bajaj A, et al. 1999. Broad spectrum antimycotic drug for the control of fungal infections in human beings. Current Science. 76(6) 836-939.

Shoji Y, Ishige H, Tamura N, et al. 1998. Enhancement of anti-herpetic activity of antisense phosphorothioate oligonucleotides 5 end modified with geraniol. Journal of Drug Targeting. 5(4) 261-273.

Susman C. 2001. Americans unaware of scope of HIV infection. www.ncm.nih.govmedlineplus/news.

Syed T, Qureshi Z, Ali S, et al. 1999. Treatment of toenail onychomycosis with 2% butenafine and 5% *Melaleuca alternifolia* (teatree in cream). Tropical Medicine & International Health. 4(4) 284-287.

Takechi M, Tanaka Y, Takehara M, et al. 1985. Structure and anti-herpetic activity among the tannins. Phytochemistry. 24(10) 2245-2250.

Tisserand R. 1992. The book that launched aromatherapy. International Journal of Aromatherapy. 4(4) 20-22.

Tong M, Altman P, Barnetson R. 1992. Teatree oil in the treatment of *Tinea pedis.* Australasian Journal of Dermatology. 33(3) 145-149.

Torok I, Stechlich G. 1986. Long term post treatment follow up of onychomycosis treated with ketoconazole. Mykosen. 29(8) 372-377.

Tubaro A, Zilli C, Redaeli C. 1984. Evaluation of anti-inflammatory activity of a chamomile extract topical application. Planta Medica. 50(4) 147-153.

Wolbling R, Leonhardt K. 1994. Local therapy of herpes simplex with dried extract from *Melissa officinalis.* Phytomedicine 1: 24-31.

18

ENDOCRINOLOGY

Without communication, no real understanding can be possible. Be sure you can communicate with yourself. If you cannot communicate with yourself, how do you expect to communicate with another person?

Tich Nhat Hanh
Anger

The endocrine system is the regulator of homeostasis (Anthony & Thibodeau 1983). This balance is maintained through some two hundred hormones in our bodies. The word *hormone* comes from the Greek *hormaein,* meaning to excite. In certain instances the nervous and endocrine systems can regulate each other's activities, as well as acting together to bring about changes in physiology. Endocrine cells in the body occur in clusters in the endocrine glands. These glands secrete hormones directly into the bloodstream. As hormones regulate our metabolism, growth, development, and reproduction, it is clear they are a fundamental necessity to life. Hormones also govern our stress response. Aromas interact with the limbic, hormonal, and endocrine systems as well as impacting prostaglandin production and cell metabolism. This makes aromatherapy a valuable tool for treating conditions related to the endocrine system (Table 18-1 introduces the main organs of the endocrine system).

Hormones play an important role in the mechanisms involving prostaglandins. Prostaglandins are a unique group of biological compounds that have a 5-carbon ring and serve important integrative functions in the body but do not fit the definition of a typical hormone. They are metabolized rapidly and so the amount in the bloodstream at one time is very low (Anthony & Thibodeau 1983). Three classes of prostaglandins—prostaglandin A (PGA), prostaglandin E (PGE), and prostaglandin F (PGF)—have been isolated and identified from a wide range of tissues. Aspirin is thought to exert its antiinflammatory action by

Table 18-1 ❧ *Main Organs of the Endocrine Systems*

Pineal gland	Regulates production of melatonin (a dark/light mechanism that affects how we sleep)
Pituitary gland	Master endocrine gland divided into two lobes:
	1) the anterior lobe governs growth, thyroid, adrenocorticotropic, and reproductive hormones, namely luteinizing and follicle-stimulating hormone
	2) the posterior lobe secretes vasopressin (antidiuretic hormone) and oxytocin (stimulates contraction of the uterus during labor)
Thyroid	Secretes thyroxin and governs metabolic rate
Parathyroid	Controls calcium and phosphate levels
Adrenal cortex	Produces corticosteroids
Adrenal medulla	Produces adrenaline and noradrenaline
Islets of Langerhans	Secretes insulin, glucagon, somatostatin, amylin, and gastrin
Female gonads	Produce estrogen and progesterone
Male gonads	Produce testosterone

inhibiting PGE synthesis. Eugenol, carvacrol, thymol, and gingerol (all compounds found within essential oils) have also been shown to influence PGE synthesis (Bennett & Stamford 1988; Wagner et al 1986). Prostaglandin F (PGF) is important in the female reproductive system (Alexander 2001).

All prostaglandins are intimately involved in endocrine regulation by influencing adenyl cyclase and adenosine 3,5-phosphate activity within the cell (Anthony & Thibodeau 1983). Anything that interferes with that cellular activity indirectly affects the hormonal and endocrine system. Calcium regulates cellular activity (Alexander 2001). Components within essential oils can interfere with the release of calcium at a cellular level. This blocking mechanism has been demonstrated for menthol, anethole, eugenol, and thymol (Melzig & Teuscher 1991). These components are found in essential oils such as peppermint, fennel, aniseed, star aniseed, bay, clove, Spanish marjoram, thyme, and oregano (Sheppard-Hangar 1995; Budavari 1996).

AROMATHERAPY AND THE FEMALE REPRODUCTIVE SYSTEM

Premenstrual syndrome (PMS) and menopausal problems are directly related to the endocrine system (Alexander 2001). The uterus makes prostagladins to help with labor, and the same prostaglandins can cause menstrual cramps. This is why medications that block the synthesis of prostaglandin are effective in dysmenorrhea. Alexander (2001) suggests it is possible that essential oils with vasodilatory or prostaglandin-antagonist properties might relieve the problem via olfaction alone, although I think this is unlikely. During menopause, 50%-70% of women experience a variety of physical and emotional symptoms (Schwingl et al 1994). Many of these symptoms can be ameliorated with certain essential oils. PMS and menopause affect many millions of women every day. Fluctuation in estrogen levels can lead to profound mental and physical symptoms. Estrogen levels drop after ovulation and at menopause.

There are three main forms of estrogen. Estradiol is the strongest form of estrogen our bodies make. Estrone is converted from estradiol in the liver, and Estriol is the weakest form of estrogen. However even estriol can have a pronounced effect (van Der 1982).

Premenstrual Syndrome

PMS became a household name in England in 1987 when Anna Reynolds was charged with the murder of her mother (a crime committed while suffering from the effects of PMS) and jailed for life. Four months later, a petition signed by 6000 people launched an appeal for her release. On June 23, 1988, the British court of appeals reduced the murder charge to manslaughter on the grounds of PMS, and Reynolds was released. This was the first time a woman had been allowed to plead diminished responsibility due to "the time of the month."

Women have known for many years that they can become irrational, irritable, weepy, and occasionally violent a few days before their menstrual period. No one quite knows why this phenomenon affects some women and not others. However, the chemistry of a woman's brain actually changes during this time and produces reactions she cannot control (Alexander 2001). The area deep within the limbic system involved with mood control has more estrogen receptors than other parts of the brain, which makes it more vulnerable to changes in estrogen levels. One in 10 women becomes irritable, depressed, and fatigued with PMS symptoms appearing 7-10 days prior to menses. However, the more violent or aggressive PMS symptoms usually appear within 5 days of the menstruation time. There is a difference in PMS behavior depending on the side of the brain involved (Alexander 2001). The left side often produces symptoms of depression and irritability. The right side is associated with anger and negative emotion.

In PMS there appears to be a fluctuation in the levels of endogenous opioids (these are abundant in the limbic system) and serotonin. In the first half of the menstrual cycle the levels of estrogen and endorphin interact with neurotransmitters serotonin, dopamine, and norepinephrine to keep mood stability. When estrogen levels first begin to drop, immediately after ovulation, serotonin receptors are primed (Rubinow et al 1998). When estrogen levels drop again prior to menstruation, the brain registers estrogen withdrawal of serotonin.

Conventional medicine treats PMS with selective serotonin reuptake inhibitors (SSRIs) such as fluoxetine, paroxetine, sertraline, and citalopram or a tricyclic antidepressant related to SSRI such as clomipramine (Reid 2002). A simpler but almost as effective method can be a large block of chocolate! Chocolate has been found to increase serotonin and has been dubbed "the Prozac of plants" by *Forbes* magazine (Bartlett 1999).

Aromatherapy can, in many instances, produce very reasonable results in PMS if regular treatments are given throughout a period of several months. The essential oils chosen are usually a combination of those thought to have estrogen-like properties, such as fennel (*Foeniculum vulgare*), sage (*Salvia officinalis*), or clary sage (*Salvia sclarea*) (Zondeck & Bergmann 1938), and those that have hormone-like properties, such as Scotch pine (*Pinus sylvestris*) and myrrh (*Commiphora myrrha*) (Franchomme & Penoel 1991). *Salvia sclarea* also has antiinflammatory properties (Moretti et al 1997). Belaiche, a French MD who devotes a whole volume of his work to female problems, suggests essential oil of sage, thyme, or geranium for PMS (Belaiche 1979). Citral (an aldehyde found in lemongrass, melissa, and verbena) demonstrates estrogen activity when applied dermally to rats, although in doses much higher than would be normally used in aromatherapy (Tisserand & Balacs 1995). Table 18-2 lists essential oils used in the treatment of PMS.

Depending on the patient's needs, another essential oil can be added to the "balancing" essential oil that will help alleviate the symptoms of the imbalance. For example, if a woman is showing symptoms of depression and is weepy, an essential oil with an antidepressant action such as bergamot (Sheppard-Hangar 1995) or rose (Rovesti & Columbo 1973) could be added to the balancing mixture. If she is

Table 18-2 ✖ *Essential Oils for PMS*

Common Name	Botanical Name	Reference
Fennel	*Foeniculum vulgare*	Zondeck & Bergmann 1938
Sage	*Salvia officinalis*	Zondeck & Bergmann 1938
Scotch pine	*Pinus sylvestris*	Franchomme & Penoel 1991
Myrrh	*Commiphora myrrha*	Franchomme & Penoel 1991
Clary sage	*Salvia sclarea*	Zondeck & Bergmann 1938
Geranium	*Pelargonium graveolens*	Belaiche 1979
Thyme	*Thymus vulgaris*	Belaiche 1979
Aniseed, fennel	rans-anethole	Albert-Puleo 1980
Lemongrass, melissa, verbena	Citral	Geldof et al 1992

violent and irrational, a sedative such as angelica (Franchomme & Penoel 1991) or ylang ylang could be used (Bucellato 1982). Geranium (*Pelargonium graveolens*) is an excellent hormonal balancer. The aqueous extract of *Pelargonium graveolens* has the added bonus of inhibiting platelet aggregation (Tzeng et al 1991), thereby possibly preventing extensive clotting during menstruation, which so often accompanies hormonal imbalance. A Korean study (Han et al 2003) indicated that 2% clary sage applied to the abdomen of menstruating women reduced the uterine . . . . and substantially reduced dysmenorrhea.

I have had some success using tarragon in conjunction with estrogen-like essential oils on women who have displayed aggressive PMS. One patient actually admitted "going for my husband with a knife." Although tarragon (*Artemisia dracunculus*) has fallen out of favor recently due to its estragole content, the research that gave rise to that view involved administering very large doses of estragole orally to rats over a period of 12 months (Tisserand & Balacs 1995). The oral route would ensure that substantially more estragole was absorbed than by the topical route, and much higher doses were used in the study than are used in aromatherapy.

Buckingham (2000) investigated the effect of essential oils on 14 women (aged 21-43) with moderate to severe PMS in a controlled study lasting 6 months. One symptom was chosen by each participant and matched to a specific essential oil. The results indicated each of the chosen essential oils, except surprisingly clary sage, had a beneficial effect on menstrual symptoms. See Table 18-3 for study findings.

Menopausal Problems

The menopause is the natural cessation of a woman's fertility. Estrogen levels fall to 40%-60% of premenopausal level, and progesterone levels fall to almost zero (Moskowitz 2001). Once looked upon with secret delight as the end of menstruation and its accompanying messy problems, menopause now seems to be viewed by many women with dismay and despair and by orthodox medicine as a condition to be fixed. Menopausal depression is thought to be one of the main symp-

Table 18-3 ❧ *Essential Oils Used in Buckingham's Study*

Essential Oil	Disorder Treated
True lavender	Anxiety
True lavender	Breast tenderness
Juniper	Fluid retention
Juniper	Breast tenderness
Clary sage	Low-back pain
Geranium	Mood swings
Geranium	Nervous tension

Table 18-4 ❧ *Essential Oils for Menopause*

Common Name	Botanical Name	Reference
Fennel	*Foeniculum vulgare*	Marini-Bettolo 1979
Geranium	*Pelargonium graveolens*	Holmes 1993
Rose	*Rosa damascena*	Buckle 1997
Clary sage	*Salvia sclarea*	Rose 1996
Sage	*Salvia officinalis*	Franchomme & Penoel 1991
Anise seed	*Pimpinella anisum*	Albert-Puleo 1980
Cypress	*Cupressus sempervirens*	Valnet 1993

toms of women seeking hormone replacement therapy (HRT) (Andrist 1998), although older women seem more concerned with osteoporosis and younger women with hot flashes (Ettinger & Pressman 1999). Between one- and two-thirds of woman discontinue HRT during the first 2 years because of weight gain and unwanted side effects such as bloating and breakthrough bleeding (Den Tonkelaar & Oddens 2000).

Hot flashes, night sweats, sleep disturbance, depression, loss of energy, and loss of concentration are all common symptoms of menopause (Schmid & Rubinow 1994). However, cessation of estrogen and progesterone production does not happen overnight, and it is the interim imbalance that is so difficult.

Essential oils such as rose (Belaiche 1979), cypress (Valnet 1993), or clary sage can be helpful when used in a hydrosol spray or spritzer sprayed around the face, neck, and shoulders during a hot flash. A few drops of peppermint added to the mix is wonderfully cooling. Essential oils that could be used for estrogen support include fennel (Marini-Bettolo 1979), sage (Franchomme & Penoel 1991), and aniseed (Albert-Puleo 1980). Geranium (Holmes 1993) and rose give added support. Using a mixture of essential oils on a daily basis can be very beneficial either on a tissue or in a bath or body lotion. I used menopausal oils in this way for several years with no ill effect. Rotating the mix of calming and estrogen-supportive essential oils will prevent the body from becoming inured to the essential oils. The combinations and permutations of some 20 essential oils can work out to be a great number of different mixes—all therapeutic and beneficial for menopausal symptoms (Table 18-4).

For night sweats, cypress, with its recognized deodorant effect and hormonal properties, is comforting (Valnet 1993). For insomnia, any of the gently relaxing and sedative oils could be added, but try also root of *Angelica archangelica* (Duke 1985). Increasing soy intake and taking daily food supplements such as red clover and black cohosh will also help tremendously as these phytoestrogens can help balance wildly fluctuating hormone levels.

Shiffman (1995) explored the effects of a selection of fragrance sprays currently on the market with 56 women aged 45-60 in a placebo-controlled study. Four groups were assigned depending on hormonal status: 1) still menstruating, 2) no longer menstruating and taking estrogen, 3) no longer menstruating and taking estrogen and progesterone, 4) no longer menstruating and not taking either estrogen or progesterone. While the scents supplied were not specified and probably were synthetic, the effects indicated that pleasant scents alleviated depression and confusion in women at midlife and were more effective in those women taking hormone replacement. Schiffman suggests the positive effects may be because pleasant aromas improve mood, thus releasing a broad range of transmitters in the limbic system.

Kozlowski (2000) explored the use of clary sage and geranium on 11 menopausal women aged 47-56 using a 5% solution applied to the reflexology point for ovaries and uterus on the feet. Clary sage produced some useful changes in hot flash intensity. One subject wrote that two nights after stopping clary sage, the hot flashes returned to their original intensity.

Both the above conditions occur exclusively in women and, fall more under gynecology than endocrinology, so perhaps a very brief mention of diabetes (an endocrine disorder that affects both men and women) and the use of essential oils might be in order.

DIABETES

Baschetti (1998) explored the hypothesis that the epidemic of diabetes in newly Westernized populations could be due to genetically unknown foods as well as a surge in calories from increased fat intake. There were no instances of diabetes in Nauru, an island in the Pacific, in a 1933 medical survey. But by 1978, 44% of the population had noninsulin-dependent diabetes mellitus (NIDDM). Similarly, there was only one possible incidence of NIDDM among Pima Indians in Arizona in 1908, but currently it is present in 50% of adults over 35 years of age (Knowler et al 1981).

These two studies, and the dramatic increase in diabetes in the United States during the last 10 years, suggest Westernized people could be adding something to their diets that their bodies cannot metabolize. The increase in diabetes has been linked to the increase in sugar consumption and to the increase in obesity.

Rosmarinus officinalis (rosemary) was shown to suppress the insulin response in a glucose-tolerance test in rabbits when plasma glucose levels remained at 55% for 2 hours. Rosemary also caused hyperglycemia in rabbits with artificially induced diabetes (Al-Hader & Hasan 1994).

Another study showed that *Eucalyptus citriodora* (lemon-scented gum) had a hypoglycemic effect on rabbits (Revoredo 1958). Valnet states that geranium has antidiabetic properties, although no clarification is given (Valnet 1993). Ylang ylang is another essential oil thought to be useful in diabetes (Franchomme & Penoel 1991; Sheppard-Hangar 1995; Price 1995), although again no research to substantiate this view was given.

REFERENCES

Albert-Puleo M. 1980. Fennel and anise as estrogenic agents. Journal of Ethnopharmacology. 2(4) 337-344.

Al-Hader A, Hasan Z. 1994. Hyperglycemic and insulin release inhibitory effects of *Rosmarinus officinalis*. Journal of Ethnopharmacology. 43(3) 217-211.

Alexander M. 2001. How Aromatherapy Works, Vol. 1: Principle Mechanisms in Olfaction. Odessa, FL: Whole Spectrum Books, 293.

Andrist L. 1998. The impact of media attention, family history, politics and maturation on women's decisions regarding hormone replacement therapy. Health Care For Women International. 19(3) 243-260.

Anthony C, Thibodeau G. 1983. Textbook of Anatomy and Physiology. St. Louis, MO: Mosby.

Bartlett J. Nov. 11, 1999. Meltdown. Forbes.com. www.forbes.com

Baschetti R. 1998. Diabetes epidemic in newly Westernized populations: is it due to thrifty genes or to genetically unknown foods? Journal of the Royal Society of Medicine. 91(12) 622-626.

Belaiche P. 1979. Syndrome premenstruel. In Traite de Phytotherapie et d'Aromatherapie. Paris: Maloine SA. 3: 60-64.

Bennett A, Stamford F. 1988. The biological activity of eugenol, a major constituent of nutmeg, on prostaglandins, the intestine and other tissues. Phytotherapy Research. 2(3) 125-129.

Buccellato F. 1982. Ylang survey. Perfumer & Flavorist. 7(4) 9-10.

Buckingham C. 2000. Effects of Aromatherapy on PMS. Unpublished dissertation. Hunter, NY: R J Buckle Associates.

Buckle J. 1997. Clinical Aromatherapy in Nursing. London: Arnold.

Budavari S (ed.). 1996. The Merck Index, 12th ed. Whitehouse Station, NJ: Merck.

Den Tonkelaar I, Oddens B. 2000. Determinants of long-term hormone replacement therapy and reasons for early discontinuation. Obstetrics & Gynecology. 95(4) 507-512.

Duke J. 1985. Handbook of Medicinal Herbs. Boca Raton, FL: CRC Press.

Ettinger B, Pressman A. 1999.Continuation of postmenopausal hormone replacement therapy in a large health maintenance organization: transdermal matrix patch versus oral estrogen therapy. American Journal of Managed Care. 5(6) 779-785.

Franchomme P, Penoel D. 1991. Aromatherapie Exactement. Limoges, France: Jollois.

Geldof A, Engel C, Rao B. 1992. Estrogenic action of commonly used fragrant agent citral induces prostatic hyperplasia. Urological Research. 20(2) 139-144.

Han S, Hur M, Buckle J. 2003. A randomized trial of effect of aromatherapy on the menstrual cramps in college students. In press.

Hahn T. 2001. Anger. New York: Riverhead.

Holmes P. 1993. The Energetics of Western Herbs. Berkeley, CA: NatTrop.

Knowler W, Pettit D, Savage P, et al. 1981. Diabetic incidence in Pima Indians: contributions to obesity and parental diabetes. American Journal of Epidemiology. 113(2) 114-156.

Kozlowski G. 2000. Use of clary sage and geranium on menopausal symptoms. Hunter, NY: R J Buckle Associates.

Marini-Bettolo G. 1979. Plants in traditional medicine. Journal of Ethnopharmacology. 1(3) 303-306.

Melzig M, Teuscher E. 1991. Investigations of the influence of essential oils and their main components on the adenosine uptake by cultivated epithelial cells. Planta Medica. 57(1) 41.

Moretti M, Peana A, Satta M. 1997. A study on anti-inflammatory and peripheral analgesic action of *Salvia sclarea* oil and its main components. Journal of Essential Oil Research. 9(2) 199-204.

Moskowitz D. 2001. Hormones and balance. In Wilson K, Moskowitz D, Thomas D (eds.), A Woman's Health Resource. Portland, OR: Transitions for Health, Inc., 3-37.

Price S, Price L. 1999. Aromatherapy for the Health Professional. London: Churchill Livingstone.

Reid R. 2002. Premenstrual syndrome. Retrieved March 17, 2003 from www.endotext.org.

Revoredo N. 1958. Hypoglycemic action of *Eucalyptus citriodora.* Monitor de la Farmacia y de la Terapeutica. 64: 37-38.

Rose J. 1992. The Aromatherapy Book. San Francisco: North Atlantic Books.

Rovesti P, Columbo E. 1973. Aromatherapy and aerosols. Soap, Perfumery and Cosmetics. 46: 475-477.

Rubinow D, Schmidt P, Roca C. 1998. Estrogen-serotonin interactions: implications for affective regulation. Bio Psychiatry. 44(9) 839-850.

Schmidt P, Rubinow D. 1991. Menopausal related affective disorders: a justification for further study. American Journal of Psychiatry. 148(1) 844-852.

Schwingl P, Hulka B, Harlow S. 1994. Risk factors for menopausal hot flashes. Obstetrics & Gynecology. 84(1) 29-34.

Sheppard-Hangar S. 1995. The Aromatherapy Practitioner's Reference Manual, Vol. 1. Tampa, FL: Atlantic Institute of Aromatherapy.

Shiffman S. 1995. Pleasant odors improve mood of women and men at midlife. In Gilbert A (ed.), Compendium of Olfactory Research. New York: Olfactory Research Fund, Ltd., 97-103.

Tisserand R, Balacs T. 1995. Essential Oil Safety. London: Churchill Livingstone.

Tzeng S, Ko W, Ko FN. 1991. Inhibition of platelet aggregation by some flavonoids. Thrombosis Research. 64(1) 91-100.

Valnet J. 1993. The Practice of Aromatherapy. Saffron Walden, UK: CW Daniels.

van Der V. 1982. The pharmacology of oestriol. Maturitas. 4(4) 291-299.

Wagner H, Wierer M, et al. 1986. In vitro-Hemmung der Prostaglandin-Biosynthese durch etherische Ole und phenolische Verbindungen. Planta Medica. 184-187.

Zondeck B, Bergmann E. 1938. Phenol methyl ethers as estrogenic agents. Biochemical Journal. 32: 641-645.

19

Hospice and End-of-Life Care

The whole natural world is scented, yet until today, no one has sought to know why.

Rene-Maurice Gattefosse
Foreword to *Gattefosse's Aromatherapy*

Hospice care may involve care of the actively dying, but it is not the same as end-of-life care. End-of-life care is just that: care of a person who is in the immediate process of dying. Hospice care (also known as palliative care) means caring for someone who may not get better, but who is nevertheless not at death's door and may live for many years (McCusker 1983). Therefore, palliative care involves alleviating the effects of disease without curing (Fowler & Fowler 1964). This may be unattractive to a medical system based on curing, and Lagay (2001) suggests patients deemed incurable may be neglected. Hospice care is a great challenge to health-care professionals because there are no set protocols; each patient is different with different needs. However, this should be health care's finest hour.

The philosophy of caring cannot be reduced to a series of actions (Drew & Dahlerg 1995). To be caring is to be holistic, so it is hardly surprising that aromatherapy is used and accepted so readily in hospice care, which sees itself as holistic—dealing with the whole person. Chapman (1998) suggest that in hospice care, professional judgement is mainly intuitive. Hillier (2001) writes hospice care is like an iceberg, with the obvious "doing" comprising less than 15% of the actual care.

Ninety percent of cancer patients spend their last year of life in their own homes (Doyle 1986), although during that last year many patients will be admitted to a hospital for a short time. Most Americans say they would like to die at home, but in reality 20%-50% of Americans die in hospitals (Wennberg 1999).

Hospice care is the process of helping patients live fully for as long as possible while alleviating suffering. Suffering can be emotional as well as physical. One of the greatest emotional shocks a person can receive is the knowledge that he or she has a terminal illness. This sets off an internal process of mourning, with the associated feelings of numbness, anger, depression, and finally acceptance (Childs-Gowell 1992). Many patients remain stuck in the second stage with the question "why me?," or they displace their anger and sense of unfairness to others and make their lives miserable (Kubler-Ross 1978). Perhaps the answer to this dilemma could be found in the following quotation:

> *The Pathless Path*
> There is no answer,
> There never has been an answer.
> There never will be an answer.
> That's the answer.   (Gertrude Stein, 1925)

Our society does little to honor the process of mourning; there is no rite of passage. The idea of mourning something other than death is given little support, but patients in palliative care are mourning the death of their future. They know there will be no happy ending, and although everyone has to die sometime, realization of the close proximity of death comes as a bitter blow to many patients. There is no way of knowing (outside a hospital) whether a person has a limited time to live unless he or she chooses to share this knowledge. Many do not share this information because they feel they cannot. Some find it difficult to put their feelings into words, and some are fearful of an uncertain response (pity and forced humor being equally unacceptable), so fear can keep patients locked in a world of their own, unable or unwilling to communicate.

AROMATHERAPY AND PALLIATIVE CARE

Gentle touch and beautiful smells can cross these barriers. Touch communicates a sense of acceptance to such patients, many of whom may have feelings of self-disapproval (Pratt & Mason 1981). Touch and smell often penetrate the despondency of a patient who is struggling to accept that life is no longer going to be as he or she had hoped. Touch is an important commodity during palliative care because patients can often feel more "skin hunger" (Simon 1976). It opens up dialogue, while smells nudge memories. Together they can help patients who may struggle with feelings of anger, denial, guilt, and frustration by allowing them to verbalize those feelings and communicate at a deeper level.

Attractive smells give pleasure and can relax a patient sufficiently to allow him or her to open up. Aromatherapy using the "m" technique allows a patient to experience pleasure, relaxation, and acceptance simultaneously. Trust can occur at a deep level between caregiver and patient. This level of intimacy allows caregivers to show their profound love of humanity in a deeply moving way and provide "comfort care" to their patients (Kolcaba 1995). Many health professionals desire to give this level of care (Montgomery 1996).

Palliative care should embrace the whole family, who may be trying to "remain brave." Smells are not easily hidden, and beautiful smells are an easy way to begin dialogue with family members. It is not unusual for aromatherapy to act as the catalyst, allowing patients and their relatives to begin talking to one another at a useful level. This period before a patient enters the terminal stage is important for a peaceful death. It is a time to clear old scores and resolve past disagreements. It is a time of completion, so the process of dying, when it finally occurs, can be as serene and dignified as possible.

Aromatherapy can aid the management of pain and nausea in a complementary way, but perhaps aromatherapy's greatest strength in palliative care lies in its ability to facilitate communication at an emotional and spiritual level, giving feelings of comfort and pleasure. For this reason, the choice of essential oils should rest with the patient. Concentrate on offering a selection that could give pleasure to the patient. If he or she is particularly withdrawn or depressed, an uplifting essential oil known for its gentle antidepressant properties, such as bergamot (*Citrus bergamia*) or frankincense (*Boswellia carterii*) would be appropriate. However, at this particular stage of illness caregivers are offering esthetic aromatherapy, rather than targeting specific problem areas.

END-OF-LIFE CARE

End-of-life care is estimated to account for up to 12% of all health-care spending in the United States (Emmanuel 1996). Annual expenditure for hospice care is about $3.5 billion (Levitt et al 2000), although hospices operate with little financial aid and are given little state or federal help. For example, New York City reimburses hospice medications at $1.50 per day, although the average cost for drugs is $12 per day (Raphael et al 2001). Of the 9.3 million Americans who are over the age of 85, 83% are women and 43% live alone. By 2060, the population over the age of 85 (both sexes) will increase by 240%. Medicare spends 40% of its budget on the last 30 days of a person's life. However, the cost of the end-of-life care for a 85-year-old is $\frac{1}{3}$ lower than the cost of a 65-75-year-old patient (Hogan et al 2000).

The Last Acts project, funded by the Robert Wood Johnson Foundation, was created in 1997 to educate the public, policymakers, and health-care professionals on end-of-life care (Cassel & Demel 2001). The Last Acts project suggests the following are fundamental to end-of-life care:

respecting patient goals, preferences, and choices;
comprehensive caring;
utilizing the strengths of interdisciplinary resources;
acknowledging and addressing caregivers' concerns;
building systems and mechanisms of support.

The physical process of dying is recognizable (Newbury 1995). Bodily functions cease, and the peripheral temperature drops as circulation fails, leaving the skin mottled and discolored. Thirst is often the last craving, with food refused. Many dying patients breathe through their mouths, which can become dry and cracked. Often their eyes are open, even though the patient may be asleep or unconscious. Rattling in the throat occurs when secretions collect in the throat and the patient is too weak to cough. Although the patient may be unaware of the sound, it is frequently distressing for relatives in the same room. A change in position may help, but aromatherapy and gentle massage may also alleviate this problem (Tattam 1992). Cheyne-Stoke breathing (irregular breathing when the patient doesn't appear to breathe for long periods) often occurs in the days prior to death. Patients may be aware someone is with them, even though they appear to be deeply unconscious. Hearing is one of the last senses to go, so what is said in front of a dying patient is important. This is the time for soothing music such as the work of Therese Schroeder-Sheker (1998).

Many people have a fear of dying alone. Abandonment is a major patient fear, and anecdotal evidence suggests patients who have "Do Not Resuscitate" orders are ignored by medical staff (Sulmasy & Rahns 2001). When patients are at the point of death, they may have been unconscious for some time, but it is still important to really be there with them. Talk gently to them, read their favorite poems, tell their favorite jokes, and play their favorite music. Tell them you are there for them, but be sure to give them permission to go. Touch and smell remain important, and aromatherapy using the "m" technique is a wonderful way to say goodbye. Pleasant smells are of particular importance in terminal nursing. The smell of death is something most people working in hospice work can recognize. Certainly if there are any suppurating lesions, the smell in a patient's room can be quite unpleasant, and patients remain aware of both smell and touch almost until the end.

Other small but highly effective ways to use aromatherapy in terminal nursing include incorporating floral waters. Currently available antiseptic mouth-care lotions can be uncomfortable or burn mouths that are fragile and sensitive (Gravett 1995). Floral waters (hydrolats) are ideal to use as they are water based, dilute, and very gentle (Kusmerik 1996). Chamomile and cornflower floral waters are useful for eye care, and linden flowers, myrtle, and orange blossom are useful for mouth care.

Floral waters provide a gentle way of using aromatherapy. Choose carefully as some, like neroli, are more astringent than geranium and rose, which are more suitable for dry, papery skin (Catty 2001). Wounds can also be cleansed with floral waters as they are antiseptic and slightly acidic. Floral waters can also be used as compresses and are a soothing way to wipe a face. They are excellent to spray around the bed and on the linen, as they are refreshing to both the dying person and relatives. Floral waters will leave a very delicate scent behind and are usually tolerated even by those with a heightened sense of smell. It is important to use true floral waters and not synthetic blends added to water. Purchase them from a reputable supplier to ensure the floral water does not contain fungal or bacterial contaminants.

Relatives learn more from what health-care professionals do than from what they say (Dossey 1994). There is a need to involve relatives in end-of-life care, and some can be encouraged to massage their loved one's hands or feet gently. Help them to choose a particular blend of aromas that has meaning for their loved one. Perhaps the patient was particularly fond of the rose garden or maybe they always potted geraniums. Perhaps they traveled extensively and enjoyed the scent of orange blossom and ylang ylang. Maybe they lived in foreign countries and walked through forests of eucalyptus or sandalwood. Perhaps they had a special herb garden. Their favorite smells can be mixed together in a "farewell blend." This highly personal blend can be used constantly during the dying process and will become identified with the person. Following death, this personalized "farewell blend" can give tremendous comfort to relatives and will help during bereavement.

Katz (1999) carried out a study on 20 patients in the active dying process experiencing terminal agitation or anxiety at her hospice in Pennsylvania. She applied 1% *Lavandula angustifolia* with the "m" technique to hands and feet. All the patients had a decreased pulse and respiration, and all demonstrated physical relaxation by unclenching their hands. In 75% of cases, family members verbalized that they had observed a decrease in agitation. Two comments from her study are haunting. "There is a sense of peace I haven't felt since the diagnosis was made," and, from a five-year-old "My granny feels better, and I helped."

O'Keefe (2000) carried out a study on 10 patients using frankincense in a foot and leg "m" technique and a drop of lavender on the pillow at her hospice in Arizona. All patients were in the active stage of dying, and some of them died within hours or days. After treatment, the restlessness of nine of the patients decreased. For most, their respiration slowed and became deeper as they became quieter. Most of them slept peacefully following the treatment. The response of the patients' relatives was one of deep appreciation for this level of caring.

Ocampo (2000) carried out a controlled study on six terminally ill patients experiencing moderate to severe pain at her hospice in New York. Eight volunteers were trained in the "m" technique and performed it on patients' hands. All patients receiving the "m" technique experienced considerable reduction in their pain perception, according to a visual analog. The treatment group slept for longer periods than the control group.

Perhaps the soul does not die but moves on, and just as a newborn child is welcomed into this world, so should a soul be welcomed into its death. Whatever the health-care provider believes, by caring for a dying patient in this way, using familiar smells and gentle touch, the transition from life as we know it is celebrated in the most supportive and holistic way possible. Health-care providers are privileged to be midwives and facilitators of this transition.

Thank you, my friend
For sharing your dying.
I can be with you
To catch a glimpse of the life you are leaving
And the life to which you return.
In the process, I can accompany your tumult,
Your fear, resistance,
And hope.
Thank you my friend
For sharing your soul.   (Dorothea Hover-Kramer, 1993; reproduced with
                                 kind permission of the author)

REFERENCES

Cassel C, Demel B. 2001. Remembering death: public policy in the USA. Journal of the Royal Society of Medicine. 94(9) 433-436.

Catty S. 2001. Hydrosols: The Next Aromatherapy. Rochester, VT: Healing Arts Press.

Chapman J. 1998. Agonising about assesssment. In Fish D, Coles C, editors: Developing Professional Judgement in Health Care: Learning through Critical Appreciation of Practice. Oxford: Butterworth-Heinemann. 157-181.

Childs-Gowell E. 1992. Good Grief Rituals. Raleigh, NC: Station Hill Press.

Dossey B. 1994. Dynamics of consciousness and healing. Journal of Holistic Nursing. 12(1) 4-10.

Doyle D. 1982. Domiciliary care: terminal care and demands on statutory services. 32(237) 285-291.

Drew N, Dahlerg K. 1995. Challenging a reductionistic paradigm as a foundation for nursing. Journal of Holistic Nursing. 13(4) 334-337.

Emmanuel E. 1996. Cost savings at the end of life: what do the data show? Journal of the American Medical Association. 275(24) 1907-1914.

Fowler H, Fowler F, editors. 1964. The Concise Oxford Dictionary of Current English, 5th ed. Oxford, UK: Oxford University Press.

Gattefosse R. 1937. (Translated in 1993 by R. Tisserand.) Aromatherapie: Les Huile Essentielles-Hormones Vegetales (Gattefosse's Aromatherapy.) Saffron Walden, UK: CW Daniels, 89.

Gravett P. July 23,1995. Medicine Now. BBC Radio 4 (broadcast transcript).

Hillier R. 2001. From cradle to grave: palliative medicine education in the UK. Journal of the Royal Society of Medicine. 94(9) 468-471.

Hogan C, Lynn J, Gable J, et al. 2000. Medicare Beneficiaries' Costs and Use of Care in the Last Year of Life: Final Report to the Medicare Payment Advisory Commission. Washington, DC: Medicare Payment Advisory Commission.

Hover-Kramer D. 1993. Thank you my friend. Journal of Holistic Nursing. 11(1) 115-116.

Katz J. 1999. Does aromatherapy enhance the dying process? Unpublished dissertation. Hunter, NY: R J Buckle.

Kolcaba K. 1995. Comfort as process and product, merged in holistic nursing art. Journal of Holistic Nursing. 13(2) 117-131.

Kubler-Ross E. 1978. To Live Until We Say Good-Bye. London: Prentice Hall.

Kusmerik J. 1996. Floral waters. Aromatherapy Quarterly. (49) 5-7.

Lagay F. 2001. Report from the Council on Ethical and Judicial Affairs, September 2001. www.ama-assn.org.

Levitt K, Cowan C, Lazenby H. 2000. Health spending in 1998: signals of change. Health Affairs. 19: 124-132.

McCusker J. 1983. Where cancer patients die: an epidemiological study. Public Health Reports. 98(2) 170-176.

Montgomery C. 1996. The care-giving relationship: paradoxical and transcendent aspects. Alternative Therapies. 2(2) 52-57.

Newbury A. 1995. The care of the patient near the end of life. In Penson J, Fisher R (eds.), Palliative care for people with cancer. London: Edward Arnold, 178-198.

O'Keefe M. 2000. The effects of *Boswellia carteri* and *Lavandula angustifolia* on the dying process. Unpublished dissertation. Hunter, NY: R J Buckle Associates.

Ocampo A. 2000. The effect of frankincense of alternation of pain perception in hospice patients. Unpublished dissertation. Hunter, NY: R J Buckle Associates.

Pratt J, Mason A. 1981. The Caring Touch. London: Heyden.

Raphael C, Ahrens J, Fowler N. 2001. Financing end-of-life care in the USA. Journal of the Royal Society Medicine. 94(9) 458-461.

Schroeder-Sheker T. 1998. The Chalice of Repose Project: prescriptive music in care of the dying. Third Annual Alternative Therapies Symposium. April 1-4. San Diego, CA: Innovision. 222.

Simon S. 1976. Caring, Feeling, Touching. London: Argus Communications.

Stein G. 1925. The pathless path. In Dossey L. (ed.). 1995. Healing Words. San Francisco: HarperSanFrancisco.

Sulmasy D, Rahns M. 2001. Time spent at the bedside of terminally ill patients with poor progress. American Journal of Medicine. 111(5) 385-389.

Tattam A. 1992. The gentle touch. Nursing Times. 88(32) 16-17.

Wennberg J (ed.). 1999. The Dartmouth Atlas of Health Care. Washington, DC: American Hospital Association Press.

20

IMMUNOLOGY

Everything we need to be whole and healthy is provided for us by nature but, somewhere along the way, most of us have lost sight of this ancient wisdom.

Dr. Mariano Spieza
Holistic Physician and CEO Speizia Organic Care, Cornwall, England

Andrew Weil, MD, (1998) wrote "There is growing evidence that adjunctive therapies can enhance immunity as well as increase the effectiveness of conventional treatments and minimize their side effects." During the last few years it has become evident that essential oils, both through topical application and inhalation, can positively impact the immune system by improving mood, increasing brain activity, and enhancing other biological functions important to health and healing (Alexander 2001). Indeed olfaction has a close link with immunology; the secret of each of our individual aromas may lie in our immunology and the way our cells communicate with each other (Lewis 1974).

Immunology is a rapidly growing field, this growth possibly having been precipitated by the HIV/AIDS epidemic and nurtured by mind-body medicine. How we feel affects how we are, and that is of particular importance in the use of aromatherapy. Candace Pert (2000) created a major conceptual shift in neuroscience with the discovery that the brain, nervous, and immune systems communicate. She discovered a "gut feeling" about something is a tangible, physiological function because the gut has opioid receptors. Recent studies indicate stress-induced neuroendocrine activation can produce profound changes in immune function (Robinson 1999).

The limbic system has the largest number of peptides and receptors, which are the substates of emotion, and these are in constant communication with the immune system. Lymphocytes also secrete endorphins and adrenocorticotropic hormone (ACTH), a stress hormone previously thought to be excreted exclusively by the pituitary gland. Cells can pick up the "scent" of a peptide on the receptors of its surface using a process known as chemotaxis (Pert 2000).

IMMUNE SYSTEM FUNCTION

The immune system is highly complicated: a sensitive balancing act linked by nerve cells that receive directions from and send directions to the brain. Psychological and emotional factors impact both antibody- and cell-mediated immune function. One important function of the immune system is its ability to distinguish between self and nonself. This allows the body to defend itself against infection without harming its own cells. Alexander (2001) draws attention to the similarity between the immune and olfactory systems: both respond instantly to vast numbers of molecules.

The organs of the immune system produce lymphocytes. These white blood cells include T cells (so called because they mature in the thymus) and B cells, which circulate antibodies. Antibodies are tiny proteins belonging to a family of immunoglobulins. Antibodies will attach themselves to the surface of an antigen (a foreign invader) much the way a key fits into a lock. Each antibody recognizes and attaches to a specific antigen.

T cells do not produce antibodies. There are four types of T cells and they attack foreign invaders in different ways.

Killer cells are constantly on the alert in the bloodstream, looking for foreign invaders. When they find them, the killer cells attach themselves and release toxic chemicals to destroy the invaders. Just like antibodies, killer cells are programmed only to kill one thing, whether it is an infective agent, a cell that has been infected, or transplanted tissue.

Nonkiller cells are also constantly on the alert. These cells can attack a broad range of targets including both tumor and infection.

Helper cells stimulate B lymphocytes to produce antibodies.

Suppressor cells shut off the helper cells when enough antibodies have been produced.

For optimum health, helper and suppressor cells should be in balance. HIV/AIDS patients have a deficiency of helper cells, whereas people with autoimmune disease have too many helper cells.

The basic role of the immune system is to defend the body. To do that, it needs to know what is body and what is not. B lymphocytes tell the body if it has been invaded, but there is another arm to the body's defense system, namely the cellular response, which involves the T lymphocytes.

Psychoneuroimmunology is the study of the reaction between the mind, the nervous system, and the immune system. In an article published in the *Lancet*, stress was linked to a depressed immune system (Cohen & Felten 1995). Research has shown changes in hormone and neurotransmitter levels alter human immune responses (Glaser & Glaser 1993). Research also indicates stress can affect the immune response (Kiecolt-Glaser & Glaser 1991), increase susceptibility to the common cold (Cohen et al 1991), adversely affect conception (Domar et al 1990), increase the incidence of skin disease (Panconesi 1984), and affect a patient's perception of pain (Turk & Nash 1993).

AROMATHERAPY AND THE IMMUNE SYSTEM

If aromatherapy elicits the "feel-good" factor, then it may well enhance the immune system. However, some essential oils may impact immune function at a cellular level. Although there is nothing clear-cut here, Penoel (1993) suggests the effects of phenols could be compared to those of human immunoglobulin M (IgM). IgM is secreted for a short period of time when the immune system encounters a pathogenic organism.

Immunoglobulin G (IgG) is secreted for long-term defense. Penoel (1993) thinks the action of IgG is mirrored by the behavior of monoterpenic alcohols. Berkarda et al (1983) reported on the ability of coumarins to increase lymphocyte transformation values in cancer patients. Coumarins are found (although only in small quantities) in citrus-peel oils and lavender. Perhaps this is why Rovesti (1973) thought lavender stimulated lymphocytosis. Lapraz is quoted as saying the presence "of essential oils in the bloodstream produces leukocytosis" (Mitchell 1993). Valnet (1990) cites Novi who demonstrated the stimulant effect of "essences of thyme, lavender, lemon, chamomile and bergamot on the white corpuscles by which curative leukocytosis is activated, enabling the body to combat toxins and to resist infectious disease." Roulier (1990) suggests clove, true verbena, niaouli, and patchouli essential oils could help to balance the immune system. However, no studies have measured the effect of aromatherapy on immunoglobulins in human blood or saliva—yet. Table 20-1 lists essential oils that may assist immune function.

Table 20-1 🐝 *Essential Oils that May Help Immune Function*

Common Name	Botanical Name	Reference
Clove	*Syzygium aromaticum*	Roulier 1990
Lemon verbena	*Lippia citriodora*	Roulier 1990
Niaouli	*Melaleuca viridiflora*	Roulier 1990
Thyme	*Thymus vulgaris* CT thymol	Valnet 1990
Lavender	*Lavandula angustifolia*	Valnet 1990
Lemon	*Citrus limon*	Valnet 1990
German chamomile	*Matricaria recutita*	Wagner 1985
Bergamot	*Citrus bergamia*	Valnet 1990
Patchouli	*Pogostemon patchouli*	Roulier 1990

Other essential oils thought to elevate levels of lymphocytes include *Matricaria recutita* (German chamomile), which increases the number of B lymphocytes (Wagner 1985), and *Citrus bergamia* (bergamot), which is thought to be an immune-system stimulant (Roulier 1990). Philippe Mailhebiau (1995) writes that *Thymus vulgaris* CT thymol has strong immunostimulant properties and is less hepatotoxic than *Satureja montana* CT thymol.

Perhaps two of the most common immunology problems encountered by health professionals are rheumatoid arthritis and HIV/AIDS. Although there is no suggestion that aromatherapy can "cure" rheumatoid arthritis or AIDS/HIV, it may have a positive impact on immune function through the feel-good factor. After all, Marette Flies, an eleven-year-old with lupus, was able to produce the same physiologic response from smelling a rose as from receiving chemotherapy when she thought she was receiving both (Olness & Ader 1992).

Rheumatoid Arthritis

Rheumatoid arthritis (RA) is a chronic, symmetrical, inflammatory polyarthritis that affects 3% of the adult population. The peak onset is between ages 25 and 55, and females are more affected than males. Juvenile RA commonly presents between ages 1-3 years. In addition to arthritis, 20%-35% of patients also manifest severe deformity of rheumatoid modules. These consist of a central area of fibrinoid necrosis surrounded by macrophages and fibrous tissue containing chronic inflammatory cells. The wrist subluxes and the radial head becomes prominent. Extensor tendons in the hand may rupture and adjacent muscles waste. RA is an autoimmune disorder affecting individuals with a genetic predisposition who are exposed to an appropriate antigenic stimulus. Once started, the disease appears to be self-perpetuating. Irreversible destruction of the joint occurs when granulation tissue invades subchondral bone, tendons, and joint capsule (Anthony & Thibodeau 1992). Conventional treatment is with nonsteroid antiinflammatory drugs, such as ibuprofen, dexamethasone drugs, and cytotoxins.

As rheumatoid arthritis affects specific joints, these areas of the body lend themselves to the use of compresses. As well as being of great topical comfort and focusing attention on the affected area of the body (unlike taking a pill), compresses allow essential oils to be absorbed through the skin directly to the site of pain and inflammation. A combination of application methods is usually beneficial, for example, a morning compress and evening bath (which can be a hand- or foot-bath). It is important to choose the application method to suit the patient. The whole process of preparing and treating an injured or painful area of the body carries with it strong placebo effects and mind-body links, which may enhance the efficacy of the treatment. Of course, some of the essential oil will also be inhaled, producing a more instant effect. Using aromatherapy in this way we are assisting the body's own self-healing mechanisms by drawing on the antiinflammatory and analgesic properties of essential oils, as well as their ability to reduce stress and thereby impact the immune system.

Essential oils have some of their most poignant antiinflammatory effects at the level of dermis and epidermis (Boyles 2000). Sawada et al (1980) explored the activity of euglobal III in a hexane extraction of *Eucalyptus globulus* and found it inhibited granulation tissue, which forms inappropriately in cases of RA. Euglobal III has the structure of a bicyclic sesquiterpene, so *Eucalyptus globulus* may be a useful essential oil to try. Inflammation in RA is caused by an increased flow of blood to the affected area, bringing with it heat, swelling, and pain (Mills 1991). (For more information please see section of Chapter 12 on inflammation.) I have found a mixture of essential oils that addresses each of these three symptoms can be helpful. Choose cooling, astringent, and analgesic essential oils, as well as those that have antiinflammatory properties (Tables 20-2 and 20-3). Sometimes heating inflammation can have a more soothing effect than cooling. Some sesquiterpene lactones have powerful antiinflammatory properties because they inhibit cellular response (Mazor et al 2000).

Table 20-2 ✎ *Antiinflammatory Components of Some Common Essential Oils*

Common Name	Botanical Name	Antiinflammatory Component(s)	Reference(s)
German chamomile	*Matricaria recutita*	Bisabolol, chamazulene	Carle & Gormaa 1992, Safayhi et al 1994
Helichrysum	*Helichrysum italicum* subsp. *serotinum*	Italidiones	Franchomme & Penoel 1991
Rosemary	*Rosmarinus officinalis* CT cineole	1,8-cineole	Juergens et al 1998
Black pepper	*Piper nigrum*	Beta-caryophyllene	Tambe et al 1996

Table 20-3 ✎ *Analgesic Components of Some Common Essential Oils*

Common Name	Botanical Name	Analgesic Component(s)	Reference
Lavender	*Lavandula angustifolia*	Linalyl acetate, linalool	Re et al 2000
West Indian lemongrass	*Cymbopogon citratus*	Myrcene	Lorenzetti et al 1991
Peppermint	*Mentha piperita*	Menthol	Tyler et al 1988
Turkish oregano	*Origanum onites*	Carvacrol	Aydin & Ozturk 1996
Brazilian mint	*Mentha X villosa*	Rotundifolene	Almeida et al 1996

Rheumatoid arthritis may be eased by cooling or by heat. Patients will know which they find most comforting. Using a cold (or hot) compress can augment the effect of essential oils. If a patient says heat helps relieve the pain, add a drop of an essential oil with vasodilatory properties such as *Piper nigrum* (black pepper) or clove to bring heat to the affected area. If the patient prefers a cooling effect, add *Mentha piperita* (peppermint) to cool the area. In all cases, it is important to allow patients to choose the essential oils. Let them smell the mixture before it is applied to their skin; after all, they will have to live with it! The "m" technique can be a useful method of applying oils.

HIV and AIDS

The prevalence of human immunodeficiency virus (HIV) and acquired immune deficiency syndrome (AIDS) continues to rise in the United States and in many other parts of the world. In June 1999, the number of people living with HIV/AIDS in the United States was 950,000 (UNAIDS 2001). It is estimated that every minute, five people between the ages of 10 and 24 become infected with HIV somewhere in the world (Sowell et al 1999). As HIV does not have to be reported in many countries, the estimate is conservative (Beal & Nield-Anderson 2000). Approximately 50% of people with HIV or AIDS are using complementary and alternative medicine (CAM) to treat their illness (Dwyer et al 1995). Initially, HIV-infected people or those who had progressed to AIDS used CAM therapies thought to have immunostimulatory or antiviral properties (Elion & Cohen 1997). However as antiretroviral drugs became more successful, patients began choosing to add CAM to their conventional regimes for specific symptom relief (Targ 2000). Commonly used therapies were acupuncture for pain (Shlay et al 1998) and massage therapy (Ironson et al 1996) and herbal supplements to boost immunity (Coss et al 1998). Although aromatherapy is a lesser-known complementary therapy, it has much to offer in HIV/AIDS treatment in terms of control of resistant infections, altering perceptions of pain, and the feel-good factor.

There has been a tremendous increase in research into plants that could be of value in the treatment of patients with HIV and AIDS. Some research has involved specific plants that could inhibit reverse transcriptase production of specific tumours (Kusumoto et al 1992), while other research has concentrated on additional antitumor and antiHIV agents (Cardellina & Boyd 1995). Many of these studies have shown encouraging results, although the research is still in its preliminary stages (Nakashima et al 1992; Mahmood et al 1993; De Tommasi et al 1991; Schols et al 1991). Water and methanol extracts (not essential oil) of *Rosa damascena* exhibited moderate antiHIV activity in a paper by Mahmood et al (1996). *Rosa damascena* was found to reduce the maturation of the infectious progeny virus due to selective inhibition of the viral protease. However, to date it is aqueous extracts rather than the essential oils that have been investigated. Yamasaki et al 1998 examined 45 aqueous herbal extracts from the Labiatae family. *Melissa officinalis*, *Mentha piperita* var. *crispa* (grapefruit mint), *Ocimum basilicum* var. *cinnamon*, and *Satureja montana* showed potent antiHIV activity (at a dilution of 16 μg/ml).

Hypericin and pseudohypericin, components of *Hypericum perforatum* (St. John's wort), were found to be effective against HIV in vitro (Meruelo et al 1988). However, the 1999 phase-1 study of 30 HIV-infected people with CD4 counts lower than 350 cells/mm^3 found 48% of the subjects could not tolerate the severe phototoxic side effects (Gulick et al 1999). This could be because the two chemical components (hypericin and pseudohypericin) had been isolated from the whole plant. In the case of essential oils (and herbs in general), when a component is removed from the whole plant and used on its own, the results can be skewed. A clear example of this is lemongrass. Citral is an aldehyde that makes up 85% of lemongrass. When citral is removed from lemongrass and used at 50% dilution on the skin, it can cause erythema. However, if the whole essential oil is used, a 50% dilution will not result in erythema. This is because lemongrass also contains d-limonene, a terpene that appears to have a "quenching effect," so no burning occurs (Tisserand & Balacs 1995).

There is no published research on the effects of essential oil of *Hypericum perforatum* on the AIDS/HIV, but the essential oil is being used for depression. New studies contraindicate the use of St. John's wort with protease inhibitors, and the essential oil might also need to be avoided (Breckenridge 2000). However, while the essential oil does not contain hypericin and pseudohypericin, it does contain quercetin, a pentahydroxyflavone (Wells 2001) that gives the essential oil its dark-red color. Quercetin is noted by Duke (1992) as having in-vitro antiHIV properties (inhibitory concentration = <1 μg/ml), which indicates the essential oil could be an interesting new avenue for antiretroviral research.

Opportunistic infections can cause morbidity and death in people with HIV (Torres 1993), but there is in-vitro evidence that candidiasis, cryptococcosis, herpes simplex, and tuberculosis (TB) are sensitive to specific essential oils. Because candidiasis, herpes, and TB have been covered in other sections, this section will concentrate on cryptococcosis.

Remember, the strength of aromatherapy lies in its feel-good factor and its ability to alleviate symptoms of HIV/AIDS and the side effects of conventional medicine rather than any ability to cure the underlying disease.

CRYPTOCOCCOSIS

This yeast infection is spread from pigeon droppings and begins as a sporadic disease manifesting with lung infestation. From the lungs, yeast cells migrate to the central nervous system and brain via the blood. Standard treatment is fluconazole, itroconazole, or amphotericin B encapsulated in liposomes (Cordonnier 1993). However, clinical resistance occurs fairly quickly.

Sixty percent of essential oils are known to possess antifungal properties (Deans et al 1989), and aromatherapy is particularly suitable for lung treatment. When essential oils are inhaled they directly target the affected area and do not need to be digested as oral medication. Electrical or battery-operated diffusers and nebulizers are the most effective ways of getting essential oils into the lungs. Nebulizers are a very suitable method of treatment for lung infestations of yeast, fungi, or bacteria as they fill the air with a very fine mist of micromolecules of essential oil, and they can be programmed to come on and off at specific times. For recommended distributors of essential oils and nebulizers, please see Appendix IV.

Effective Essential Oils

Voillon and Chaumont (1994) tested the susceptibility of a strain of *Cryptococcus neoformans* isolated from the blood of a patient with AIDS to 25 essential oils and 17 separate chemical constituents found in essential oils. Antifungal activity was tested by dilution method on solid Sabouraud dextrose agar DIFCO with chloramphenicol 0.005%. (The presence of chloramphenicol assured the inhibition of possible pollution by bacteria that could confound the results.) Ten μl of *Cryptoccocus neoformans* from the patient's blood was spread on the culture. (A μl is a microliter or a millionth of a liter.) Cells were counted and the plates incubated at 37° C for 48 hours. Then the minimum inhibitory concentration was measured.

Many of the essential oils used showed good fungistatic action. The best effects were from palma rosa, geranium, savory, sandalwood, thyme, marjoram, and lavender. These are all common, inexpensive essential oils. What was interesting about this study was that lavender and sweet marjoram, two essential oils previously been found to be ineffective against *Cryptococcus neoformans* on fungal growth in vitro, were very effective when the fungus was isolated from infected human tissue. This appeared to agree with the findings of Dr. Jean Valnet (1990), who said the terrain of the patient is very important in control of infection.

Due to the high volatility, Voillon and Chaumont (1994) hypothesized essential oils would be effective against pulmonary cryptococcosis, would easily penetrate into the tissues due to their low molecular weight, and would easily reach the cerebral spinal fluid in cases of meningitis. The researchers further hypothesized essential oils would be less toxic than conventional drugs as they have fewer side effects.

Lemongrass, *Eucalyptus globulus*, palma rosa, and peppermint were the most effective essential oils tested against *Cryptococcus* by Pattnaik et al (1996). Lemongrass was effective not only against *Cryptococcus* but against 11 other fungi tested in low dilutions. Minimum inhibitory concentration for each of the four essential oils against *Cryptococcus* was $5\mu l/ml^{-1}$. While the way essential oils work as fungicides is not completely clear, it seems metabolism and growth of the fungus is inhibited, often with a breakdown in the lipid part of the membrane, resulting in increased permeability and/or rupture (Larrondo & Calvo 1991). The main constituent of lemongrass is citral, and Larrondo and Calvo (1991) have compared the topical and inhaled action of citral to the systemic effects of clotrimazole.

Patchouli was found to be effective against *Cryptococcus* and 16 other pathogenic fungi and commensal bacteria in a study by Yang et al (1996). In this invitro study, essential oil of patchouli from three different countries, China, Indonesia, and India was compared. Interestingly, only the Chinese patchouli was effective against *Cryptococcus neoformans*. This was attributed to the higher content of patchouli alcohol (41%) as compared to 20%-23% in the Indonesian and Indian essential oils. These findings underline the importance of knowing the chemistry of the essential oil. In this case, the chemistry was directly related to where the plant was grown.

Soliman et al (1994) tested essential oil of rosemary (*Rosmarinus officinalis*). They investigated the essential oil distilled from two plants growing in different climatic conditions. They found both rosemary essential oils were effective against *Cryptococcus neoformans* in vitro and recommended either essential oil as an effective treatment in AIDS patients with cryptococcal meningitis and pneumonia. While both rosemarys were effective, it could have been a different chemical component in each oil that contributed to the success of the study.

Eugenol is a phenolic component found in several essential oils. An in-vitro study found it to be effective against 33 strains of *Cryptococcus neoformans* using isolates from human patients (Boonchild & Flegel 1982). The researchers concluded eugenol would be effective against cutaneous mycoses, but toxicity tests excluded the use of eugenol as a systemic agent. As a phenol, eugenol would not be suitable for extensive use on the skin as it can be irritating and is hepatotoxic (Schnaubelt 1999). Eugenol is found in clove and savory, two essential oils to be used with caution on the skin but they could be used in small amounts in a nebulizer. Table 20-4 lists essential oils used in the treatment of infections of *Cryptococcus neoformans*.

Table 20-4 ❧ *Essential Oils for Treating Infections of* Cryptococcus neoformans

Common Name	Botanical Name	Reference
Rosemary	*Rosmarinus officinalis*	Soliman 1994
Palma rosa	*Cymbopogon martini*	Viollon 1994
Geranium	*Pelargonium graveolens*	Voillon & Chaumont 1994
Marjoram	*Origanum majorana*	Voillon & Chaumont 1994
Sandalwood	*Santalum album*	Voillon & Chaumont 1994
Lemongrass	*Cymbopogon citratus*	Voillon & Chaumont 1994
Eucalyptus	*Eucalyptus globulus*	Voillon & Chaumont 1994
Patchouli	*Pogostemon cablin*	Voillon & Chaumont 1994
Basil	*Ocimum basilicum*	Voillon & Chaumont 1994
Cypress lavender	*Santolina chamaecyparissus*	Suresh 1995

Patients with HIV and AIDS are especially appreciative of touch and smell. I have found that *Boswellia carterii* (frankincense) is particularly useful. It seems to help even the most defensive patient to open up, often with tears of release. *Citrus aurantium* (neroli) and *Rosa damascena* (rose) both have wonderful aromas that most patients like. However, if the aroma seems too flowery, *Origanum marjorana* (sweet marjoram), *Angelica archangelica* (angelica root), or *Santalum album* (sandalwood) are often acceptable alternatives.

Diarrhea is often a problem in the immune-compromised patient. Several studies have indicated the oral use of essential oils might be one way of controlling this debilitating symptom. Hajihashemi et al (2000) found essential oil of *Satureje hortentis* (given orally) was effective against diarrhea in mice. Orafidiya and Elujoba (2000) conducted a controlled, in-vivo study with mice and found *Ocimum gratissimum* (Holy basil) to be an effective agent against diarrhea. The essential oil reduced fecal output in a dose-dependent manner, with the highest dose of 7.91 µg/ml similar to the action of the control, loperamide (an opioid that inhibits perastalsis), but at a fraction of the cost.

In a study on humans, a British physician (Gravett 2001) found that oral doses of essential oils were as effective as conventional medication (codeine phosphate 120 mg and Buscopan 20 mg) in high-dose chemoinduced diarrhea. Eighty patients were randomly allocated into two groups. The experimental group took an essential oil blend: 15 drops of geranium, 10 drops of German chamomile, and 10 drops of patchouli which were mixed with tumeric phytol and divided into three portions. The three portions were blended into warm water and honey and taken three times a day. There was no difference in overall duration of hospitalization but the diarrhea in patients who took the essential oils was marginally less. The cost of the aromatherapy treatment was about 40 cents a day compared to more than $4 a day for conventional treatment. Finally, *Lavandula intermedia* CT grosso was found to be effective against nontubercular opportunistic mycobacterum in a sternal wound (Gabrielli et al 1988).

References

Ader R, Cohen N, Felten D. 1995. Psychoneuroimmunology: interactions between the nervous system and the immune system. Lancet. 345(8942) 99-103.

Alexander M. 2001. How Aromatherapy Works. Odessa, FL: Whole Spectrum Books.

Almeida R, Hiruma C, Barbosa-Filho J. 1996. Analgesic effect of rotundifolene in rodents. Fitoterapia. 67(4) 334-339.

Beal M, Nield-Anderson L. 2000. Acupuncture for symptom relief in HIV positive adults: lessons learned from a pilot study. Alternative Therapies in Health and Medicine. 6(5) 33-42.

Berkarda B, Bouffard-Eyuboglu H, Derman U. 1983. The effect of coumarin derivatives on the immunological system of man. Agents and Actions. 13(1) 50-52.

Boonchird D, Flegel T. 1982. In vitro activity of eugenol and vanillin against *Candida albicans* and *Cryptococcus neoformans*. Canadian Journal of Microbiology. 28(11) 1235-1241.

Boyles J. 2000. The Basic Chemistry of Aromatherapeutic Essential Oils. Sydney, Australia: Pirie Printers.

Breckenridge A. Important news from the committee on safety of medicine. Retrieved March 28, 2003 from www.cascade-drugs.org.uk/.

Cardellina J, Boyd M. 1995. Pursuits of new leads to antitumour and anti-HIV agents from plants. Proceedings of the Phytochemical Society of Europe. Oxford, UK: Oxford Science Press, 81-93.

Carle R, Gormaa K. 1992. The medicinal use of *Matricaria flos.* British Journal of Phytotherapy. 2(4) 147-153.

Cohen S, Tyrrell D, Smith A. 1991. Psychological stress and susceptibility to the common cold. New England Journal of Medicine. 325(9) 606-612.

Cordonnier C. 1993. Les traitment preventifs et curatifs des mycoses en oncohematologie. In Euromedicine 1993. Monpelier-Le corum. Rencontres internationals de recherches et de technologies medicales et pharmaceutiques. Paris: 10-13 November.

Coss R, McGrath P, Caggiano V. 1998. Alternative care: patient choices for adjunct therapies within a cancer center. Cancer Practice. 6(3) 176-181.

De Tommasi N, De Simone F, De Feo V. 1991. Phenylpropanoid glycosides and rosmarinic acid from *Momardica balsamina.* Planta Medica. 57(2) 201.

Deans S, Svoboda K, Kennedy A. 1989. Biological activity of plant volatile oils and their constituents. Planta Medica. 55(1) 588.

Domar A, Seibel M, Benson H. 1990. The mind/body program for infertility. A new behavioural treatment approach for women with infertility. Fertility and Sterility. 53(2) 246-249.

Duke J. 1992. Handbook of biologically active phytochemicals and their activities. Boca Raton, FL: CRC Press.

Dwyer J, Salvato-Schille A, Coulston A. 1995. The use of unconventional remedies among HIV positive men living in California. Journal of the Association of Nurses in AIDS Care. 6(1) 17-28.

Elion R, Cohen C. 1997. Complementary Medicine and HIV infection. Complementary and Alternative Therapies in Primary Care. 24(4) 905-919.

Gabrielli G, Loggini F, Cioni P, et al. 1988. Activity of lavandino essential oil. Pharmacological Research Communications. 20(Suppl. V) 37-41.

Glaser J, Glaser R. 1993. Mind and immunity. In Mind-Body Medicine. New York: Consumer Report Books, pp. 39-59.

Gravett P. 2001. Treatment of gastrointestinal upset following high-dose chemotherapy. International Journal of Aromatherapy. 11(2) 84-86.

Gulick R, McAuliffe V, Holden-Wiltse J, et al. 1999. Phase 1 studies of hypericin, the active compound in St John's Wort, as an antiretroviral agent in HIV-infected adults. Annals of Internal Medicine. 130(6) 510-514.

Hajihashemi V, Sadraei H, Ghannadi A, et al. 2000. Antispasmodic and anti-diarrhoeal effect of *Satureja hortensis* essential oil. Journal of Ethnopharmacology. 71(1-2) 187-192

Ironson G, Field T, Scafadi F, et al. 1996. Massage therapy is associated with enhancement of the immune system's cytotoxic capacity. Int Journal of Neuroscience. 84(1-4) 205-217.

Juergens U, Stober M, Schmidt-Schilling L, et al. 1998. Anti-inflammatory effects of eucalyptol (1,8 cineole) in bronchial asthma: inhibition of arachidonic acid metabolism in human monocytes ex vivo. European Journal of Medical Research. 2(9) 407-412.

Kiecolt-Glaser J, Glaser R. 1991. Stress and the immune system: human studies. In Tasman A, Riba M. (eds.), Annual Review of Psychiatry, Vol. 11. Washington, DC: American Psychiatric Press, 169-180.

Kusumoto I, Shimada E. 1992. Inhibitory effects of Indonesian plant extracts on reverse transcriptase of an RNA tumour virus. Phytotherapy Research. 6: 241-244.

Larrondo J, Calvo M. 1991. Effect of essential oils on *Candida albicans:* a scanning electron microscope study. Biomedical Letters. 46(184) 269-272.

Lewis T. 1974. The Lives of a Cell: Notes of a Biology Watcher. New York: Viking.

Mahmood N, Piacente S, Pizza C, et al. 1996. The anti-HIV activity and mechanism of action of pure compounds isolated from rosa damascena. Biochemical and Biophysical Research Communications. London: Academic Press. 229(1) 73-79.

Mailhebiau P. 1995. The thymus folder. Les Cahiers de l'Aromatherapie. 1: 38-60.

Mazor R, Menendez I, Ryan M, et al. 2000. Sesquiterpene lactones are potent inhibitors of interleukin 8 gene expression in cultured human respiratory epithelium. Cytokine. 12(3) 239-245.

Meruelo D, Lavie G, Lavie D. 1988. Therapeutic agents with dramatic antiretroviral activity and little toxicity at effective doses: Aromatic polycyclic diones hypericin and pseudohypericin. Proceedings of the National Academy of Sciences. 85:5230-5234.

Mills S. 1991. Out of the Earth. London:Viking Arkana.

Mitchell S. 1993. Dementia. International Journal of Aromatherapy. 5(2) 20-23.

Nakashima H, Murakami T, Yamamoto N. 1992. Inhibition of human immunodeficiency viral replications by tannins and related compounds. Antiviral Research. 18(1) 91-103.

Olness K, Ader R. 1992. Conditioning as an adjunct in the pharmacotherapy of Lupus Erythematosus. Developmental and Behavioral Pediatrics 13(2) 127-127.

Panconesi E (ed.). 1984. Clinics in Dermatology, Vol. 2: Stress and skin diseases: psychosomatic dermatology. Philadelphia: JB Lippincott.

Pattnaik S, Subramanyam V, Kole C. 1996. Antibacterial and antifungal activity of essential oils in vitro. Microbios. 86(349) 237-246.

Penoel D. 1993. The immune system of mankind. In Aroma 93 Conference Proceedings. Brighton, UK: Aromatherapy Publications.

Pert C. 2000. Molecules of Emotion. New York: Scribner.

Re L, Barocci S, Sonnino S, et al. 2000. Linalool modifies the nicotinic receptor-ion channel kinetics at the mouse neuromuscular junction. Pharmacological Research. 42(2) 177-182.

Robinson F. 1999. Stress and HIV disease progression: psychoneuroimmunolgocial framework. Journal of the Association of Nurses in AIDS Care. 10(1) 21-31.

Roulier G. 1990. Les Huiles Essentielles Pour Votre Sante. St Jean-de-Braye, France: Dangles.

Rovesti P, Columbo E. 1973. Aromatherapy and aerosols. Soaps, Perfumery and Cosmetics. 46: 49-54.

Safayhi H, Sabieraj J, Sailer E, et al. 1994. Chamzulene: an antioxidant-type inhibitor of leukotriene B4 formation. Planta Medica. 60(5) 410-413.

Sawada T, Tozuka M, Komiya T, et al. 1980. A novel granulation inhibiting agent from *Eucalyptus globulus.* Chemical & Pharmaceutical Bulletin. 28(8) 2546-2548.

Schnaubelt K. 1999. Medical Aromatherapy. Berkeley, CA: Frog Ltd., 179.

Schols D, Wutzler P, Klocking R. 1991. Selective inhibitory activity of polyhydroxycarboxylates derived from phenolic compounds against human immunodeficiency virus replication. Journal of Acquired Immune Deficiency Syndrome. 4(7) 677-684.

Shlay J, Chaloner K, Max M. 1998. Acupuncture and amitriptyline for pain due to HIV related peripheral neuropathy. Journal of the American Medical Association. 280(18) 1590-1595.

Sowell R, Moneyham L, Arnada-Naranjo B. 1999. The care of women with AIDS. Nursing Clinics of North America. 34(1) 179-198.

Spieza M. 2002. Mission Statement. Retrieved October 10, 2001 from www.spiezaorganics.org.

Tambe Y, Tsujiuchi H, Honda G, et al. 1996. Gastric cytoprotection of the non-steroidal anti-inflammatory sesquiterpene, beta-carylophyllene. Plant Medica. 62(5) 469-470.

Targ E. 2000. CAM and HIV/AIDS: The importance of complementarity. Alternative Therapies in Health and Medicine. 6(5) 30-31.

Tisserand R, Balars T. 1995. Essential Oil Safety. London: Churchill Livingstone.

Torres G. 1993. Treatment issues. Gay Men's Health Crisis: Newsletter of Experimental AIDS Therapies. 7: 1-2.

Turk D, Nash J. 1993. Chronic pain. New ways to cope. In Goleman D, Gurin J, editors: Mind-Body Medicine. New York: Consumer Reports Books. 111-131.

Tyler V, Brady L, Robbers J. 1988. Pharmacognosy. Philadelphia: Lea & Febiger. 113-119.

Valnet J. 1990. The Practice of Aromatherapy. Saffron Walden, UK: CW Daniels.

Viollon C, Chaumont J. 1994. Antifungal properties of essential oil components against *Cryptococcus neoformans.* Mycopathologia. 128(3) 151-153.

Wagner H. 1985. Economic and medicinal plant research, Vol. 1. London: Academic Press.

Wells C., Director, Essentially Oils Ltd., Chipping Norton, UK. 1991. Personal communication.

Yamasaki K, Nakano M, Kawahata T, et al. 1998. Anti-HIV-1 activity of herbs in Lamiatae. Biological & Pharmaceutical Bulletin. 21(8) 829-833.

Yang D, Micehl D, Mandin D, et al. 1996. Antifungal and antibacterial properties in vitro of three *Patchouli* essential oils of different origins. Acta Botanica Gallica. 143(1) 29-35.

21

OBSTETRICS AND GYNECOLOGY

Aromatherapy is a relatively modern name for an ancient holistic practice. Aromatherapy gives us something that is sometimes lacking in other alternative practices: quite simply, it has the power to make us feel good.

Romy Rawlings (1999)
Healing Gardens

AROMATHERAPY AND PREGNANCY

The use of essential oils during pregnancy is controversial, but most fears are unfounded (Guba 2002). Some aromatherapy schools condone the use of essential oils in pregnancy during the first trimester, and some question their use at all. Since the thalidomide tragedy, expectant mothers and their physicians have been extra cautious of using anything that could have an adverse effect on the unborn child or the security of the pregnancy. However, essential oils have been used safely for hundreds of years by thousands of pregnant women in the form of perfumes, bath essences, and scented soap.

There are no records of abnormal fetuses or aborted fetuses due to the "normal" use of essential oils, either by inhalation or topical application. There are no records of a few drops of essential oil taken by mouth causing any problems either. However, there are a handful of records that link two specific essential oils, pennyroyal and parsley seed, to abortion. The amount of essential oil (taken by mouth) was extremely high—several milliliters at one time—which caused hepatotoxicity. This meant the body was unable to maintain the pregnancy. However, there were two other cases recorded where the same amount of pennyroyal taken by mouth did not result in the fetus being aborted, and the mothers recovered. The amounts taken varied from 10 ml (in the case of pennyroyal) and 1.5-6 ml for 8 consecutive days (parsley seed). This is between 100 to 200 times greater than the normal amount of essential oil used in aromatherapy. (Usually only one to five drops are applied topically to the skin or inhaled.) For internal use, the normal amount is 0.5-10 ml per day (Brinker 2000). The volume of one drop of essential oil is equivalent to 0.05 ml. This works out to between 10 and 20 drops per day. There are approximately 20 drops in a milliliter.

There is only one essential oil compound, sabinyl acetate, that has been shown to have teratogenic effect in laboratory animals (Guba 2002). Sabinyl acetate comprises 20% of savin (*Juniperus sabina*) and less than 10% of Spanish sage (*Salvia lavandulifolia*). Both essential oils should be avoided in pregnancy and have no aromatherapeutic use. More information on these oils is given in Chapter 4.1 on toxicity.

There are several books available that cover the use of essential oils in pregnancy, including two good ones written by midwives: *Aromatherapy in Midwifery Practice* by Tiran (1996) and *Aromatherapy for the Mother and Baby* by England (1994). England attends 2500 deliveries annually, and Tiran is a lecturer in midwifery at the University of Greenwich. In the United Kingdom, essential oils have been used during pregnancy and delivery at many hospitals for approximately 15 years, and expectant mothers often appear at the delivery suite with their own box of essential oils especially chosen for the birth of their child. Essential oils have been used at Hinchingbrooke Hospital, Huntingdon, St John's, and St Elizabeth's Hospitals in London and at the Radcliffe Infirmary in Oxford, England, since 1987. It would be expected that any adverse effects would have appeared by now. However, it is always best to err towards caution, and there is no need to use large amounts of essential oils. Nonetheless, when used correctly, essential oils are very safe in pregnancy. These substances can give the expectant mother a sense of empowerment, reduce the annoying side effects of pregnancy, and can help make her feel beautiful. If there is a choice between a synthetic chemical (with no studies on long-term effects) or an essential oil (with hundreds of years of use) it would be judicious to choose the latter. Aromatherapy can be helpful for many symptoms of pregnancy: general tiredness, aches and pains, nausea, insomnia, and backache.

Some essential oils are thought to have emmenagogic actions, meaning they cause tiny uterine contractions and can bring on a menstrual period early. However the hormonal and physical effects of pregnancy are quite different from those of the menstrual cycle, and Guba (2002) suggests the topical or inhaled effect of emmenagogic essential oils will not compromise a stable pregnancy. There is conflicting information on exactly which essential oils are emmenagogic. Some authors believe *Lavandula angustifolia* is emmenagogic but also state it is safe to use in the first trimester (England 1994).

It is extremely unlikely that a secure pregnancy will be compromised because a mother has used an emmenagogic essential oil. Babies are difficult to dislodge in a secure pregnancy. However, if the mother has had a previous miscarriage, it would be prudent to avoid aromatherapy especially after the first trimester. Brinker (2000) suggests avoiding angelica, Roman chamomile, cinnamon, any citrus, myrrh, lemongrass, hyssop, lavender, German chamomile, melissa, peppermint, basil, oregano, black pepper, rosemary, sandalwood, vetiver, and ginger. However, I have several friends who used aromatherapy throughout their pregnancies. They have all been uneventful and have produced beautiful babies.

One of the most significant medical events for a pregnant woman is the development of pregnancy-induced hypertension (PIH) and its more severe complications: preeclampsia and HELLP syndrome (hemolysis, elevated liver enzymes, and low platelets). The patient usually presents with epigastric pain and blood pressure may or may not be elevated. HELLP is a variant of preeclampsia and eclampsia.

Pregnancy-Induced Hypertension (PIH)

This condition occurs in 7%-10% of all pregnancies and causes 15% of maternal deaths. Women who have a history of hypertension before pregnancy are twice as likely to develop PIH. PIH can also lead to intrauterine fetal death through placental insufficiency. Orthodox treatment is bed rest with the feet elevated and intravenous magnesium sulphate. If the blood pressure does not come down to levels below 150-110/110, labetalol, an alpha- and beta-adrenergic blocking agent, is given. A blood pressure of 150-160/100-110 constitutes severe preeclampsia, calling for antihypertensives (hydralazine or labetalol). Common side effects are drowsiness, fatigue, pulse slower than 50 beats per minute, and nausea. The mother is kept quiet in a darkened room. However, her mind is unlikely to be quiet! At such a terrifying time, smell and touch can do much to help reassure a woman, and reassurance can play an important role in this situation.

Nathan (2000), a midwife on Long Island, New York, used aromatherapy to help a mother whose blood pressure remained above 200/100 despite intravenous medication. The patient was continuously monitored for blood pressure and pulse. Unable to control the hypertension, the attending physician asked Nathan if she would try aromatherapy. After verbal consent from the patient, Nathan used a 2% solution of *Lavandula angustifolia* in a hand "m" technique. Slowly the blood pressure began to come down. After 15 minutes it was 150/85. The fetal heart rate also improved, from mid 150s to mid 130s. Within 1 hour, the mother's blood pressure was 140/85. The patient was given 5 minutes of "m" technique with dilute lavender every hour during the night, and her blood pressure was maintained at 140/85. The mother was discharged 2 days later and went on to full term. As a result of this case study, Nathan carried out a small project on eight hypertensive patients in her maternity unit in 2000. Each patient chose rose or lavender essential oil and received a 5-minute "m" technique on the hand. This resulted in a measurable drop in blood pressure for each patient.

Essential Oils in Labor

Swingle (2001) carried out a study at the Newborn Family Center in Chenango Memorial Hospital in Norwich, New York, on 25 laboring mothers. Four essential oils, lavender, geranium, frankincense, and clary sage, were used in 1% dilution. The oils were used from early labor through delivery. Each essential oil was used for specific reasons. Lavender was used for relaxation, to relieve backache, and to help expel the placenta, and was successful on all counts. Geranium was used to decrease perineal swelling and to relieve hemorrhoids; it was also successful. Clary sage was used to stimulate contractions but was not found successful. Frankincense was used successfully for extreme anxiety between transition and the second stage of labor. There were no side effects from any of the essential oils used and everyone commented on their nice aromas.

Adams (2000) carried out a controlled study on the use of lavender to reduce patient anxiety when labor was induced at Desert Samaritan Hospital in Mesa, Arizona. One or two drops of lavender were inhaled continuously, or at will, from a cotton ball. Each of the 23 patients self-evaluated her anxiety level before the lavender and 30 minutes after the lavender. The levels of evaluation were as follows: very nervous, nervous, OK, calm, and very calm. The lavender group had a greater perception of reduced anxiety than the control group. Two subjects commented that their headaches went away when they inhaled lavender. All had positive comments. The attending nurses' comments ranged from "patient slept after lavender," to "more calm, much more mellow," to "less anxious, physician very pleased with effects of lavender."

Burns et al (2000) evaluated the effect of aromatherapy on 8058 mothers during an 8-year period (see Table 21-1 for a list of the essential oils used). Mothers in labor were offered aromatherapy to relieve pain, anxiety, or nausea or to strengthen contractions. Data from the unit audit were used to provide a comparison group of mothers not given aromatherapy (n = 15.799). Aromatherapy was offered by a core group of midwives who followed guidelines laid down by a qualified aromatherapist.

Table 21-1 🐾 *Essential Oils Used in Burns et al (2000) Study*

Common Name	Botanical Name
Rose	*Rosa centifolia*
Lavender	*Lavandula angustifolia*
Jasmine	*Jasminum grandiflorum*
Roman chamomile	*Chamaemelum nobile*
Blue gum	*Eucalyptus globulus*
Mandarin	*Citrus reticulata*
Clary sage	*Salvia sclarea*
Frankincense	*Boswellia carteri*
Peppermint	*Mentha piperita*
Lemon	*Citrus limonum*

More than 50% of the mothers found aromatherapy useful. Only 14% of mothers found it unhelpful. The number of adverse symptoms reported was low (1%) and included symptoms commonly found in labor such as headache, nausea, and itchy rash. Aromatherapy was typically used by mothers in established labor (60%) or in the latent stage (29%). Of the women who used aromatherapy, 32% had their labor induced. Fewer women needed pain relief in the aromatherapy group than the control group, and fewer epidurals were given. During the 8 years of study, the use of pethidine declined. In 1990, 13% of mothers used pethidine. By 1997, use had dropped to less than 0.2%. Frankincense was found to be the most effective essential oil for pain. Rose was found to be the most helpful for anxiety (71%). Peppermint was found to be the most effective for nausea (96%). Aromatherapy did not appear to augment contractions. However, 70% of multigravidae in dysfunctional labor did not require an oxytocin infusion, and 92% of the mothers went on to spontaneous vaginal delivery. This is an unusually high figure. Only 36% of women said they found aromatherapy helped strengthen their contractions, and the most commonly offered essential oil for this was clary sage (87%).

VAGINAL INFECTIONS

Yeast Infections

Vaginal yeast infection, caused by *Candida albicans,* is a common nuisance factor in many women's lives. It thrives in an acid environment and is sometimes the side effect of antibiotics, or it may occur during pregnancy or when a woman is immune compromised. It is often messy, uncomfortable, and embarrassing and can reappear with depressing regularity. Antifungal drugs such as Terazol and Femstat may only bring temporary relief. Other over-the-counter preparations can be purchased, although some forms of this yeast infection have become resistant to many of the orthodox preparations on the market (Goldway et al 1995). Candidiasis is uncomfortable and often makes the sufferer feel powerless to cope with it. However there is one essential oil that may eradicate this fungal infection permanently and within only a few days (Belaiche 1985). It is called tea tree. Belaiche (1985) wrote about its effect on vaginal infections 15 years ago.

Tea tree is the name of all species of *Melaleuca, Leptospermum, Kunzea,* and *Baeckea* plants (Guenther 1972). In other words, specifying tea tree is not enough, as it covers several hundred different plants. In New Zealand, *Leptospermum flavescens* is also known as tea tree, but this is a completely different genus, although it belongs to the same family (Myrtaceae) as tea tree. The tea tree needed to treat vaginal infections is *Melaleuca alternifolia.* The Australian government has set standards for the amount of terpineol (an alcohol) and 1,8-cineole (an oxide) in tea tree. Some tea tree imitations are available that contain high levels of 1,8-cineole. Occasionally oxides can be uncomfortable when applied to irritated or abraded vaginal tissue. To avoid this, make sure the bottle of essential oil includes the botanical name, and purchase it from a reliable source. The functional group, alcohols, is kinder on abraded vaginal tissue. The levels of 1,8-cineole and terpineol will show up on a gas chromatograph/mass spectrometer.

Mix two or three drops of *Melaleuca alternifolia* in 5 ml of cold-pressed vegetable oil, like oil of evening primrose or sweet almond oil. Roll a tampon in the mixture and then insert into the vagina. The simplest method is to mix the essential oil and vegetable oil on a saucer and then roll the tampon in the mixture until it is saturated. The tampon should be changed three times a day for a new tampon with a fresh dilution of carrier oil and tea tree. The tampon also needs to remain in situ overnight. It will not lead to toxic shock syndrome. This is a very safe and effective method of eradicating candidiasis and many other vaginal infections, and there appear to be no adverse side effects. However, a word of caution should be given. If the yeast infection has exposed, raw areas in the vaginal wall, *Lavandula angustifolia* diluted in vegetable oil should be used first. It can be applied in exactly the same way, on a tampon, for 1 or 2 days until the excoriated area has healed. This method has been used successfully in pregnancy with no adverse effects to the mother or baby. Having suggested this treatment to many patients and colleagues over the last 10 years, I am confident *Melaleuca alternifolia* should remove the infection within 3 days, regardless of how long the patient has had the infection. Table 21-2 lists essential oils effective against *Candida albicans*.

Table 21-2 ❧ *Essential Oils Effective against* **Candida albicans**

Common Name	Botanical Name	Reference
Tea tree	*Melaleuca alternifolia*	Belaiche 1985, Pena 1962
Peppermint	*Mentha piperita*	Carson & Riley 1994
Palma rosa	*Cymbopogon martinii*	Pattnaik et al 1996
Eucalyptus	*Eucalyptus globulus*	Pattnaik et al 1996
Lemongrass	*Cymbopogon citratus*	Pattnaik et al 1996
Geranium	*Pelargonium graveolens*	Pattnaik et al 1996
Bay	*Pimenta racemosa*	Chaumont & Bardy 1989, Viollon et al 1993
Vetiver	*Vetiveria zizanoides*	Chaumont & Bardy 1989
Santolina	*Santolina chamaecyparisus*	Suresh et al 1997
Melissa	*Melissa officinalis*	Suresh et al 1997
Rosemary	*Rosmarinus officinalis*	Larrondo & Calvo 1991
Lippia	*Lippia alba*	Soliman et al 1994
Austrian pine	*Picea albies*	Stiles et al 1995, Kartnig et al 1991

Bacterial Infections

Bacterial Vaginosis

Bacterial vaginosis (BV) is a polymicrobial vaginal infection that affects women of reproductive age (Cook et al 1992). Many of the bacteria, such as *Peptostreptococcus*, are anaerobic and appear to replace the normally predominant *Lactobacilli*. One of the main symptoms is copious, smelly discharge, often reducing a woman to tears of frustration. The fishy smell is from the amine compounds produced by anaerobes. There is no inflammatory reaction, so there are no white blood cells in the discharge. Orthodox treatment is oral Metronidazole, which usually results in normal flora and reduction of symptoms but often produces unpleasant side effects such as gastrointestinal upsets or unpleasant taste. A second treatment is topical clindamycin cream (Cleocin). The cost of a tube of Cleocin vaginal cream is high, approximately $50 for one-week supply. In 40% of cases treated with oral Metronidazole, BV recurs within 3 months (Cook et al 1992).

Walsh and Longstaff (1987), Shapiro et al (1994), and Carson and Riley (1993), tested tea tree against fusobacteria, *Prevotella*, and *Peptostreptococcus* bacteria by agar and broth dilution, and all came up with comparable data. Whereas the previously mentioned bacteria were susceptible, *Lactobacilli* were more resistant to tea tree, suggesting that *Melaleuca alternifolia* could help restore the acid of the vagina and make it more resistant to pathogenic bacteria. Blackwell (1991) treated a patient with BV using *Melaleuca alternifolia* vaginal pessaries with good results. Self-medication with alternative medicine is common among women with chronic vaginal symptoms (Nyirjesy et al 1997), and diluted tea tree in cold-pressed carrier oil on a tampon can be a very effective treatment. Diluted tea tree is pleasant to use and empowering to the patient. It smells pleasantly antiseptic, and the tampon application makes the vagina feel fresh. Usually, symptoms will disappear within one week.

Trichomonasas

Trichomonas vaginalis is a bacterial infection that causes inflammation of the vaginal mucosa accompanied by an unpleasant, pungent discharge. The sufferer is embarrassed and frequently complains of "feeling dirty." Conventional treatment is with systemic or cream Metronidazole. This is expensive. Humphrey suggested tea tree for trichomonasas as long ago as 1930, and it was found effective by Pena (1962). Diluted tea tree in cold-pressed carrier oil on a tampon is an effective treatment. Usually, the bacteria will be gone within one week.

Because the vagina is situated closer to the urethra and essential oils are absorbed through the walls of the vagina, this is an excellent way of treating cystitis. Essential oils can be absorbed systemically from vaginal application.

DYSMENORRHEA

The menstrual cycle is delicately balanced and can easily be thrown out of equilibrium by stress, illness, or a poor diet. Primary dysmenorrhea manifests symptoms such as low-abdominal cramping that starts just before or with the menstrual flow. This is often associated with nausea, vomiting, headache, and faintness. Secondary dysmenorrhea usually affects older women who have symptoms of congestion and aching associated with low-abdominal cramps that typically start up to one week prior to menstruation (McFerren 1996). There are two ways to approach dysmenorrhea using aromatherapy, physically and psychologically.

To address physical symptoms, use a mix of essential oils known for their antispasmodic, hormonal balancing, or analgesic properties (Table 21-3). Many essential oils have antispasmodic properties. Roman chamomile contains more esters than any other essential oil (up to 310 including those from angelic and tiglic acid) and is thought to be one of the most antispasmodic essential oils available (Evans 1994). It is also a recognized analgesic (Wren 1988). Han et al (2002) carried out a placebo-controlled study on 85 nurses with dysmenorrhea, using rose, clary sage, and lavender in 3% dilution applied to the abdomen. The mixture reduced the severity of symptoms significantly.

Some essential oils have topical analgesic effect (Table 21-4). Those that are high in phenols such as clove may be too aggressive to apply to the skin of the lower abdomen except in very low dilutions and are best avoided.

Geranium is thought to encourage regular ovulation (Belaiche 1979a) and has been used for generations to balance fluctuating hormonal levels during menopause through its action on the adrenal cortex (Holmes 1993). Add a few drops of geranium (*Pelargonium graveolens*) to the mixture and rub it gently into the lower abdomen and lumbar area. The best geranium oil comes from Reunion Island and is usually called Bourbon. For optimum results, repeat the mixture every hour until dysmenorrhea symptoms have subsided.

Compresses can bring great comfort when applied to the low abdomen. A hot-water bottle has been an effective remedy for period pains for eons. Placed on

Table 21-3 ❧ *Antispasmodic Essential Oils for Dysmenorrhea*

Common Name	Botanical Name	Reference
Roman chamomile	*Chamaemelum nobile*	Franchomme & Penoel 1991
Petitgrain	*Citrus amara fol*	Reiter & Brandt 1985
Spearmint	*Mentha spicata*	Bulat et al 1999
Rosemary	*Rosmarinus officinalis*	Al-Sereiti et al 1999
Peppermint	*Mentha piperita*	Taddei et al 1988
Sage	*Salvia officinalis*	Taddei et al 1988
Lavender	*Lavandula angustifolia*	Lis-Balchin & Hart 1999
Summer savory	*Satureja hortensis*	Hajihashemi et al 2000

Table 21-4 ❧ *Analgesic Essential Oils for Dysmenorrhea*

Common Name	Botanical Name	Reference
Lavender	*Lavandula angustifolia*	Ghelardini et al 1999
Lemongrass	*Cymbopogon citratus*	Viana et al 2000
Peppermint	*Mentha piperita*	Gobel et al 1994

top of an essential oil compress, it will encourage more rapid absorption of the essential oils, as well as giving the added comfort of heat. This can really help painful cramps. The whole process of tending a painful area topically brings with it strong placebo and mind-body links that can only enhance the efficacy of the therapy.

Psychologically relaxing essential oils can be given in a full body massage or "m" technique. This will focus attention on the body and its state of relaxation (unlike taking a tablet). Of course, some of the essential oil will also be inhaled, producing a psychological effect. Severe dysmenorrhea sometimes brings with it nausea. Inhaling a little essential oil of peppermint or spearmint will alleviate this. Aromatherapy, used in this way, works along with the body's own self-regulating mechanisms.

REFERENCES

Adams A. 2000. Does *Lavandula angustifolia* reduce patient anxiety during induced labor? Unpublished dissertation. Hunter, N.Y.: R J Buckle Associates.

Al-Sereiti M, Abu-Amer K, Sen P. 1999. Pharmacology of rosemary and its therapeutic potential. Indian Journal of Experimental Biology. 37(2) 124-130.

Belaiche P. 1979a. Syndrome premenstruel. In Traite de Phytotherapie et d'Aromatherapie, Vol. 3. Paris: Maloine SA, 60-64.

Belaiche P. 1979b. Traite de Phytotherapie et d'Aromatherapie, Vol.1. Paris: Maloine SA.

Belaiche P. 1985. Treatment of vaginal infections of *Candida albicans* with essential oil of *Melaleuca alternifolia.* Phytotherapie. 15:13-15.

Blackwell R. 1991. Teatree oil and anaerobic (bacterial) vaginosis (letter). Lancet. 337(8736) 300.

Brinker F. 2000. The Toxicology of Botanical Medicine, 3rd ed. Sandy, OR: Eclectic Medical Publications.

Bulat R, Fachnie E, Chauehan U, et al. 1999. Effect of spearmint on lower oesophageal sphincter function and acid reflux in health volunteers. Alimentary Pharmacology & Therapeutics. 13(6) 805-812.

Burns E, Blamey C, Ersser S, et al. 2000. An investigation into the use of aromatherapy in intrapartum midwifery practice. The Journal of Alternative & Complementary Medicine. 6(2) 141-147.

Carson C, Riley T. 1993. Antimicrobial activity of the essential oil of *Melaleuca alternifolia.* Letters in Applied Microbiology. 16:49-55.

Carson C, Riley T. 1994. The antimicrobial activity of teatree. Medical Journal of Australia. 160:236.

Chaumont J, Bardy I. 1989. The in-vitro antifungal activities of seven essential oils. Fitoterapia. 60(3) 263-266.

Cook R, Redondo-Lopez V, Schmitt C, et al. 1992. Clinical, microbiological and biochemical factors in recurrent bacterial vaginosis. Journal of Clinical Microbiology. 30(4) 870-877.

England A. 1994. Aromatherapy for the Mother and Baby. Rochester, VT: Healing Arts Press.

Evans W. 1994. Trease and Evans' Pharmacognosy, 13th ed. London: Bailliere Tindall.

Franchomme P, Penoel D. 1991. Aromatherapie Exactement. Limoges, France: Jollois.

Gobel H, Schmidt G, Soyka D. 1994. Effect of peppermint and eucalyptus oil preparations on neurophysiological and experimental algesimetric headache parameters. Cephalagia. 14(3) 228-234.

Goldway M, Teff D, Schmidt R, et al. 1995. Multidrug resistance in *Candida albicans.* Antimicrobial Agents and Chemotherapy. 39(2) 422-426.

Guba R. 2002. Toxicity Myths. International Society of Professional Aromatherapists. London: Regents College. (Handout from conference presentation in March of 2002)

Guenther E. 1972. The Essential Oils. Melbourne, FL: Krieger Publishing.

Hajhashemi V, Sadraei H, Ghannadi A, et al. 2000. Antispasmodic and anti-diarrhoeal effect of *Satureja hortensis.* Journal of Ethnopharmacology. 71(1-2) 187-192.

Han S, Hur M, Buckle J, et al. 2002. Randomized controlled trial on the effect of aromatherapy on menstrual cramps in college students. Unpublished dissertation. Seoul, Korea: School of Nursing.

Holmes P. 1993. The Energetics of Western Herbs. Berkeley, CA: NatTrop.

Humphrey E. 1930. A new Australian germicide. Medical Journal of Australia. 1:417-418.

Kartnig T, Still F, Reinthaler F. 1991. Antimicrobial activity of the essential oil of young pine shoots (*Picea albies*). Journal of Ethnopharmacology. 35(92) 155-157.

Larrondo J, Calvo M. 1991. Effect of essential oils on *Candida albicans:* a scanning electron microscope study. Biomedical Letters. 46(184) 269-272.

Lis-Balchin M, Hart S, Roth G. 1997. The spasmolytic activity of the essential oils of scented *Pelargoniums.* Phytotherapy Research. 11(8) 583-583.

Lis-Balchin M, Hart S. 1999. Studies on the mode of action of essential oil of lavender, *Lavandula angustifolia.* Phytotherapy Research. 13(6) 540-542.

McFerren T (ed.). 1996. Oxford Dictionary of Nursing, 2nd ed. Oxford, UK: Oxford University Press.

Nathan E. 2000. Aromatherapy for pregnancy induced hypertension. Unpublished dissertation. Hunter, NY: R J Buckle Associates.

Nyirjesy P, Weitz M, Grody M, et al. 1997. Over-the-counter and alternative medicines in the treatment of chronic vaginal symptoms. Obstetrics & Gynecology. 90:50-53.

Pattnaik S, Subramanyam V, Kole C. 1996. Antibacterial and antifungal activity of essential oils in vitro. Microbios. 86(349) 237-246.

Pena E. 1925. *Melaleuca alternifolia* oil. Its use for trichomanal vaginitis and other vaginal infections. Proceedings of the Royal Society of Medicine. New South Wales, Australia. 60:167-170.

Pena E. 1962. Melaleuca alternifolia oil. Its use for trichomonal vaginitis and other vaginal infections. Obstet Gynecol. 19(6) 793-795.

Rawlings R. Healing Gardens. Minocqua, WI: Willow Creek Press, 125.

Reiter M, Brandt W. 1985. Relaxant effect on the trachea and ilea of smooth muscle of the guinea pig. Arzneimittel-Forschung Drug Research (Aulendorf). 35:408-414.

Shapiro S, Meier A, Guggenheim B. 1994. The antimicrobial acitivy of essential oils and essential oil components towards oral bacteria. Oral Microbiology and Immunology. 9:202-208.

Soliman F, El-Kashoury E, Fathy M, et al.1994. Analysis and biological activity of the essential oil of *Rosmarinus officinalis* from Egypt. Flavour and Fragrance Journal. 9:29-33.

Stiles J, Sparks M, Ronzio B, et al. 1995. The inhibition of *Candida albicans* by oregano. Journal of Applied Nutrition. 47(4) 96-102.

Suresh B, Siram S, Dhanarj S, et al. 1997. Anticandidal activity of *Santolina chamaecyparisus* volatile oil. Journal of Ethnopharmacology. 55:151-159.

Swingle J. 2001. Use of essential oils in intrapartum care. Unpublished dissertation. Hunter, N.Y.: R J Buckle Associates.

Taddei I, Giachetti E, Taddei P. 1988. Spasmolytic activity of peppermint, sage and rosemary essences and their major constituents. Fitoterapia. 59(6) 463-468.

Tiran D. 1996. Aromatherapy in Midwifery Practice. London: Bailliere Tindall.

Viana G, Vale T, Pinho R, et al. 2000. Antinociceptor effect of the essential oil from *Cymbopogon citratus* in mice. Journal of Ethnopharmacology. 70(3) 323-327.

Viollon C, Leger D, Caumont J. 1993. The antagonistic properties in vitro of specified natural volatile compounds with respect to the germs of the vaginal flora. Plantes Medicinales et Phytotherapie. 16(1) 17-22.

Walsh L, Longstaff J. 1987.The antimicrobial activity of an essential oil on selected oral pathogens. Periodontology. 8:11-15.

Wren R. 1988. Potter's New Cyclopaedia of Botanical Drugs and Preparations. London: Churchill Livingstone.

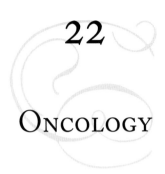

22

ONCOLOGY

If one learns from others but does not think, one will be bewildered. If on the other hand, one thinks but does not learn from others, one will be in peril.

Confucius
Analects, Book II

Cancer affects approximately one person in three (Stevenson 1996) and is the general term applied to a series of malignant diseases that may affect different parts of the body (Dewick 1989). The possible causes of cancer are many and range from electromagnetic and chemical pollution to genetic predisposition and severe stress. According to the American Cancer Society, approximately 550,000 Americans die each year from cancer (Lam 2001). At least half of them are thought to suffer symptoms such as pain, nausea, and emotional distress that conventional medicine either does not or cannot treat (Okie 2001). Cancer has been around for a million years; traces of it were found in mummies from the Great Pyramid at Giza (Lewis & Elvin-Lewis 1977). Humans do not have a monopoly on the disease, as higher-order animals also suffer from cancer.

The three main orthodox treatments for cancer are surgery, radiation, and chemotherapy agents. These treatments have saved lives but have been hard to endure. Now, some of those treatments are being questioned. On May 17, 1999, bone-marrow transplants received controversial press following an announcement at the annual meeting of the American Society of Clinical Oncology in Georgia that a multinational research program found "no evidence that bone marrow transplants were any more beneficial than chemotherapy in breast cancer" (Porter 1999). Five hundred twenty-five women in Scandinavia, 154 in South Africa, 553 in Philadelphia PA, and 61 in France took part in the randomized studies. The researchers found that survival after bone-marrow transplants was 40%, not much higher than a placebo.

Cancer-drug research has also had its share of bad publicity. Barlow (2001) of the British *Financial Times,* wrote "clinical research into cancer drugs was found to be eight times more likely to reach a positive conclusion when funded by a drug company than when publicly funded."

AROMATHERAPY AND CANCER TREATMENT

Many plants and plant materials have been used to treat malignant diseases for centuries. It is fascinating how the same plants keep being cited all over the world for the treatment of cancer. For example, Dr. Fell completed a study of 25 cases of breast cancer using the herb bloodwort at the Middlesex Hospital in London in 1857. He chose bloodwort (*Sanguinaria canadensis*) because he learned it had been used by American Indians for hundreds of years. Fell found all his cases went into remission (Fell 1857). It is difficult to establish whether this really happened, although *Sanguinaria* also has a long history of use in Russia for the treatment of cancer (Lewis & Elvin-Lewis 1977).

Madagascan periwinkle (*Catharanthus roseus*) contains the alkaloids vinblastine and vincristine, which have been useful in treating cancer (Dewick 1989). More recently, *Centella asiatica,* sometimes called gotu kola or South African Pennywort, was featured in an in-vitro study of cultured cancer cells. *Centella* appeared to destroy 100% of the cultured cancer cells. When the study was conducted on mice, *Centella* doubled the life span of mice with tumors. *Centella* has virtually no toxic effect on normal human lymphocytes (Foster 1995). *Centella asiatica* can also be obtained as an infused oil (phytol). Phytols are often used in aromatherapy and are supplied by many essential-oil distributors.

Some essential oils, or components found within essential oils, have been found to have antitumoral activity. Sclareol, a diterpenol in *Salvia sclarea* (clary sage), was found to kill cell-lines of human leukemia and had an inhibitory concentration of lower than 20 (μg/ml) (Dimas et al 1999). Delora et al (1994) found myrrh had an anticarcinogenic effect on tumors induced in mice. Bergamottin, a furanocoumarin found in bergamot (5%) and lemon (0.2%) was one of several coumarins found to inhibit in-vitro tumor promoters (Miyake et al 1999).

Limonene is metabolized into perillyl alcohol by the body. Perillyl alcohol, a monoterpenol also found in lavandin, peppermint, and spearmint, inhibited more than 80% of all chemically induced breast cancers in animal studies (Haag & Gould 1992) and was also found to regress pancreatic, mammary, and liver tumors (Belanger 1998). Perillyl alcohol was found to have chemopreventative activity against colon, skin, and lung cancer and to revert tumor cells to a differentiated state. However, preliminary human trials have not demonstrated tumor regression as of yet, but this could be because only part of an essential oil has been used in isolation. It would be interesting to run the study using the complete essential oil.

Treating Conventional Side Effects

The side effects of some conventional treatments for cancer can be very hard to endure. Several of my friends are cancer survivors. I also had a small aromatherapy private practice in England. My patients came by doctor's referral or word of mouth. Almost half of them had cancer, and the role of aromatherapy in their treatment was one of support. The cancer patients were mainly undergoing chemotherapy and radiation therapy following surgery and, without exception, they found the going very tough. Many expressed their despair that conventional medicine did not adequately address the unpleasant side effects of the cancer treatment.

Several years ago, there was some controversy about the use of massage on cancer patients, with the suggestion that massage could actually spread the disease (Goodman 1995). However, a study and rigorous review of the published literature indicates massage should not be contraindicated (McNamara 1994). Bernie Siegel, MD, also states massage therapy is not contraindicated in a cancer patient (Siegel 1996). Deep massage is rarely requested by an oncology patient. What oncology patients usually prefer is a very light touch, more like stroking. The "m'" technique can be really valuable, particularly as it is so quick to learn and to do and could be taught to family members and friends who are eager to help but don't know how.

Conrad (2000) investigated the effects of aromatherapy on a cancer support group to see if diffused essential oils could decrease anxiety and encourage communication. Ten to 12 cancer patients met weekly. The preponderance was women, but there were some men in the support group. Some individuals were receiving chemotherapy or radiation therapy and some were 3- to 10-year survivors. Three essential oils were chosen for their ability to calm and soothe. The study took six weeks. During weeks one and two no essential oils were diffused, although the diffuser was placed in the room and switched on. During weeks three and four, two drops of a mixture of six drops lavender and four drops mandarin were diffused. During weeks five and six, six drops of lavender and four drops of frankincense were diffused. The diffuser was an AromaStream electric fan. Questionnaires were given to each of the support group members with five simple questions. The questions ranged from whether they could smell anything to whether they found communication more or less difficult. A Likert scale was used to tally the responses. The facilitator did not know when the essential oils were being diffused or which ones were being used. However the facilitator noticed major changes in the group when the essential oils were diffused. During the lavender/mandarin week, there was more laughter and sharing. The sessions seemed more fluid and effortless. During the lavender/frankincense week, the group seemed more emotional and labile. There were more tears than usual, and the group was challenging to facilitate. The participants recorded they felt more relaxed when talking about difficult subjects during the aromatherapy weeks, particularly when the lavender/mandarin mixture was diffused.

Gravett (2001) reported on the effects of topically applied essential oils to an infected Hickman arterial line. He used tea tree, *Eucalyptus globulus,* and lavender (*Lavandula angustifolia*) in a 10% cream applied to the site twice a day. The control group received Povidone iodine spray, which is the standard treatment for an infected line. Gravett notes that chemical antiseptic sprays can lead to cutaneous sensitivity as well as to direct chemical damage and resistant organisms. Gravett found that economically the essential-oil treatment was preferable and appeared to work as well as the Povidone spray.

Researchers at Memorial Sloane Kettering Cancer Center in New York used aromatherapy to reduce anxiety attacks of patients undergoing magnetic resonance imaging. They diffused heliotropin and found it relieved anxiety (Castleman 1996). Heliotropin is a close relative to vanilla. A pilot survey conducted in 1995 showed a wide variety of cancer patients sought complementary care therapy (Clover et al 1995). In a study involving two London hospitals, 16% of patients who had received complementary therapies said they had wanted them to gain emotional support and hope (Downer et al 1994). Perhaps aromatherapy can help during the "dark times," and enhance the quality of care as well as quality of life.

Nausea, constipation, depression, exhaustion, shooting pains, "feeling my bones might break," lymphedema, postradiation burns, hair loss, and insomnia are possibly the most common side effects of radiation therapy and chemotherapy. Of these symptoms, nausea, postradiation burns, hair loss, and lymphedema have been selected for discussion in this chpater. As Dobbs, a British nurse, wrote "complementary therapies may enrich our interventions and bring comfort and better health to patients with cancer" (Dobbs 1985).

Nausea

The cytotoxic drugs used in chemotherapy for cancer have two well-known side effects: nausea and immune supression (Bovbjerg et al 1990). One-third of patients with cancer experience nausea and vomiting (Finlay 1995). Nausea is common during radiation or chemotherapy treatment, and 24%-75% of patients develop anticipatory nausea and vomiting during the course of repeated chemotherapy (Bovbjerg et al 1990). Patients frequently report that everything tastes different. They also say they are very sensitive to odors, often smelling something they had not noticed before or feeling great distaste for a smell that had not bothered them previously. While conventional medicine can be used in the form of antiemetics, there are also essential oils that can reduce nausea. See Table 22-1 for suggestions.

Just a few drops of one of the oils in Table 22-1 on a tissue can bring relief. Sipping hot water with a sliver of ginger root can also frequently bring relief from nausea and is a well-known remedy for morning sickness during pregnancy. A more in-depth review of essential oils for nausea can be found in Chapter 11 on nausea.

Table 22-1 ❧ *Essential Oils for Nausea*

Common Name	Botanical Name	Reference
Peppermint	*Mentha piperita*	Briggs 1993, Williams 1998, Williamson & Evans 1988
Ginger	*Zingiber officinale*	Mowry 1982
Cardamom	*Elettoria cardamomum*	Nadkarani 1992, Cabo & Crespo 1986
Patchouli	*Pogostemon cablin*	Yang et al 1999
Spearmint	*Mentha spicata*	Buckle 1997

Patients receiving bone-marrow transplants frequently have to endure the smell of dimethyl sulfoxide (DMSO). DMSO causes differentiation of malignant bone-marrow cells (Toren & Rechavi 1993) and can help deliver anticancer substances to the site of the cancer (Wilner 1994). It also seems to enhance the effects of various cytotoxic agents while simultaneously reducing the toxicity of conventional medication (Pommier et al 1988). Citrus essential oils such as lemon and grapefruit are being used successfully to hide this aroma at Columbia Presbyterian Medical center in New York, according to my students. The essence of oranges is a traditional treatment in Sicily for sea sickness.

Postradiation burns

Although most radiologists request nothing be put on the skin during radiation, this is mainly to ensure the marks for radiation will not be removed (Sheppard-Hanger 2000). It is extremely important that nothing should disturb the marks. Maiche et al (1990) conducted their study (see following description) throughout irradiation by applying a cream to the area before and after each radiation treatment.

Before the area is marked, the skin can be prepared with undiluted naiouli (*Melaleuca viridiflora*). This seems to toughen the skin and results in fewer and less severe burns. Apply naiouli to the area three times a day for a week. Roulier (1990) and Penoel and Franchomme (1990) both suggest using 50% naiouli immediately before each radiation session and 50% in a St. John's wort-infused oil or rosehip carrier oil after each session. Sheppard-Hanger (2000) also used spritzers of everlasting (*Helichrysum italicum*) and blue tansy (*Tanacetum annum*) immediately following each radiation treatment. Blue tansy is dark blue in color and high in chamazulene, an antiinflammatory. Do not mistakenly use *Tanacetum vulgare,* another species of *Tanacetum. Tanacetum vulgare* is yellow to pale blue and contains 60% thujone, a ketone, and is not recommended for use in oncology or aromatherapy in general.

My patients have used tansy and everlasting in spritzers and also spritzers of lavender and rose with good results. Yarrow and blue chamomile are also good choices. Table 22-2 lists essential oils that can be used in post-radiation spritzers.

To make a spritzer, add 4 ml of essential oils to 4 oz of water and put in a spray bottle. Shake well before using. Anything to be used topically that has been stored in an aluminum container or contains aluminum (such as antiperspirants) cannot be used during radiation therapy as aluminum can interfere with the treatment.

When radiation therapy is finished, apply a compress. Mix antiinflammatory essential oils like German chamomile, frankincense, or rose into a base of either aloe vera gel or tamanu (*Calophyllum inophyllum*). An infused oil of gotu kola (*Centella asiatica*) or comfrey (*Symphytum officinale*) can also bring rapid relief and help promote healing.

Maiche et al (1990) carried out a controlled, single-blind study on 50 women ages 30-79 who had been operated on for breast cancer and who had received radiation therapy. Kamillosan Ointment, a proprietary cream containing chamomile that is widely available in Europe, was applied 30 minutes before radiation and just before bed. Measurements were made by a physician using a four-point scale (no change through moist desquamation). A comparison between the control group and the Kamillosan group showed no statistical significant changes overall, but skin deterioration appeared to happen later in the Kamillosan group, and there were fewer patients who presented with Grade 2 (dark erythema) reactions. In a further controlled study on leg ulcers, Kamillosan appeared to enhance standard treatment of corticosteroids and antihistamines (Nasemann 1975).

Hair loss

In a randomized, double-blind, controlled study, hair loss due to alopecia responded well to topically applied essential oils (Hay et al 1998). Eighty-six patients took part in the study. The active group massaged thyme, rosemary, lavender, and cedarwood in a mixture of jojoba and grapeseed oil into their scalps daily. The control group massaged their scalps with vegetable oils only. Measurement

Table 22-2 ❧ *Spritzers for Postradiation Burns*

Common Name	Botanical Name	Reference
Lavender	*Lavandula angustifolia*	Tisserand 1993
German chamomile	*Matricaria recutita*	Maiche et al 1990, Williamson & Evans 1988
Roman chamomile	*Chamaemelum nobile*	Maiche et al 1990, Grieve 1931
Rose	*Rosa damascena*	Brud & Szydlowska 1991
Everlasting	*Helichrysum italicum*	Sheppard-Hanger 2000
Blue tansy	*Tanacetum annum*	Sheppard-Hanger 2000
Yarrow	*Achillea millefolium*	Sheppard-Hanger 2000

was taken three ways: through a standardized, professional photograph taken initially, and then again after 3 and 7 months. Measurement was on a four-point scale and with a map of the alopecia traced onto transparent film. This was converted into a computerized image so exact calculations could be made. Nineteen (44%) of the 43 patients in the active group showed improvement compared with six (15%) of the control group (p = 0.008).

When chemotherapy stops, usually the patient's hair begins to grow again, often more luxuriantly.

Lymphedema

Lymphedema occurs frequently following mastectomy but is also fairly common following lumpectomy if there has been removal of lymph glands. It stands to reason that the lymph system will have more difficulty returning excess interstitial fluid to the blood if there has been a reduction in the number of lymph pathways. The large, lymphatic vessel walls are contractile (so progress is in one direction only), and when one or more of the lymph glands has been removed via surgery or damage, lymph accumulates in the subcutaneous tissue causing the affected limb to become swollen and tender (Badger 1995).

Lymph contains large protein molecules, and build-up of protein in the tissue leads to chronic inflammation and, over a period of time, thickened, leathery looking skin. After the initial phase of soft skin and pitting, chronic lymphedema is characteristically nonpitting. Because of chronic inflammation, local immunity is compromised, with subsequent bouts of cellulitis and poor resistance to insect bites or minor cuts.

Lymphatic drainage should be carried out regularly, as there is no pumping action by the lymph system itself. Normal lymphatic drainage relies on muscular activity during exercise to move the lymph in the right direction. When this no longer happens, the lymph needs a little extra help. However, because the problem occurs at a subcutaneous level, the pressure needed is extremely light and only in the direction of the lymph. This is one instance where normal massage is contraindicated. The pressure of an ordinary massage can cause spasm in the lymph vessels, temporarily suspending the lymphatic flow (Idoux 1996), and most massage strokes are not suitable.

Lymphatic drainage is a completely different technique and needs to be learned. Perhaps the most famous and accepted method is the Vodder method, which was developed in Austria 50 years ago. Rather than a massage stroke, which tends to be a two- directional movement with both hands working in opposite directions, lymphatic drainage works in one direction only: the direction of flow of the lymph, which is toward the main lymph ducts, away from the peripheries, and toward the thoracic duct. Regular sessions, daily if possible, can reduce the size of a lymph-enlarged limb quite dramatically. The limb will feel lighter and the skin more supple. The elbow (or other joint) will become more clearly defined, and there will be more tactile sensation. I have had success using "tramlines," running my fingers gently, slowly, and repeatedly in the direction of the lymph. With a bit of practice it was possible to feel the lymph move.

Aromatherapy can play an important role when the skin loses its elasticity and infections become more frequent. However, it is unlikely that essential oils could help the lymph to move. Table 22-3 lists carrier and infused oils used in the treatment of lymphedema.

Essential oils can be useful to protect the engorged limb from bacterial or fungal infection (Table 22-4). Choose an essential oil the patient likes, and avoid those with an astringent action like *Cupressus sempervirens* (cypress).

Kirshbaum (1996) carried out a small study with eight patients with lymphedema using diluted lavender in a massage. She found aromatherapy massage reduced pain and swelling and improved movement, a finding that seems to contradict the conclusion of Idoux (1996). Casley-Smith (1999) found topically applied coumarins reduced edema, but not as effectively as when taken orally.

Benefits of Aromatherapy for Cancer Patients

Aromatherapy is often used to enhance the quality of life of cancer patients. In a study at the Marie Curie Center in Liverpool, England, patients received a massage with or without Roman chamomile. The group that received the aromatherapy massage was found to have statistically significant improved quality of life and reduced anxiety (Wilkinson 1995). In another study conducted to assess the acceptability of using aromatherapy in palliative care, doctors, nurses, paramedics, and volunteers were reported to be extremely enthusiastic about the concept (Arnold 1995).

Corner et al (1995) used a premade mixture of lavender, rosewood, lemon, rose, and valerian in their randomized controlled study of 52 patients with a variety of cancers. Just over half of the patients received chemotherapy, radiation, or surgery during the 8-week study. Patients were randomly assigned to a group to receive a weekly massage with or without essential oils. A matching control group was selected from patients who were unable to attend the 8-week course of massage. The

Table 22-3   *Carrier and Infused Oils for Treating Lymphedema*

Common Name	Botanical Name	Reference
Gotu kola	*Centella asiatica*	Price et al 1999
Oil of evening primrose	*Oenothera biennis*	Earle 1991
Passionflower	*Passiflora incarnata*	Earle 1991

Table 22-4   *Skin-Friendly Essential Oils with Antibacterial or Antifungal Actions*

Common Name	Botanical Name	Reference
Lavender	*Lavandula angustifolia*	Valnet 1991
Frankincense	*Boswellia carterii*	Duwiejua et al 1993
Sweet marjoram	*Origanum majorana*	Ross et al 1980

results showed a statistical difference in anxiety between the two groups receiving massage, but pain and mobility showed almost equal improvement.

Evans (1995) conducted an audit into aromatherapy massage in cancer patients in a palliative-care setting. The study lasted 6 months and involved 69 patients. Participants were offered an aromatherapy session with an aromatherapy massage and therapist advice on symptom control using aromatherapy. Eighty percent of the patients felt they benefited, although it is difficult to assess whether this was due to the essential oils, massage, or the one-on-one care. Everson (2002) found that while her white-blood-cell (WBC) count fell with each chemotherapy treatment, the WBC rebounded faster when she added bergamot to her daily regimen. Table 22-5 lists isolates believed to have anticarcinogenic properties.

Essential Oils to Avoid in Oncology

Recent studies have indicated that phytoestrogens, once thought to be contraindicated in cancer, may actually reduce the risk of cancer and could therefore be beneficial. However, as the jury is still out and until more definite information emerges, it might be prudent to avoid essential oils with estrogen-like properties in tumors that are estrogen dependent. Estrogen-dependent cancers are breast, uterine, and ovarian. It is extremely unlikely that the tiny amounts of estrogen-like compounds used in aromatherapy would impact cancerous growth. As early as 1938, Zondeck and Bergmann wrote about the estrogenic properties of phenol methyl ethers. Essential oils thought to have an estrogen-like effect include fennel and aniseed as they contain anethole (Albert-Puleo 1980). Anethole is a phe-

Table 22-5   *Isolates Thought to Have Anticarcinogenic Properties*

Isolate	Source	Botanical Name	Reference
Sclareol	Clary sage	*Salvia sclarea*	Dimas et al 1999
Bergamottin	Bergamot	*Citrus bergamia*	Miyake et al 1999
Perillyl alcohol	Peppermint Spearmint Lavandin	*Mentha piperita* *Mentha spicata* *Lavandula intermedia*	Belanger 1998
D-limonene, geraniol	Lemongrass	*Cymbopogon citratus*	Zheng et al 1993
Carvone, anethufuran, limonene	Dill	*Anethum graveolens*	Zheng et al 1991
Carvone, anethufuran, limonene	Caraway	*Carum carvi*	Zheng et al 1991

nol methyl ether. Scareol (found in clary sage) and viridifloral (found in niaouli) are other components of essential oils that have structures similar to estrogen (Franchomme & Penoel 1991). Therapists using aniseed and fennel on a daily basis found that their periods came earlier than usual. The link to geranium and rose is really too tenuous, and both essential oils should be fine to use in estrogen-dependent tumors.

In-vitro studies on rat skin indicated that some essential oils enhance the penetration of 5-fluorouracil (5FU) (Abdullah et al 1996). Peppermint increased penetration by 46 times, and *Eucalyptus globulus* increased penetration by 60 times. It might be advisable to avoid using these two essential oils topically near the intravenous site during chemotherapy with 5FU.

Conclusion

In summary, aromatherapy is a way to "enrich interventions and bring comfort and better health to patients with cancer" (Penson & Fisher 1995). Such actions demonstrate *caring*. Perhaps this is the caring referred to by the nursing theorist Orem as "a moral idea of nursing" (Leddy & Pepper 1993). However, caring is a moral issue for all health-care professionals.

References

Abdullah D, Ping Q, Liu G. 1996. Enhancing the effect of essential oils on the penetration of 5-fluorouracil through rat skin. Yao Xue Xue Bao. 31(3) 214-221.

Albert-Puleo M. 1980. Fennel and anise as estrogenic agents. Journal of Ethnopharmacology. 2(4) 337-344.

Arnold L. 1995. The use of aromatherapy and essential oils in palliative care: risk versus research. Positive Health. 32-34.

Badger C. 1995. Lymphoedema. In Penson J, Fisher R (eds.), Palliative Care for People with Cancer. London: Edward Arnold, 81-90.

Barlow T. 2001. When the devil invites you to dine. Financial Times. May 26/27, 11.

Belanger J. 1998. Perillyl alcohol: applications in oncology. Alternative Medicine Review. 3(96) 448-457.

Bovbjerg D, Redd W, Maier L, et al. 1990. Anticipatory immune suppression and nausea in women receiving cyclic chemotherapy for ovarian cancer. Journal of Consulting and Clinical Psychology. 58(2) 153-157.

Briggs C. 1993. Peppermint: medicinal herb and flavouring agent. Canadian Pharmaceutical Journal. 126:89-92.

Cabo J, Crespo M. 1986. The spasmolytic activity of various aromatic plants from Granada: the activity of the major components of their essential oils. Plantes Medicinales et Phytotherapie. 20(3) 213-218.

Casley-Smith J.1999. Benzo-pyrones in the treatment of lymphedema. International Journal of Angiology. 18(1) 31-41.

Castleman M. 1996. Aromatherapy: Nature's Cures. Emmaus, PA: Rodale Press, 39.

Clover A, Last P, Fisher P. 1995. Complementary cancer therapy: a pilot study of patients, therapies and quality of life. Complementary Therapies in Medicine. 3(3) 129-133.

Conrad P. 2000. Aromatherapy and the cancer support group. Unpublished dissertation. Hunter, N.Y.: R J Buckle Associates.

Corner J, Cawley N, Hildebrand S. 1995. An evaluation of the use of massage and essential oils on the well being of cancer patients. International Journal of Palliative Nursing. 1(2) 67-73.

Delora P, Luceri C, Gherlandini C, et al. 1994. Anticarcinogenic effect of *Commophora momol* on solid tumors induced by Ehrlich carcinoma cells in mice. Chemotherapy. 40:337-347.

Dewick P. 1989. Tumour inhibitors from plants. In Evans W (ed.), Trease and Evan's Pharmacognosy, 13th ed. London: Bailliere Tindall, 634-656.

Dimas K, Kokkinopoulos D, Demetzos C, et al. 1999. The effect of sclareol on growth and cell cycle progression of human leukemic cell lines. Leukemia Research. 23(3) 217-234.

Dobbs B. 1985. Alternative health approaches. Nursing Mirror. 160:41-42.

Downer S, Cody M, McCluskey P. 1994. Pursuit and practice of complementary therapies by cancer patients receiving conventional treatment. British Medical Journal. 309(6947) 86-89.

Duwiejua M, Zeitlin I, Waterman P, et al. 1993. Anti-inflammatory activity of resins from some species of the plant family Burseraceae. Planta Medica. 59(5) 12-16.

Earle L. 1991. Vital Oils. London: Vermilion.

Evans B. 1995. An audit into the effects of aromatherapy massage and the cancer patient in palliative and terminal cancer. Complementary Therapies in Medicine. 3(4) 239-241.

Everson C. 2002. Personal communication.

Fell J. 1857. A Treatise on Cancer and Its Treatment. London: J & A Churchill.

Finlay I. 1995. The management of other frequently encountered symptoms. In Penson J, Fisher R (eds.), Palliative Care for People with Cancer. London: Edward Arnold, 57-80.

Foster S. 1995. Anti-cancer effects of Gotu Kola (*Centella asiatica*). HerbalGram. 36:17-18.

Franchomme P, Penoel D. 1990. Aromatherapie Exactement. Limoges, France: Jollois.

Gattefosse R. 1937. (Translated in 1993 by R. Tisserand.) Aromatherapie: Les Huile Essentielles-Hormones Vegetales (Gattefosse's Aromatherapy.) Saffron Walden, UK: CW Daniels, 89.

Goodman S (ed.). 1995. Book review: Massage for People with Cancer. Positive Health. 26.

Gravett P. 2001. Aromatherapy treatment for patients with Hickman line infection following high-dose chemotherapy. Int J of Aromatherapy. 11(1) 18-20.

Grieve M. 1931. A Modern Herbal. Harmondsworth, UK: Penguin Books.

Haag J, Gould M. 1992. Mammary carcinoma regression induced by perillyl alcohol, an hydroxylated analog of d-lmonene. Cancer Chemother Pharmacog. 34(6) 477-483.

Hay I, Jamieson M, Ormerod D. 1998. Randomized trial of aromatherapy: successful treatment for alopecia areata. Archives of Dermatology. 134(11) 1349-1352.

Idoux M. 1996. Treatment for lymphoedema following mastectomy or lumpectomy. Holistic Nurses' Association Newsletter. 3:4-5.

Kirshbaum M. 1996.Using massage in the relief of lymphedema. Professional Nurse. 11(4) 230-232.

Lam M. 2001. Annual cancer deaths in USA. Retrieved March 17, 2003 from www.LamMD.com.

Leddy S, Pepper J. 1993. Conceptual Bases of Professional Nursing. Philadelphia: Lippincott.

Lewis W, Elvin-Lewis M. 1977. Medical Botany. New York: Wiley Interscience.

Maiche A, Grohn P, Maki-Hokkonen H. 1990. Effect of chamomile cream and almond ointment on acute radiation skin reaction. Acta Oncologica. 30(3) 395-396.

McNamara P. 1994. Massage for People with Cancer. London: Wandsworth Cancer Support Centre.

Miyake Y, Murakami A, Sugiyama Y, et al. 1999. Identification of coumarins from lemon fruit (*Citrus limon*) as inhibitors of in vitro tumor promotion and superoxide and nitric oxide generation. Journal of Agricultural and Food Chemistry. 47(8) 3151-3157.

Mowrey D. 1982. Motion sickness, ginger and psychophysics. Lancet. 1(8273) 655-657.

Nadkarni K. 1992. Indian Material Medica, Vol. 1. Prakashan, India: Bombay Popular.

Nasemann T. 1975. Kamillosan therapy in dermatology. Z Allgemeinmed. 25:1105-1106.

Okie S. 2001. Report faults priorities of cancer care in the US. Albany, N.Y.: Times Union, A5.

Penson J, Fisher R. 1995. Palliative Care for People with Cancer. London: Edward Arnold.

Pommier RF, Woltering EA, Milo G, 1988. Cytotoxicity of DMSO and antineoplastic combinations against human tumors. American Journal of Surgery. 155(5) 672-675.

Porter C. 1999. Business thrives on unproven care, leaving science behind. New York Times. CXLIX A1.

Price L, Smith I, Price S. 1999. Carrier Oils. Stratford-upon-Avon, UK: Riverhead.

Ross S, El-Keltaw N, Megella S. 1980. Antimicrobial activity of some Egyptian aromatic plants. Fitoterapia. 51:201-205.

Roulier G. 1990. Les Huiles Essentielles Pour Votre Sante. St. Jean-de-Braye, France: Dangles.

Siegal B. 1996. Letter to the editor. Massage Therapy Journal. 35:12-13.

Sheppard-Hanger S. 2000. Use of essential oils and natural extracts to help counter side effects of radiation during cancer treatment. Proceedings of the 3rd Scientific Wholistic Aromatherapy Conference. San Francisco. Nov 10-12, 174-191.

Stevenson C. 1996. Disease. In Vickers A (ed.), Massage and Aromatherapy. London: Chapman & Hall, 193-202.

Toren A, Rechavi G. 1993. What really cures in autologous bone marrow transplantation? A possible role for dimethylsulfide. Medical Hypotheses. 41(6) 495-498.

Weil A. 1998. Complementary Care for Cancer. Dr. Andrew Weil's Self- Healing. 1, 6.

Wilkinson S, Aldridge J, Salmon I. 1999. An evaluation of Aromatherapy massage in palliative care. Journal of Palliative Medicine. 13(5) 409-417.

Williamson E, Evans F (eds.). 1988. Potter's New Cyclopedia of Botanical Drugs and Preparations. Saffron Walden, UK: CW Daniels.

Wilner J. 1994. DMSO. The Cancer Solution. Boca Raton, FL: Peltec Publishing.

Yang Y, Kinoshita K, Koyama K, et al. 1999. Anti-emetic principles of *Pogostemon cablin*. Phytomedicine. 6(2) 89-93.

Zheng G, Kenney P, Lam K. 1991. Anethofurna, carvone and limonene: Potential cancer chemopreventive agents from dill weed oil and caraway oil. Planta Medica. 58(4) 338-341.

Zheng G, Kenney P, Lam K. 1993. Potential anticarcinogenic natural products isolated from lemongrass oils and galanga root oil. Journal of Agricultural and Food Chemistry. 41(2) 153-157.

Zondeck B, Bergmann E. 1938. Phenol methyl ethers as estrogenic agents. Biochemical Journal. 32:641-645.

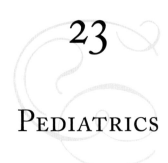

PEDIATRICS

And when you crush an apple with your teeth, say to it in your heart:
"Your seeds shall live in my body.
And the buds of your tomorrow shall blossom in my heart.
And your fragrance shall be my breath,
And together, we shall rejoice through all the seasons."

Kahil Gibran
The Prophet

There is a Chinese saying that "Children get sick easily, and sickness can quickly become serious," and another saying that "Children easily ill, easily cured." There is no doubt that children in the hospital are very vulnerable. They do indeed deteriorate or improve rapidly, and they need a tremendous amount of love and support, particularly if their families cannot visit. Although children are more adaptable than adults and often face very intimidating procedures with wide-eyed interest and no apparent fear, many do display behavioral problems just because they have become institutionalized.

Some of the most distressing aspects of hospitalization are the invasive medical procedures, like venipuncture and the placing of nasogastric tubes. Aromatherapy can help soothe the child prior to these interventions. A few moments of hand or face "m" technique can help relax children while you explain what is going to happen, how long it will last, and how it will help them. Anxiety about being hurt has been identified as one of a child's greatest fears (Kurfit Stephens et al 1999). Sweet orange oil was found to be helpful in the induction of 120 unpremedicated children aged 5-14 years in a study by Mehta et al (1998). Children in the essential oil group were significantly more likely to say they would like to have a similar anaesthetic technique again in the future ($p<0.05$). As nausea is frequently a symptom of fear in children, lavender might be another useful essential oil to use. Lavender straw (the discarded by-product of stream distillation) still retains some aroma and was found to alleviate stress and travel sickness in 40 pigs being transported by road (Bradshaw et al 1998).

Aromatherapy is a natural thing to a child, whose early life revolves around smell and touch. Babies identify their mothers through the mother's smell (Russell 1976). This is easy to understand when one realizes that babies are born with structurally mature olfactory systems (Humphrey 1940). Young children up to the age of 5 years are not repelled by smells that most adults dislike, such as feces. However, by the age of seven, many children are beginning to establish similar "tastes" in smells to adults (Engen 1974). Children also display the facility of "learned memory" early on, gravitating toward the smell of a perfume worn by their mother, rather than another unknown perfume (Schleidt & Genzel 1990). Therefore, familiar smells are more acceptable to children than other smells. This is particularly important in the case of children from other cultures, who may respond to exotic aromas with which Western children might not identify, such as spices. Children can be extremely sensitive to smell. Schilcher (1997), head of the Institute of Pharmaceutical Biology at Berlin's Independent University, suggests inhalation of volatile oils is an excellent method of choice for pediatrics.

Most of us find it an instinctive action to cuddle and stroke a child. Aromatherapy takes that instinct a little further and adds some extra therapeutic value. Parents and relatives can be taught very easily how to use the "m" technique on a sick child, and they relish the feeling of being empowered to do something in a situation most parents fear. This experience of empowerment can be made more potent by the addition of an aroma with which both mother or father and child are familiar and which they both like. Gentle aromas can soothe a child, but the emphasis is on gentleness. It is necessary to use only half the normal number of drops of an essential oil required for an adult. Please see Table 23-1 for dosage recommendations for children.

Bear in mind that some children may have been subjected to abuse and will not be receptive to touch, finding it more threatening than comforting. If this is

Table 23-1 ❧ Doses for Children and Babies

Premies	Floral waters only	N/A
Newborn-6 months	1 drop in 20 ml	0.25%
6 months-2 years	1 drop in 10 ml	0.5%
2-5 years	1 drop in 5 ml	1%
5-10 years	1-2 drops in 5 ml	1-2%
More than 10 years	1-5 drops in 5 ml	1-5%

*unless treating specific infections, for example onychomycosis (toenail fungus) or hair lice.

the case, merely using the appropriate aroma can still be beneficial. Children quite like to be involved in choosing an aroma, especially if the choice is small. More than four essential oils will demand too much effort from a sick child. Sometimes a choice of just two will make aromatherapy acceptable, whereas if only one smell is offered it might be refused. However, it is important never to insist; children are patients with patients' rights, no matter how old they are.

Of the possible problems that might be helped by aromatherapy, hyperactivity, attention deficit hyperactivity disorder (ADHD), and head lice have been chosen for discussion in this chapter. Clinical aromatherapy has an important role in pediatrics alongside orthodox medicine. Aromatherapy can also bring comfort to both child and parent and give a sense of empowerment to staff. Caring for sick children is an emotionally draining experience, and caring for a dying child is one of the most daunting tasks faced by any health professional (Hodson 1985).

HYPERACTIVITY

Hyperactivity in children who have become hospitalized is common. This form of excitable behavior is different from attention deficit/hyperactivity disorder (ADHD), which is a recognized mental disorder and will be covered in a later section (McFerran 1996).

Every child will have a unique response to being hospitalized. Some children become withdrawn, some become placatory, and others become hyperactive. It is the hyperactive children who can become a source of irritation to staff and other children. Aromatherapy can often help. The cause underlying the behavior may be the strange environment and smells, which make the child feel threatened. Hyperactivity may be a means of asking for more attention or a means of communicating a child's sense of ill ease. The "m" technique with a familiar smell (Table 23-2) may soothe a child and reduce hyperactivity. Sometimes mixing aromas to produce a new but faintly familiar aroma can be beneficial (Worwood 2000).

Table 23-2 ✖ *Essential Oils to Relax a Hyperactive Child in the Hospital*

Common Name	Botanical Name
Roman chamomile	*Chamaemelum nobile*
Mandarin	*Citrus reticulata*
Lavender	*Lavandula angustifolia*
Neroli	*Citrus aurantium flos*
Rose	*Rosa damascena*
Geranium	*Pelargonium graveolens*
Sweet marjoram	*Origanum majorana*

A foot or hand "m" technique is usually acceptable to a sick child. Teaching parents to help their sick children is one of the most rewarding things I have ever done. A mother's touch, no matter how unfamiliar she is with any technique or stroke, is what a child will usually recognize and respond to. Gentleness and slow strokes are what matters. This is particularly important to remember if the child is unconscious. If the mother wears a lot of bracelets, do not ask her to remove them, as her child will remember how they sounded and how they felt.

Sometimes the smallest amount of a compound in an essential oil can have a profound effect. One example is the smell of rose caused by an oxide present at a concentration of only 0.1 parts per million. Another example is a compound called indole present at trace levels in citrus oils, honeysuckle, and jasmine (Collin & Hoeke 1993). In large amounts, indole smells vile and would make most people gag because it contributes to the smell of rotting meat! However, indole has a remarkable relationship with tryptophan and appears to aid its synthesis (Clark 1995). Tryptophan is found in various foodstuffs like chicken, milk, bananas, and rice and is the chemical precursor of serotonin, the "feel-good" neurochemical (Parish 1991). Using an essential oil containing a trace of indole may help a child relax.

ATTENTION DEFICIT/HYPERACTIVITY DISORDER

ADHD is a combination of inattention, hyperactivity, and impulsive behavior that is classified as a disorder when these behaviors are severe. ADHD is thought to be a developmental failure in the brain circuitry that underlies inhibition and self control (Tucker 1999). During the last 10 years, an increasing number of children have been diagnosed with ADHD. It is the most commonly diagnosed behavioral disorder in children and the fastest growing disorder in adults. Since 1990, the number of children in the United States diagnosed with ADHD has increased from 900,000 to more than 5.5 million. ADHD is thought to affect 5-10% of all school-aged children. One and a half million adults also have been diagnosed with ADHD.

Charles Bradley first noticed that amphetamine (Benzedrine) calmed hyperactive children in 1937 (Gainetdinov & Caron 2001). Numerous studies carried out since that time have shown that stimulants such as amphetamines interact with plasma-membrane monoamine transporters (dopamine, serotonin, and norepinephrine transporters) (Gainetdinov et al 1999). The current treatment for ADHD is with a stimulant medication such as Ritalin. Sales of Ritalin have increased 700% since 1990 (Haislip 2002). Little is known about the long-term effect of stimulants on brain chemistry, and there is increasing concern about the long-term use of Ritalin (Breggin 1998).

Some research on ADHD suggests many different contributing factors are involved, including sensitivity to the yellow dye tartrazine. However, no definite cause for the disorder has been found. Recent research at Harvard and Massachusetts General Hospital shows adult subjects with longstanding ADHD have an abnormal elevation in their number of dopamine transporters. Ritalin was thought to work by altering levels of dopamine. However, studies with rats suggest Ritalin works by boosting serotonin levels in the brain. The researchers concluded that ADHD may occur when the chemical balance between dopamine and serotonin is thrown off (Caron 1999).

I have found that children with ADHD become more stimulated with sedative essential oils such as Roman chamomile and lavender. So, I tried essential oils with stimulant properties and found they had a relaxing effect. Because of this finding, two of my students carried out two separate studies on ADHD using two different essential oils. The first study, by Sorenson (1999), was very simple and involved observing four children with ADHD who were attending piano lessons. When lavender (*Lavandula angustifolia*) was diffused into the air, all four children became more inattentive and restless. When rosemary (*Rosmarinus officinalis*) was diffused into the air, three of the four children became more attentive and less restless.

Sptizer (2000) carried out a study on 10 children (aged 7-9 years) attending a school for children with special needs. Children who were prone to seizures were excluded from the study. Two occupational therapists conducted the experiment at the school and used a Likert scale for analysis. Baseline data were recorded for four separate visits. This included the number of times the children got out of their chairs, the number of times the children needed directions repeated, the number of times the children engaged in self stimulation (rocking), and the number of minutes the children sustained attention to a particular task. During the experimental stage, two drops of *Rosmarinus officanalis* were placed on an aromastone before each of the four occupational therapy sessions. (An aromastone is a ceramic stone that uses electricity to gently heat a few drops of essential oil placed on the stone.)

As each child was so different, the data were discussed individually. In the best case scenario, child six managed to focus with rosemary and sustained attention for up to 23 minutes, instead of 18 without the oil. Child one sustained focused attention for 9 minutes instead of 3 minutes. Child three was able to remain seated longer. Child four, who was prone to tantrums, did not have any tantrums during the aromatherapy sessions. Child five did not have any self-regulating problems, and therefore there was no room for improvement. Three other children had slight improvements overall, two children had no difference, and one child performed worse. Although this study is inconclusive, both occupational therapists felt the findings warranted further study.

Pitman (2000) invited a group of 11 children with ADHD to choose three essential oils from a selection of 15 oils that included stimulant and sedative essential oils. The three were then mixed together, diluted in vegetable oil, and applied to the children's wrists. The same mixture was sometimes used at home in a bath or diffused into the air. The oils appeared to relax the children, increase their concentration in class, and decrease disruptions, and the children all appeared calmer. The parents agreed the essential-oil mixtures had helped their children calm down. However, one parent said the child became hyperactive when a citrus aroma was vaporized for too long.

PEDICULOSIS (HEAD LICE)

Head-louse infestation is common worldwide. In developed countries the infestation rate is increasing, especially in the 4- to 13-year-old age group (Mumcuoglu 1999). This increased infestation could be due to the incorrect use of effective agents that has led to lice strains becoming resistant to insecticides. Compounds such as Permethrin, malathion, and DDT are no longer sucessful (Combescot et al 1996). Izri and Briere (1995) report on the first case of resistant head lice in France in Paris and Tours, citing that resistance had already occurred in the United Kingdom. Most pediculicides are only partially ovicidal, resulting in another batch of new lice after 10 days. It is important that a special lice comb is used and all the eggs are removed after treatment, as some nits can remain glued to the hair for several months, even if they are dead. Suffocating agents such as olive, soya, or sunflower vegetable oil can be effective if used for more than 12 hours. While some studies have shown that essential oils can be pediculicidal, there is no evidence that essential oils repel lice (Mumcuoglu 1999).

Veal (1996) tested seven essential oils and three blends (by Shirley Price) in vitro. Aniseed, oregano, cinnamon leaf, red thyme, and tea tree all performed well when tested in an alcoholic solution using overnight exposure. Veal concluded it would be important to use the same essential oil in the rinse that was contained in the original application. She recommended using an essential oil, vinegar, and water solution but alcohol and water could also be effective. Phenols and phenolic ethers, ketones, and 1,8-cineole appeared to be the compounds most likely to kill lice.

Laurent et al (1997) reported that linalol, menthone, menthol, and limonene were also effective larvicides and ovicides. Gauthier et al (1989) showed that a-pinene was another effective compound against head lice in his study on the effectiveness of Myrtle.

Lahlou et al (2000) investigated the effectiveness of 24 essential oils and 15 of their isolated compounds against human head lice in vitro using microatmosphere and direct application. *Mentha pulegium* (pennyroyal), *Thymus broussonetti*, *Chenopodium ambrosioides* (American wormseed), and *Ruta chalepensis* were found to be the most effective. Unfortunately, these essential oils are not the most suitable for children. (It was interesting that they did not include tea tree in their study.) The lice died within 15 minutes of direct application by the essential oils. However, the nits were a little more difficult. At a 1:4 dilution of *Thymus broussonettii* applied directly, 20% of the nits hatched. Of the isolated compounds, phenols and phenolic ethers, ketones, and 1,8-cineole were the most effective.

Oladimeji et al (2000) investigated the effects of *Lippa multiflora* essential oil on head and body lice and scabies and found it effective. In the study, 0.02 ml of a 25% solution of *Lippia* in liquid paraffin was sufficient to kill head lice within

2 hours. (The lice had been removed from the children to a petri dish.) *Lippia multiflora* was more effective than benzyl benzoate at the same concentration, but not as effective as kerosene.

References

ADD/ADHD research. Jan. 11, 2001. ADD/ADHD Online Support Group. www.adders.org.

Bradshaw R, Marchant J, Meredith M, et al. 1998. Effects of lavender straw on stress and travel sickness in pigs. Journal of Alternative & Complementary Medicine. 4(3) 271-275.

Breggin P. 1998. Report to the plenary session of the NIH consensus conference on ADHD and its treatment. www.breggin.com.

Caron M. 1999. Role of serotonin in the paradoxical calming effect of psychostimulants on hyperactivity. Science. 283:397-401.

Clark G. 1995. An aroma chemical profile: indole. Perfumer & Flavorist. 20(2) 21-31.

Collin G, Hoeke H. 1993. Ullman's Encyclopedia of Industrial Chemistry, Vol. 14, 5th ed. Weinheim, Germany: VCH.

Combescot C, Combescot-Lang C, Remy-Kristensen A, et al. 1996. Tests for evaluating the effectiveness of pediculicides: importance and limitations. Bulletin de l'Academie Nationale de Medecine. 180(6) 1315-1323.

Engen T. 1974. Method and theory in the study of odor preferences. In Johnston J (ed.), Human Response to Environmental Odors. New York: Academic Press, 121-141.

Gainetdinov R, Wetzel W, Jones S, et al. 1999. Role of serotonin in the paradoxical calming effect of psychostimulants on hyperactivity. Science. 283(5400) 397-401.

Gainetdinov R, Caron M. 2001. Genetics of Childhood Disorders: XXIV, Part 8: Hyperdopaminergic mice as an animal model of ADHD. Journal of the American Academy of Child Psychiatry. 40(3) 380-382.

Gauthier R, Agoumi A, Gourai M. 1989. Activite d'extraits de *Myrtus communis* contre *Pediculus humanis capitis*. Plantes Medicinales et Phytotherapie. 23(2) 95-108.

Haislip G. 2002. Ritalin: the smart drug? www.vanderbilt.edu/AnS/psychology. Accessed September 2002.

Hodson D. 1995. The special needs of children and adolescents. In Penson J, Fisher R (eds.), Palliative Care for People with Cancer, 2nd ed. London: Edward Arnold, 198-229.

Howard Hughes Medical Institute News (Jan 15, 1999 newsletter). Nov. 4, 1999. Serotonin may hold key to hyperactivity disorder. www.hhmi.org/news/caron2.html.

Humphrey T. 1940. The development of the olfactory and the accessory olfactory formations in human embryos and fetuses. Journal of Comparative Neurology. 73:431-468.

Izri M, Briere C. 1995 First cases of resistance of Pediculus capitis Linne 1758 to malathion in France. La Presse Medicale. 24(31) 1444.

Kurfit Stephens B, Barkey M, Hall H. 1999. Technique to comfort children during stressful procedures. Advances in Mind-Body Medicine. 15(1) 49-60.

Lahlou M, Berrada R, Agoumi A, et al. 2000. The potential effectiveness of essential oils in the control of human head lice in Morocco. International Journal of Aromatherapy. 10(3/4) 108-123.

Laurent D, Vilaseca L, Chantraine J, et al. 1997. Insecticidal activity of essential oils on *Triatoma infestans*. Phytotherapy Research. 11(4) 285-290.

McFerran T. 1996. A Dictionary of Nursing, 2nd ed. Oxford, UK: Oxford University Press.

Mehta S, Stone D, Whitehead H. 1998. Use of essential oil to promote induction of anesthesia in children. Anaesthesia. 53(7) 720-721.

Mumcuoglu K. 1999. Prevention and treatment of head lice in children. Pediatric Drugs. 1(3) 211-218.

Oladimeji F, Orafidlya O, Ogunniyi T, et al. 2000. Pediculocidal and scabicidal properties of *Lippia multiflora* essential oil. Journal of Ethnopharmacology. 72(1-2) 304-311.

Parish P. 1991. Medical Treatments: The Benefits and Risks. Harmondsworth, UK: Penguin Books.

Pitman V. 2000. Aromatherapy and children with learning difficulties. Aromatherapy Today. 15:20-23.

Russell M. 1976. Human olfactory communication. Nature. 260:520-522.

Schleidt M, Genzel C. 1990. The significance of mother's perfume for infants in the first weeks of their life. Ethology and Sociobiology. 11(1) 145-150.

Schilcher H. 1997. Physiotherapy in Pediatrics. Stuttgart, Germany: Medpharm.

Sorenson K. 1999. Effects of aroma with poor attention span in music lessons. Unpublished dissrtation. Hunter, N.Y.: R J Buckle Associates.

Sptizer H. 2000. Special needs children and aromatherapy: rosemary oil. Unpublished dissertation. Hunter, N.Y.: R J Buckle Associates.

Tucker S. 1999. Attention deficit hyperactivity disorder. Journal of the Royal Society of Medicine. 92(5) 217-219.

Veal L. 1996.The potential effectiveness of essential oils as a treatment for headlice, *Pediculus humanus capitis*. Complementary Therapies in Nursing & Midwifery. 2(4) 97-102.

Worwood V. 2000. Aromatherapy for the Healthy Child. Navato, CA: New World Library.

24

PSYCHIATRIC CARE

The use of scents is not practiced in modern physic but might be carried out with advantage seeing that some smells are so depressing and others so inspiring and reviving.

Sir William Temple (1701)
Essay on Health and Long Life

Anyone who believes scent does not have a profound impact on the human psyche should read *Perfume: The Story of a Murderer* (Suskind 1987). The novel is set in 18th-century France, and Grenouille, the lead character, is born with a heightened sense of smell but without body odor himself. These two factors rule his life and impact those around him with devastating consequences. Pickover (1998) quotes Hippocrates, who wrote, "Men ought to know that from nothing else but the brain come joys, delights, laughter and sports, and sorrows, griefs, despondency and lamentations."

Wiener (1966) of the New York Medical College suggested our bodies have an internal and external communicating system that uses our nervous system without alerting us to its existence. Such a system is made up of chemicals and interacts with the other systems in the body by means of odor. He further suggests that if someone had the ability to communicate consciously in this system it could be distressing. Subsequent to this theory was the discovery that schizophrenics give out a persistent aroma discernible to dogs and rats. This aroma becomes more pronounced when they are in crisis (Smith & Sines 1960).

Certainly there is a link between depression and the inability to smell (anosmia) (Douek 1988). Aristotle noted that pleasurable aromas could contribute to the well being of humans, and both malodors and bad odors impact on our health. Stand next to a garbage dump downwind for just a few moments and you get a good sense of this! Malaria literally means "bad air" as it was believed that odor emanating from marshes caused the disease (King 1988).

The use of psychoactive products evolved along two related paths: for religious or recreational pursuits and to modify normal behavior (Alexander 2001). The effects of aromas on the brain were first tested by Moncrieff (1966) using an electroencephalograph to monitor changes in brainwave patterns. He found that basil, black pepper, cardamom, and rosemary induced mainly beta patterns and that jasmine, neroli, and rose induced mainly delta patterns (Moncrieff 1977). Beta brain patterns (13-40 cycles per second) are concerned with attention and alertness. Delta brain patterns (0-4 cycles per second) are concerned with euphoria and calmness (Mureriwa 2001). Dodd and Van Toller (1983) compared the action of chemical components found in essential oils to the action of psychotropic drugs such as antidepressants. Torii et al (1988) reported on the electrical changes of the brain and the similarities between emotion and the sense of smell. King (1988) postulated the relation between odor and olfaction was probably a two-way relationship.

A report in the *Journal of the American Medical Association* suggests a study of smell could shed light on some of the symptoms of schizophrenia. Dr. Daniel O'Leary from the University of Iowa Hospitals and Clinics exposed 18 people with schizophrenia and 15 healthy volunteers to a pleasant smell (vanilla) and an unpleasant smell (O'Neil 2001). An imaging device was used to track blood flow to different areas of the brain, and subjects were asked to rate each smell. The mental imaging showed big differences between the two groups in the mental processing of the unpleasant smell. The limbic system appeared to be highly active in healthy subjects but largely unused with people with schizophrenia. The latter depended more on frontal cortical areas usually reserved for functions such as decisionmaking. This misuse of brain circuits could play a role in paranoia.

Insanity or mental illness is an area of fear for many people, and yet almost everyone has experienced insanity at some time in their life: a crazy decision, a wrong choice, a mad moment, a dark time. I remember when my son went missing. He was only 2 years old and my daughter was a newborn. One moment he was there next to the cheese counter in the supermarket, and the next moment he was gone. During the following 2 hours I experienced a sense of insanity and all reality appeared put on hold.

During times like this, one's link with reality can seem blurred as sensory perception becomes skewed and basic physical needs are forgotten. This is when familiar smells and reassuring touch may help find a way out of the fog and back to reality. Patients with mental-health problems are a constant reminder just how fragile sanity is.

AROMATHERAPY AND MENTAL ILLNESS

"Components within essential oils that alter brain chemistry and relieve psychiatric symptoms have brought great hope and help to many people" (Alexander

2001). Sugano (1992) suggests natural fragrances can provide a cost-effective and efficient alternative to many common drug treatments, especially stimulants and sedatives. Tisserand (1988) suggests olfactory "ecstasy" was discovered by man at a very early age, and that aromatics can be perceived as drugs. Alexander (2001) suggests that "EOs [essential oils] for the brain that have antidepressant, mood-balancing, anxiolytic and hormone regulating properties are nourishment at the biochemical level."

Most synthetic psychotropic medications have limited efficacy and significant side effects, and preliminary findings suggest several treatments based on natural substances are as effective and safe as the synthetic pharmaceuticals in current use (Lake 2000). Lake's review article on the use of herbs for neurological problems is a must-read. However, the number of herbs he covers is limited by space. The Napralert database (which I have used extensively for this book) contains more than 1000 citations on herbs useful for psychiatry.

Many health professionals working in psychiatric units have been grateful for strong sedatives when patients have become psychotic and unmanageable. However, there are some people who are may just have a poor ability to cope with life. This could be due to genetics, environmental issues, or just one of those unexplainable things. However, with the demand for a cure, or at least medicine, seems to be a growing group of people who take antidepressant drugs but who are not clinically depressed. They are just life depressed. In the words of Patch Adams, MD (1997), "Prozac has replaced a hug." It is this shadowy area in which aromatherapy may help. While all the hi-tech advances in the world cannot rewire the brain, something as simple as an essential oil can enable the brain to reregulate itself (Alexander 2001).

Addiction

Today's society is an addictive one, and it often rewards socially acceptable addictions like workaholism, in addition to accepting shopaholics and nicotine addiction, condoning alcohol addiction, and prosecuting drug addiction. Yet the ethos behind addiction—instant gratification—is at the very core of today's society. People want things instantly. Large portions are required even if they cannot be eaten. Everything must be big. It is as though people feel too small in a world that undervalues them. Reassurance of worth is sought from external sources rather than from within. It is as though people have a hole in their wholeness and are hungry for anything that will stop the feeling of emptiness. Health professionals are often presented with evidence of a sick society in which individuals who do not fit in or are unable to cope are isolated, ridiculed, or forgotten.

A few detoxification programs have included herbal treatment protocols for the management of acute benzodiazepine or opiate withdrawal with positive effects (Rasmussen 1996). But there is scant if any published literature on the use of essential oils for alcohol or benzodiazepine withdrawal. However, some anecdotal success with weaning patients from antidepressants and night sedation using both nontouch modality (diffusers at night and face tissues during the day) and the "m" technique has been achieved. The process was very gradual and under physician control. This is not recommended unless physician support is given. Limited success with helping reduce the cravings of women withdrawing from alcohol has also been achieved using specific inhaled essential oils (Lundgren 1999). A protocol that has been used is shown in Table 24-1.

The idea that an olfactory stimuli might reduce craving for nicotine was investigated by Seyette and Parrott (1999). They found that both negative and positive aromas decreased cravings against a nonodoriferous control in nicotine addiction. The sense of smell is lessened in a heavy smoker; nevertheless, aromatherapy has achieved some modest success. DaCosta (1999) explored inhaling essential oil as a means to reduce the craving of nicotine withdrawal. The three essential oils tested were lavender (*Lavandula angustifolia*), *Helicrysum italicum,* and *Angelica archangelica.* Four male subjects who smoked at least 10 cigarettes a day and had tried to stop smoking in the past were recruited. The period immediately after breakfast, lunch, and supper were chosen as those were the hardest times to abstain from smoking. The normal period the test subjects could wait before smoking (baseline) was minimal, less than 2 minutes. Each essential oil was then tested separately for 5 consecutive days, divided by a dry-out period of 2 days, and the subjects timed how long they could last without a cigarette. Angelica root appeared to be the most helpful, with subjects able to wait an average of 53 minutes before having a cigarette. This was considerable improvement on 2 minutes, although inhaling angelica did not prevent them from smoking after 53 minutes.

Table 24-1 ❧ *Protocol for Coming Off Benzodiazepine or Night Sedation with Aromatherapy*

Week 1	Choose aroma(s) from a selection of six. Choose touch or nontouch application. Apply oil in office. Give written instructions on when and how to use aromatherapy.
Week 2	Reduce medication by $\frac{1}{4}$.
Week 3	Reduce medication by further $\frac{1}{4}$.
Week 4	Remain on $\frac{1}{2}$ medication .
Week 5	Reduce medication to $\frac{1}{4}$.
Week 6	Remain on $\frac{1}{4}$ medication.
Week 7	$\frac{1}{4}$ medication alternate days.
Week 8	Remain on $\frac{1}{4}$ alternate days.
Week 9	$\frac{1}{4}$ medication twice a week.
Week 10	$\frac{1}{4}$ medication once a week.

Rose and Behm (1994) used black pepper essential oil as an aid in a smoking-cessation program. They hypothesized that clients needed to experience the respiratory-tract sensations that accompany cigarette smoking to quit successfully, and they believed black pepper essential oil could simulate those sensations. They found "the vapor of black pepper essential oil, when inhaled, partially reproduces the respiratory tract sensations experienced when smoking, thereby reducing the craving for cigarettes."

Newsham (2001) explored the effect of aromatherapy as an adjunct to auricular acupuncture for drug detoxification at Yonkers General Hospital in New Jersey. This was a study compared to a historical control. Two hundred eighty-two auricular treatments (some subjects received more than one treatment) were given with ambient odor of lavender in the room. The comparison group received 230 auricular treatments without lavender. Two standard aromatherapy diffusers were used to diffuse a room of approximately 400 square feet. Twenty drops of lavender were placed in the nebulizer. All patients routinely completed a short questionnaire before and after treatment. Analysis was done to see if there was any difference between the aromatherapy group and the comparison group. Fifty percent of patients did not complete the full 21 days of treatment. The actual treatment range was 1-14 with an average of 4. Data were collected monthly and aggregate data were used. Questions ranged from "How are you feeling right now?" to "How would you rate any cravings you have right now?" The choice of answers was on a 0-5 scale.

There was no difference between the aromatherapy group and the comparison group in the number of patients who said they felt "very good" physically or emotionally after the treatment. There was a difference in those who felt "good" physically and emotionally. Physically, there was 6% change in the comparison group and a 24.8% change in the aromatherapy group. Emotionally, there was 4.6% change in the comparison group and a 24.9% change in the aromatherapy group. However, there seemed to be no difference in the cravings. More than half the patients said they were unable to smell the essential oils diffused into the room.

Caldwell (2001) explored the effects of ylang ylang (*Cananga odorata*) in a small, controlled study of 10 women suffering from cravings following withdrawal of substance abuse. All women were taking orthodox medication. The participants were randomly split into two groups: an experimental group and a control group. The experimental group was given essential oil of *Cananga odorata* (ylang ylang) to inhale, and the control group received plain almond oil. Both groups were told that they were using ylang ylang oil. The participants were self-selecting and limited to women dealing with chemical addiction. All 10 participants had either stopped using and were still experiencing cravings, or were trying to stop using and were experiencing cravings.

Each participant put two drops of the oil on a cotton square and put the square in her pillowcase every night for seven nights. The participants were also asked to put two to three drops of oil on a cotton hanky, carry the hanky with them for seven days, and smell it if they experienced a craving. The participants were asked to record the number of cravings, their intensity, and any other comments.

The results showed the number of cravings for the essential oil group went down more than for the control group. However, ylang ylang did not prevent cravings completely. Four out of 5 women in the experimental group believed "smelling the oil relieved the stress and anxiety of that moment." None of the participants using the almond oil expressed this feeling. Caldwell (2001) notes that ylang ylang's positive effect might be enhanced by using a diffuser at night.

Olfactory loss is common in alcoholics (Shear et al 1992), cocaine users (Schwartz et al 1998), and heroin addicts (Perl et al 1997). Loss of smell is not thought to affect the transfer of the volatile molecules unless there is damage to the olfactory nerve. Loss of smell in addicts is thought to be due to damage to the cortical and subcortical brain regions (Shear et al 1992), but it is possible there is nerve damage due to snorting or sniffing cocaine, heroin, and glue.

Bipolar Disorder

Approximately 2.5 million Americans are thought to be affected with bipolar disease. Originally named manic-depression, the disease was discovered by German psychiatrist Emil Kraepelin after carefully observing many patients in the 19th century (DRADA 2001). Kraepelin found many patients had spontaneous remission of symptoms that could last for months or years before relapsing and that patients who had suffered episodic periods of illness in their 20s were more likely to have them in their 40s. Psychiatrists today conclude that bipolar disease is a relapsing illness that may recur more frequently as the patient ages. Bipolar disease is thought to run in families, and recent research is concentrating on chromosome 18 in an attempt to locate the gene responsible (Stine et al 1995). However, bipolar disease is quintessentially a disease of the Western world. The World Health Organization conducted studies over a 25-year period and found that in underdeveloped countries, psychotic disorders such as bipolar were fewer, less severe, and resolved more rapidly (Sartorius 1990).

People, and in particular scientists, have a fascination with putting things in categories. Since manic-depressive disorder became bipolar disorder, bipolar has been divided into seven subcategories:
1. Pure mania;
2. Mixed mania (symptoms of mania and depression appearing simultaneously);
3. Rapid cycling (four or more episodes a year);
4. Secondary mania (appearance of mania after another illness);
5. Bipolar disorder with coexisting substance abuse;
6. Bipolar disorder type II (mildly manic states); and
7. Cyclothymia (chronic mood cycles with depression or mania too mild to be classified).

Because mental illness is thought of as a brain disorder, magnetic resonance imaging is frequently used as a diagnostic tool (DRADA 2001), although there are inconsistent findings. The areas of the brain examined are the amygdala, the entorhinal cortex, and the asymmetries—areas of the brain bigger on one side than the other. In the brain of a normal, right-handed person, the brain area for language is much bigger on the left side (Pearlson 1996). Pearlson also found schizophrenic patients had greatly shrunken entorhinal cortexes and striking reversal of some key brain asymmetries. In bipolar patients these structures looked normal, although the amygdala was slightly shrunken. In mood-disorder patients, the amygdala was significantly shrunken on the left side.

Many neurological problems are a function of altered brain pattern and a change in neurochemicals. Conventional drug treatment is with Lithium, divalproex (Depakote), and carbamazepine (Tegretol). However, all three have significant side effects. Bowden (1996) suggests Lithium has a narrow band of effective blood levels before reaching toxicity. However, Purol-Hershey (2002), a psychiatric nurse and teaching professor, states that the band 0.5-1.2 mg is pretty broad for lithium. The information on Tegretol suggesting precautions for "emotional or mental problems" could be perceived as rather strange as the drug is prescribed for bipolar disorder (Winter Griffith 1997). However, Tegretol is also an antiseizure medication with mood-stabilizing features. Table 24-2 has been created from information in *Treatment Options in Bipolar Disorder* by Bowden (1996)

Table 24-2 ✖ *Commonly Used Medications for Bipolar Disorder:*
Benefits and Common Side Effects

Lithium	Pure mania, history of depression, family history of bipolar disorder, previous favorable response to Lithium, few previous episodes, full relief between symptoms	May correct chemical imbalance in brains' transmission of nerve impulses that influence mood and behavior	Weight gain, dry mouth, confusion, poor concentration, shakiness, tremor, increased urination
Depakote	Mixed mania, nonfavorable response to Lithium, mood swings, adverse effects less severe, attention deficit hyperactivity disorder, substance abuse	Increases gamma aminobutyric acid, which inhibits nerve transmission to parts of the brain	Loss of appetite, nausea, diarrhea, tremor, unusual weight gain (or loss), menstrual changes
Carbamazepine	No family history of bipolar disorder, bipolar disorder is a secondary condition, lack of response to other medication	Analgesic, anticonvulsant	Dizziness, blurred vision, headaches, back-and-forth eye movement (nystogmus)

and the *Complete Guide to Prescription and Nonprescription Drugs* (Winter Griffith 1997).

The human body is controlled by extremely delicate mechanisms that rely on hormonal and chemical communication. Each person has a slightly different body chemistry that requires different things to achieve homeostasis. Like herbs, essential oils are therapeutically multifaceted. Therefore, the components within an essential oil may produce a different reaction in one person than in another, depending on the availability of receptor sites (Mills 1991). For example, an essential oil may work to reduce blood pressure (acting as a hypotensor) if that is what is required for homeostasis, or it may not if the blood pressure is normal for that person. When a plant has the ability to change function it is called adaptogenic. Many essential oils also have a balancing effect on the emotions.

Various antipsychotic agents have antagonistic interactions toward a whole selection of receptor sites including serotoninic, adrenergic, and histaminic. Therefore their ongoing effects on the autonomic nervous system are complex and unpredictable (Alexander 2001). This is the case with each of the hundreds of components in essential oils that interact with many receptor sites. While antidepressants work by making the neurotransmitter serotonin linger in the gaps between brain cells, essential oils are thought to work as serotonin agonists, which can push the serotonin system into overdrive. This makes the brain more sensitive, rather like turning up the volume on a radio so very weak stations can be heard.

There is no suggestion that bipolar patients should give up medication in favor of aromatherapy. There is little if anything published on bipolar disorder and aromatherapy. However, essential oils may enhance orthodox medication so dosages may be kept sufficiently low and reduce side effects. However, a few psychiatric nurses who were my students have had some success with stabilizing patients using aromatherapy. As these were case studies it is difficult to say whether the patients' stability would have happened anyway. Other case studies by psychiatric nurses have indicated aromatherapy may help reduce the need for orthodox medication and still retain stability (Table 24-3).

A set ritual or protocol is useful when working with bipolar patients. This is worked out in detail with the patient: the when, where, and how of treatment. Essential oils need to be experienced for the first time in a stable, calm, balanced situation with supervision. When this pattern is well established, the essential oils can be experienced in the patient's own setting. This is akin to preparing a "psychological comfort blanket." This setting of a psychological trigger is similar to Bett's research (1994) with epilepsy. He found massage with ylang ylang set a precedent so strong that ultimately patients had only to think about the aroma of ylang ylang to prevent a seizure occurring.

Tisserand and Balacs (1995) suggest several essential oils should be avoided with patients who are prone to seizure. It might be a good idea to avoid them in bipolar patients as well. These oils are listed in Table 24-4.

The flowers of *Matricaria recutita* (German chamomile) contain apigenin, which can completely inhibit central nervous system benzodiazepine binding

Table 24-3 ✥ *Balancing Essential Oils that May Be Useful in Cases of Bipolar Disorder*

Common Name	Botanical Name
Geranium	*Pelargonium graveolens*
Lavender	*Lavandula angustifolia*
Sandalwood	*Santalum album*
Angelica root	*Angelica archangelica*
Rose	*Rosa damascena*
Patchouli	*Pogostemon cablin*
Ylang ylang	*Cananga odorata* var. *genuina*
Valerian	*Valeriana fauriei*
Vetiver	*Vetiveria zizanoides*
Spikenard	*Nardostachys jatamansi*
Melissa	*Melissa officinalis*
Bergamot	*Citrus bergamia*
Clary sage	*Salvia sclarea*

Table 24-4 ✥ *Essential Oils to Avoid in Bipolar Disorder*

Essential Oil	Suspect Component	Amount (approximate)
White camphor	Camphor	30%-50%
Hyssop	Pinocamphone	70%
Nutmeg	Myristicin, Elemicin	3%-14% 0.1%-4.6%
Pennyroyal	Pulegone	55%-95%
Tansy	Thujone	66%-81%

without sedation. There are no known negative side effects (Viola et al 1995). Apigenin occurs in the CO_2 extract but not in the steam-distilled extract of German chamomile. Valerian root (*Valeriana officinalis*) has been shown to reduce mild to moderate anxiety and may be useful in substance withdrawal (Brown 1994). Essential oil of valerian root is available and could be combined with *Melissa officinalis* essential oil for an enhanced sedative effect. Valerian is safe to inhale in pregnancy, and long-term use does not produce dependency. The therapeutic effects are thought to be through gamma-aminobutyric acid-antago-nistic action (Lake 2000).

Lake (2000), a board-certified psychiatrist, reports the oral intake of St John's wort (*Hypericum perforatum*) is effective in certain mild depression, seasonal affective disorder, and other neurological malfunctions. Essential oil of *Hypericum perforatum* offers a more concentrated version that so far has not shown any of the photosensitivity problems connected with the oral intake of St. John's wort. This could be an interesting area for further research.

REFERENCES

Adams P. 1997 (June). Lecture at AHNA conference, Burlington, VT.

Alexander M. 2001. How Aromatherapy Works. Odessa, FL: Whole Spectrum Books.

Bett T. 1994. Sniffing the breeze. Aromatherapy Quarterly. 40:19-22.

Bowden C. 1996. Treatment of bipolar disorder. The American Psychiatric Press Textbook of Psychopharmacology. Chapter 29:603-614.

Brown D. Fall 1994. Valerian root: non addictive alternative for insomnia and anxiety. Review of Natural Medicine. 221-224.

Caldwell N. 2001. Effects of ylang ylang on cravings of women with substance abuse. Hunter, N.Y.: R J Buckle Associates.

DaCosta R. 1999. Nicotine withdrawal and aromatherapy. Unpublished dissertation. Hunter, N.Y.: R J Buckle Associates.

DePaulo JR. Sept. 4, 2001. Recent findings in the genetics of bipolar disorder, Smooth Sailing, 1996. Depression and Related Affective Disorders Association. www.med.jhu.edu/drada.

Dodd G, Van Toller S. 1983. The biology and psychology of perfumery. Perfumer & Flavorist. 8:1-14.

Douek E. 1988. Abnormalities of smell. In Van Toller S, Dodd G (eds.), Perfumery: The Psychology and Biology of Fragrance. London: Chapman and Hall, xvii-3.

King J. 1988. Anxiety reduction using fragrances. In Van Toller S, Dodd G (eds.), Perfumery: The Psychology and Biology of Fragrance. London: Chapman and Hall, 147-167.

Lake J. 2000. Psychotropic medications from natural products: a review of promising research and recommendations. Alternative Therapies in Health & Medicine. 6(3) 36-60.

Lundgren W. 1999. Clary sage for withdrawal cravings in alcoholic women. Unpublished dissertation. Hunter, N.Y.: R J Buckle Associates.

Mills S. 1991.Out of the Earth. London: Viking Arkana.

Moncrieff R. 1966. Odor Preferences. New York: Wiley.

Moncrieff R. 1977. Emotional response to odors. Soap, Perfumery and Cosmetics. 50:24-25.

Mureriwa J. Jan. 2001. EEG Biofeedback. Retrieved March 17, 2003, from www.biofeedback.co.2a/biofeedback-eeg.htm

Newsham G. 2001. Lavender for auricular acupuncture support in detoxification. Unpublished dissertation. Hunter, N.Y.: R J Buckle Associates.

O'Neil J. Jan. 2001. Smells used to explore schizophrenia. www.schizophrenia.com.

Pearlson G. Sept. 4, 2001. Excepts from schizophrenia vs. mood disorder: a puzzle solved. Smooth Sailing, 1-2, 1996. Depression and Related Affective Disorders Association. www.med.jhi.edu/drada/pearlson.html.

Perl E, Shufman E, Vas A, et al. 1997. Taste and odor reactivity in heroin addicts. Israel Journal of Psychiatry and Related Sciences. 34(4) 290-299.

Pickover C. 1998. Strange Brains and Genius. New York: Plenum.

Purol-Hershey S. Sept., 2002. Personal communication.

Rasmussen P. 1996. A role for phytotherapy in the treatment of benzodiazepine and opiate drug withdrawal. European Journal of Herbal Medicine. 3(1) 12-21.

Rose J, Behm F. 1994. Inhalation of vapor from black pepper extract reduces smoking withdrawal symptoms. Drug and Alcohol Dependence. 34(3) 225-229.

Sartorius N. 1990. Cultural factors in the etiology of schizophrenia. In Stefanis C (ed.), Psychiatry: A World Perspective, Vol. 4. New York: Elsevier Science, 33-40.

Schwartz R, Estroff T, Fairbanks D, et al. 1998. Nasal symptoms associated with cocaine abuse during adolescence. Archives of Otolaryngology-Head & Neck Surgery. 115(1) 63-64.

Seyette M, Parrott D. 1999. Effects of olfactory stimuli on urge reduction in smokers. Experimental and Clinical Psychopharmacology. 7(2) 151-159.

Shear P, Butters N, Jernigan T, et al. 1992. Olfactory loss in alcoholics: correlations with cortical and subcortical MRI indices. Alcohol. 9(3) 247-255.

Smith K, Sines J. 1960. Demonstration of a peculiar odor in the sweat of schizophrenic patients. Archives of General Psychiatry. 2:184.

Stine O, Xu J, Koskela R, et al. 1995. Evidence for linkage of bipolar disorder to chromosome 18 with a parent-or-origin effect. American Journal of Human Genetics. 57(6) 1384-1394.

Sugano H. 1992. Psychophysical studies of fragrances. In Dodd G, Van Toller S (eds.), Fragrance: The Psychology and Biology of Perfume. London: Elsevier Science, 227.

Suskind P. 1987. Perfume: The Story of a Murderer. London: Penguin Books.

Temple W. 1701. Essay on Health and Long Life, 1701. In Cornaro L, 1915, The Art of Living Long, Kessinger Publishing, www.kessinger-publishing.com.

Tisserand R, Balacs T. 1995. Essential Oil Safety. London: Churchill Livingstone.

Tisserand R. 1988. Essential oils as psychotherapeutic agents. In Van Toller S, Dodd G (eds.), Perfumery: The Psychology and Biology of Fragrance. London: Chapman and Hall, 167-180.

Torii S, Fukada H, Kanemoto H, et al. 1988. Contingent negative variation (CNV) and the psychological effects of odor. In Van Toller S, Dodd G (eds.), Perfumery: The Psychology and Biology of Fragrance. London: Chapman and Hall, 107-118.

Viola H, Wasowski C, Levi de Stein M. 1995. Apigenin. A component of *Matricaria recutita* flowers that is a central benzodiazepine receptor ligand with anxiolytic effects. Planta Medica. 61:213-216.

Wiener H. 1966. External chemical messengers I. New York State Journal of Medicine. 66:3153.

Winter Griffith H. 1997. Complete Guide to Prescription and Nonprescription Drugs. New York: Berkeley Publishing.

25

RESPIRATORY CARE

Scent has a persuasive power stronger than words, appearances, feelings and wishes.
There is no defense against the persuasive power of scent; it looks into us, like the air
we breathe enters our lungs, it fulfils us perfectly and there is no antidote to it.

Patrick Suskind (1987)
Perfume: The Story of a Murderer

Of all the clinical specialties, perhaps respiratory care is the most obvious candidate for aromatherapy, for when we inhale to smell, we inhale to breathe as well. Why bother with digesting essential oils and "first pass" (metabolizing them via the liver) when inhaled oils may work as well? Falk et al (1990) noted the high solubility of α-pinene in human volunteers. Alpha pinene (22%) is found in rosemary essential oil, camphor chemotype. Falk et al found 60% of α-pinene was absorbed through inhalation, but only 8% was exhaled. The rest was excreted in the urine, suggesting inhaled essential oils could also treat cystitis. Some essential oils taken by mouth are exhaled. Some essential oils given rectally are excreted through respiration. Pulmonary excretion of 1,8-cineole, menthol, and thymol was demonstrated following rectal application in rats, although the percentage exhaled was extremely small (Grisk & Fischer 1969).

Air pollution has become more prevalent, especially in cities and especially during the summer. Inner-city air seems to contain less and less oxygen and more and more environmental toxins. In fact, for more than 30 years, environmental influences have been linked to chest problems (Cruz-Coke 1960). Environmental pollutants range from dust mites to cockroaches and latex to second-hand smoke.

Cases of asthma and chronic bronchitis doubled between 1982 and 1994, and more than 14 million Americans are now diagnosed with asthma (Weil 1997). Three in 10 people consult their doctor at least once a year about a respiratory disease, with the most common complaint being upper-respiratory tract infection (Newman-Taylor 1995). In the United Kingdom, 10% of all prescriptions are for drugs to treat respiratory problems (Lung and Asthma Information Agency 1995), and one in seven children has asthma. In 1995, 5600 deaths in the United States were attributed to asthma (Weil 1997).

While some kinds of asthma could be exacerbated by essential oils, other kinds can be greatly ameliorated. *Eucalyptus radiata* and *Styrax benzoin* (benzoin) have been used by health professionals to treat respiratory infections for many years (Stevenson 1995). Essential oils to avoid in asthma are those high in alpha- and beta-pinene or delta-3-carene, as they were found to cause airway and breathing discomfort during a study by Filipsson (1996) on turpentine. Bowles (2000) also notes that inhalation of pinene-rich essential oils could cause this problem in asthma. Alpha-pinene is found in Scotch pine (*Pinus sylvestris*), at a level of 42%.

There are two chronic respiratory problems becoming endemic in the United States, namely recurrent bronchitis and tuberculosis. These will be discussed in this chapter.

CHRONIC BRONCHITIS, ASTHMA, AND SINUSITIS

Recurrent chest infections, or chronic bronchitis, are on the increase. Each outbreak of the disease begins with a dry cough followed by a mucolytic stage with a productive cough. The underlying problem may be infection, viral or bacterial, or it may be chronic inflammation similar to an allergy.

Essential oils have been used in cough medicines for many years (Boyd 1954). The expectorant action of a cough medicine is mainly due to the local action of aromatics on the lining of the respiratory tract during exhalation, after the medicine has been swallowed (Boyd & Sheppard 1970). Boyd (1967) found systemic expectorants (including glyceryl guaiacolate) have little pharmacological expectorant action. but some inhaled expectorants, such as cedar leaf, have an effect, even at a subliminal level (Boyd and Sheppard 1968). Kendig et al (1967) found water vapor (steam) to be the most effective means of liquefying secretions, and Boyd and Sheppard conclude in their 1970 paper that "inhaled expectorants may be superior to systemic expectorants." This certainly opens the way for aromatherapy as a useful modality for upper-respiratory infections.

Boyd and Sheppard (1970) found the expectorant effect of inhaled nutmeg oil was due to its high camphene content (60%). However, the amount of camphene may be adversely affected if the nutmeg has been irradiated (Wilmers & Grobel 1990). According to The Merck Index (Budavari 1996) camphene is found (to a lesser degree) in the oils listed in Table 25-1.

An ointment containing camphene and menthol was found to be effective in reducing bronchospasms by 50% when it was insufflated through the respiratory system of laboratory animals, but it was only slightly effective when applied cutaneously (Schaefer & Schaefer 1981). Applying essential oils to an airway with

Table 25-1 ✖ *Essential Oils Containing Camphene*

Common Name	Botanical Name
Neroli	*Citrus aurantium*
Citronella	*Cymbopogon nardus*
Bergamot	*Citrus bergamia*
Cypress	*Cupressus sempervirens*
Ginger	*Zingiber officinale*

nasal ointment has also been shown effective in stimulating airway secretary glands and reducing mucus. However, caution is needed in pediatrics. In another study, children were mistakenly given nosedrops that contained menthol or euca-lyptol (constituents of essential oils) instead of saline drops. Adverse effects ranged from irritated mucous membrane to tachycardia (Melis et al 1989).

In a randomized trial involving 182 institutionalized patients, "essence" drops containing mint, clove, thyme, cinnamon, and lavender appeared to reduce the frequency of bouts of chronic bronchitis (Ferley et al 1989). The essential oils most effective in this study were clove, lavender, lemon, marjoram, mint, niaouli, pine, rosemary, and thyme. This could be because some essential oils are known to destroy airborne *Staphylococcus aureus* and *Streptococcus pyogenes* within hours, and these would be an effective way of preventing ailments such as bronchitis (Bardeau 1976). Other essential oils frequently used to treat chest infections are *Boswellia carterii* (frankincense) and *Pinus sylvestris* (Scotch pine) (Sheppard-Hanger 1995; Abdel Wahab et al 1987).

Charron (1997) carried out an exploratory study on 40 patients with bronchial and sinus congestion. Patients inhaled two drops of Spike lavender floating in a bowl of hot water. All patients cleared their mucus immediately with results lasting from 20 minutes to 2 hours. Some patients who had been on yearly repeat antibiotics no longer needed them.

A 3% solution of frankincense, Spike lavender, and lavender was used in an exploratory study of eight patients with asthma (Spear 1999). Application was topical to chest and back. The age of patients ranged from 14-70 years. Four pa-tients registered a moderate improvement in their peak-flow meters, and three registered a substantial improvement. Six patients noticed a change in their emo-tional attitude, and the same six felt their sleep was much improved. No patient became worse, but one patient noticed no improvement.

Lockhart (2000) used inhaled essential oil of Frankincense on eight subjects (20-52 years of age), five females and three males, throughout a period of 6 weeks. Following patch testing and assessment for allergies, the subjects were given a bottle of pure essential oil from the same supplier (same batch number) and asked to inhale it when they felt an asthma attack coming. A Likert scale was used at the end of 6 weeks. All subjects felt their anxiety levels decreased when they inhaled the frankincense, and all subjects decreased the use of their normal inhalers.

Pitcher (2001) studied the effects of inhaled *Mentha piperita* on 20 adult patients (age range 18-90) with chronic sinusitis. Five of the 20 patients had a history of medically diagnosed asthma. Four patients used inhalers daily. No patients were using prescription decongestants daily, although 12 patients used over-the-counter decongestants as necessary. Smokers were excluded from the study. Undiluted peppermint was inhaled for 10 minutes at a time. A small cushion with two drops of peppermint on it was kept by the bedside to assist with night breathing. Measurements of nasal congestion, sense of smell, headache, and postnasal drip were taken. There was a significant improvement in all symptoms. Inhaler users reported a decline in the number of times they used their inhaler. No side effects were reported. When the symptoms returned at a later date, each participant reached for the peppermint bottle again!

Machon (2001) carried out a controlled study to evaluate the effects of a mixture of *Eucalyptus globulus*, *Ravansara aromatica*, *Pinus sylvestris*, and *Mentha piperita* essential oils on sinus infections. Eight subjects (five females and three males) used three drops of the mixture in a steam inhalation for 10 minutes, three times a day for 5 days. Three subjects (both male and female) acted as controls and received only steam inhalation. Baseline measurements of pain, sense of wellness, color of mucus, and amount of mucus were taken using a visual analog scale of 0-10. The essential-oil group was consistently more improved with three of the five members completely clear of congestion and two nearly free. By the fifth day, their mucus was clear. In the control group, the congestion remained the same, and the mucus remained green in color.

Rudansky (2000) used *Eucalyptus globulus* to good effect to aid expectoration in a patient with cystic fibrosis. The subject, a 36-year-old woman, had pneumonia and plural edema and was being treated with intravenous antibiotics (6 weeks on and 3 weeks off). She was also dependent on an oxygen-concentrator machine. Her mucus was thick, dense, and flecked with blood. Working with the woman's physician, Rudansky was able to increase the subject's lung elasticity causing a measurable reduction in pulse and oxygen demand. She used regular inhalations and body treatments to help the woman relax. The cycle of intravenous antibiotics was reduced, and at the time of writing the patient had received no antibiotic cover for 2 months and was doing well. The patient felt the heaviness in her lungs had decreased substantially, and she was sleeping better.

Mattys et al (2000) carried out a randomized, double-blind study to explore the effects of myrtol. Myrtol is a standardized distillate marketed under the brand name Gelomyrtol and contains α-pinene, 1,8-cineole, and d-limonene. Six hundred seventy-six patients were divided into four groups. The experimental group received myrtol orally (4×300 mg daily) for two weeks. The two control groups received either cefuroxine (2×250 mg daily) or ambroxol (a mucolytic agent), and the fourth group received placebo capsules (four daily) for 14 days. Patients receiving myrtol experienced a significant reduction in coughing. Lung auscultation improved significantly. Myrtol was found to be comparable to the other medications (and superior to the placebo) and carries no risk of causing bacterial resistance.

Essential oils with expectorant properties may be unable to fight the infection causing the problem, in which case the cause of the symptom is not being addressed. An aromatogram would be needed to culture the bacteria and find out to which essential oil it was sensitive. There are laboratories that can do this (see Appendix 3 and Chapter 7 on infections for more details). In many instances the infection may linger in sinuses (Belaiche 1979a). Some infections that are resistant to antibiotics can be alleviated with the use of the correct essential oil (Carson et al 1995). Table 25-2 lists essential oils I have used to treat respiratory problems.

Belaiche (1979a) found thyme (*Thymus vulgaris*) and cinnamon (*Cinnamomum zeylanicum*) were effective against *Streptococcus aureus* and lavender (*Lavandula angustifolia*), marjoram (*Origanum majorana*), and winter savory (*Satureja montana*) effective against *Staphylococcus aureus* (Belaiche 1979). *Eucalyptus globulus* (2%) will kill 70% of ambient *Staphylococcus aureus* within hours. Duke writes that in Cuba essential oil of *Eucalyptus globulus* is used to treat all lung ailments (Duke 1985).

Table 25-2 ❧ *General Respiratory Aid Essential Oils Used by the Author*

Common Name	Botanical Name
Ravansara	*Ravansara aromatica*
Gully gum	*Eucalyptus smithi*
Spike lavender	*Lavandula latifolia*
Sweet marjoram	*Origanum majorana*
Lavender	*Lavandula angustifolia*
Niaouli	*Melaleuca viridiflora*
Scots pine	*Pinus sylvestris*
Rosemary	*Rosmarinus officinalis* CT cineole
Thyme	*Thymus vulgaris* CT linalol, CT thujanol
Tea tree	*Melaleuca alternifolia*
Blue gum	*Eucalyptus globulus*
Cypress	*Cupressus sempervirens*

TUBERCULOSIS

Tuberculosis (TB) is a mycobacterial disease spread by droplet infection. Primary TB is usually pulmonary. A peripheral lesion forms, and its draining nodes are infected, so there is early spread of the bacillus throughout the body. Immunity rapidly develops, and the infection becomes quiescent at all sites. The most common nonpulmonary primary infection is in the ileocecal junction and associated lymph nodes (Hope et al 1993). Postprimary TB occurs when any form of immunocompromise allows reactivation. The lung lesions progressively fibrose, particularly in the upper lobe. Sometimes the bacilli can spread to other parts of the body, setting up nodular lesions called tubercules (McFerran 1996). Sometimes bone, brain, or genitourinary tract is involved.

TB was relatively well controlled in the Western world by Bacille Calmette-Guerin (BCG) vaccine, and infection numbers fell to 10 in 100,000 people by the end of the 1980s (MacSween & Whaley 1992). In 1996, the Centers for Disease Control recommended the BCG vaccine be used only for health workers in whom there was a high likelihood of multiple drug-resistant (MDR) TB. The incidence of the disease has increased quite dramatically throughout the last 15 years. This trend is directly related to immigrant communities who were not vaccinated in their country of origin, and also to the spread of AIDS.

One-third of the world's population is infected with TB. Annual global deaths are approximately one million, and TB is the leading cause of death due to an infectious agent in the world (NIAID 2002). Recently, MDR TB has appeared. Outbreaks have occurred in hospitals, correctional institutions, residential-care facilities, and homeless shelters. In the United States, several hundred people have contracted TB at their workplace. TB has also caused concern in the aviation industry as commercial pilots and crew have been infected by passengers (WHO 1998).

Although there still are antibiotics to treat MDR TB, these medications are expensive, have side effects, and are slowly becoming ineffective. MDR TB is more difficult to treat than TB, as it requires expensive second-line drugs to be taken for at least 18 months compared with cheaper, first-line drugs taken for only 6 months in cases of TB. The cost of first-line treatment is approximately $120 for a 6-month course. The cost of second-line treatment is approximately $10,000 (Davies 2001).

Before the advent of para-aminosalicylic acid and isoniazid, patients with TB were sent to sanatoriums, often located high in the mountains and frequently close to pine forests, because it was thought that breathing mountain air laced with pine essence would aid recuperation. Sanatorium windows contained no panes of glass so air could flow freely through the facility.

There is no suggestion that aromatherapy should replace conventional treatment for TB. However, essential oils can enhance a patient's quality of life. Some essential oils have been found effective against TB in vitro, and some have been found to increase the potency of orthodox medicines. Valnet (1993) was one of the first physicians to document the use of aromatherapy in the treatment of TB. He found essential oil of hyssop neutralized the TB bacillus at a concentration of 0.2 parts per 1000 (Valnet 1993). This finding was similar to that of Hilal et al (1980). Hilal found the volatile oil of hyssop was effective using different chromatograph and spectral methods. Hyssop is eliminated through the lungs. Due to the high percentage of the ketones iso-pinocamphone and pinocamphone (70%), this essential oil should not be taken orally and many feel it is contraindicated in epilepsy. It also has a pronounced hypertensive action (Valnet 1990). However, in view of Valnet's findings of hyssop's effectiveness as such a very low percentage (0.002%), hyssop could play a part in TB control if used in low dosages.

Despite the fact that most of the research on TB and essential oils has been conducted on animals, there are a few papers that suggest essential oils might be effective against TB in humans. A Russian paper reports the results of a 2-month study on the effects of inhaled essential oils. The symptoms of 81.8%-95.6% patients disappeared, and their body masses increased (Petrosian et al 1999). Unfortunately, only the abstract is in English and the name of the essential oil is not given. TB is rampant in Russian correctional facilities where a virulent, resistant strain is endemic.

Lall and Meyer (1999) found that 14 out of 20 South African-plant extracts (extracted with acetone) were effective against isoniazid- and riampin-resistant strains of TB at 0.5mg/ml using the agar-plate method. A further rapid-radiometric method often used for drug susceptibility testing confirmed inhibitory activity. Eight of the plants showed activity against the resistant strain at 1.0mg/ml. One of the plants belonged to the *Helichrysum* genus (spp. *melanacme*), although the other plants were unfamiliar. Gupta and Viswanathan (1955) reported on the tuberculostatic activity of *Occimum sanctum* (Holy basil) and *Piper betle* (betle juice). In a further paper they found that *Occimum canum* inhibited the growth of TB in dilution of 1: 50,000 (Gupta & Viswanathan 1955a).

Kufferath and Mundualgo (1954) found *Eucalyptus globulus* enhanced the activity of streptomycin, isoniazid, and sulfetrone in the treatment of TB (Kufferath & Mundualgo 1954). Schaubelt (1994) wrote that *Cupressus sempervirens* (cypress) and *Pinus sylvestris* (Scotch pine) are also effective against TB.

The essential oils should be diffused continuously over several months and are best used in rotation. Steam inhalation and/or use of a nebulizer will help get the essential oils deep into the lungs. Sputum tests will indicate if the infection is being contained. Hopefully further in-vitro research will show that other essential oils also have TB activity, and these can be added to a general mix of four essential oils. It might be helpful to add *Lavandula angustifolia* and/or tea tree to enhance immune function. In addition, the patient should take steam inhalations with four drops of the essential oil mix three times daily to get the essential oils deep inside the lungs. Adding an antiinflammatory essential oil such as *Helichrysum italicum,* German chamomile, or frankincense will help soothe the mucous membrane. Table 25-3 lists inhaled essential oils of use in the treatment of pulmonary TB.

Table 25-3 ✖ *Inhaled Essential Oils to Use with Pulmonary TB*

Botanical Name	Common Name	Reference
Blue gum	*Eucalyptus globulus*	Kufferath & Mundualgo 1954
Niaouli	*Melaleuca viridiflora*	Kufferath & Mundualgo 1954
Marjoram	*Origanum majorana*	Valnet 1993
Holy basil	*Occimum sanctum**	Gupta & Viswanathan 1955
Hyssop	*Hyssopus officinalis*	Hilal et al 1978
Juniper	*Juniperus communis*	Duke 1985

* low doses; suggested amount below 0.5%

REFERENCES

Abdel Wahab S, Adoutabl E, El-Zalabani S, et al. 1987. The essential oil of *Olibanum*. Planta Medica. 53(4) 382-384.

Bardeau F. 1976. Use of essential aromatic oils to purify and deodorise the air. Le Chirurgien-Dentiste de France. 46:53.

Belaiche P. 1979. Traite de Phytotherapie et d'Aromatherapie, Vol.1. Paris: Maloine SA.

Belaiche P. 1979a. Traite de Phytotherapie et d'Aromatherapie, Vol. 2. Paris: Maloine SA.

Boyd E. 1954. Expectorants and respiratory tract fluid. Pharmacological Review. 6:521-542.

Boyd E, Sheppard E, Boyd C. 1967. The pharmacological basis of the expectorant action of glyceryl guaiacolate. Applied Therapies. 9(1) 55-59.

Boyd E, Sheppard E. 1968. The effect of steam inhalation of volatile oils on the output and composition of respiratory tract fluid. Journal of Pharmacology and Experimental Therapeutics. 163(4) 250-256.

Boyd E, Sheppard P. 1970. Nutmeg and camphene as inhaled expectorants. Archives of Otolaryngology (Chicago). 92:372-378.

Budavari S (ed). 1996. The Merck Index, 12th ed. Whitehouse Station, NJ: Merck & Co Ltd.

Carson C, Cookson B, Farrelly H, et al. 1995. Susceptibility of MRSA to the essential oil of *Melaleuca alternifolia*. Journal of Antimicrobial Chemotherapy. 35(3) 421-424.

Centers for Disease Control and Prevention. 1996. Notifiable diseases and deaths in selected cities. Morbidity and Mortality Weekly Report. 45(4) 1-27. www.cdc.gov/mmwr.

Charron J. 1997. Use of *Lavandula latifolia* as an expectorant. Journal of Alternative & Complementary Medicine. 3(3) 211.

Cruz-Coke R. 1960. Environmental influences and arterial blood pressure. Lancet. 2(345) 295-296.

Davies P. 2001. Drug resistant tuberculosis. Journal of the Royal Society of Medicine. 94(6) 261-263.

Duke J. 1985. Handbook of Medicinal Herbs. Boca Raton, FL: CRC Press.

Falk A, Gullstrand E, Lof A. 1990. Liquid/air partition coefficients of four terpenes. British Journal of Industrial Medicine. 47(1) 62-64.

Ferley J, Poutignat N, Mirou D. 1989. Prophylactic aromatherapy for supervening infections in patients with chronic bronchitis. Statistical evaluation conducted in clinics against a placebo. Phytotherapy Research. 3(3) 97-100.

Filipsson A. 1996. Short term inhalation exposure to turpentine, toxicokinetics and acute effects in men. Occupational and Environmental Medicine. 53(2) 100-105.

Grisk A, Fischer W. 1969. On the pulmonar excretion of cineole, menthol and thymol in rats following rectal application. Zeitschrift fur Arztliche Fortbilding. 63(4) 233-236.

Gupta K, Viswanathan R. 1956. A short note on antitubercular substance from *Occimum sanctum*. Antibiotics and Chemotherapy. 6(3) 247.

Gupta K, Viswanathan R. 1956a. Antitubercular substances from plants. Antibiotics and Chemotherapy. 6(2) 194-195.

Kendig E, Chernick V (eds.). 1983. ed 4. Disorders of the Respiratory Tract in Children. Philadelphia: WB Saunders.

Kufferath F, Mundualgo G. 1954. The activity of some preparations containing essential oils in TB. Fitoterapia. 25:483-485.

Lall N, Meyer J. 1999. In vitro inhibition of drug-resistant and drug-sensitive strains of *Mycobacterium tuberculosis* by ethnobotanically selected South African plants. Journal of Ethnopharmacology. 66(3) 347-354.

Lockhart N. 2000. Inhalation of frankincense and its affect on asthmatics. Unpublished dissertation. Hunter, N.Y.: R J Buckle Associates.

Lung and Asthma Information Agency. 1995. Factsheet. London: Department of Public Health Sciences, St. George's Hospital Medical School.

Machon L. 2001. Use of four essential oils in the treatment of sinus infections. Unpublished dissertation. Hunter, N.Y.: R J Buckle Associates.

MacSween R, Whaley K (eds.). 1992. Muir's Textbook of Pathology. London: Edward Arnold.

Mattys H, de Mey C, Carls C, et al. 2000. Efficacy and tolerability of myrtol. Standardized in acute bronchitis. A multi-centre, randomised, double-blind, placebo-controlled parallel group clinical trial vs. cefuroxime and ambroxol. Arzneimittel-Forschung Drug Research. 50(8) 700-711.

McFerran T. 1996. A Dictionary of Nursing, 2nd ed. Oxford, UK: Oxford University Press.

Melis K, Bochner A, Hanssens G. 1989. Accidental nasal eucalyptol and menthol instillation. European Journal of Pediatrics. 148(8) 786-788.

National Institute of Allergy and Infectious Diseases. 2002. One third of the world's population has tuberculosis bacterium. Oct., 2002. NIAID News, 2002. www.hivandhepatitis.com.

Newman-Taylor A. 1995. Environmental determinants of asthma. Lancet. 345(8945) 296-299.

Petrosian F, L'vov S, Levchenko G. 1999. The methods of traditional medicine in the treatment of tuberculosis. Voenno-Meditsinskii Zhurnal. 320(10) 45-48.

Pitcher L. 2001. The Effects of *Mentha piperita* on chronic upper respiratory symptoms in adults. Unpublished dissertation. Hunter, N.Y.: R J Buckle Associates.

Rudansky R. 2000. *Eucalyptus globulus* and cystic fibrosis: a case-study. Unpublished dissertation. Hunter, N.Y.: R J Buckle Associates.

Schafer D, Schafer W. 1981. Pharmacological studies with an ointment containing menthol, camphene and essential oils for broncholytic and secretolytic effects. Arzneimittelforschung. 31(1) 82-86.

Schnaubelt K. 1993. Aromatherapy Course, Part 3. San Rafael, CA: Pacific Institute of Aromatherapy.

Sheppard-Hanger S. 1995. The Aromatherapy Practitioner Reference Manual, Vol. 11. Tampa, FL: Atlantic Institute of Aromatherapy.

Spear B. 1999. Essential oils and their effectiveness in the relief of symptoms of asthma. Unpublished dissertation. Hunter, N.Y.: R J Buckle Associates.

Stevenson C. 1995. Aromatherapy. In Rankin-Box D (ed.), The Nurses' Handbook of Complementary Therapies. London: Churchill Livingstone, 52-58.

Suskind P. 1987. Perfume: The Story of a Murderer. London: Penguin Books.

Valnet J. 1990. The Practice of Aromatherapy. Saffron Walden, UK: CW Daniels.

Varga E, Hajdu Z, Veres K, et al. 1998. Investigation of variation of the production of biological and chemical compounds of Hyssopus officinalis L. Acta Pharm Hung May. 68(3) 183-188.

Wagner T. 1999. Looking to make death a little less painful. Times Union. B1.

Weil A. 1997. Breathing Easier with Asthma. Dr. Andrew Weil's Self-Healing. 6-7.

Wilmers K, Grobel W. 1990. Chemometric evaluation of GC/MS profiles for the detection of g-irradiated spices as exemplified by nutmeg. Deutsch Lebensen. Rundsch. 86: 344-348.

World Health Organization. 2002. Tuberculosis and air travel: guidelines for prevention and control. Oct. 2002 WHO Press Release, 1998. www.who.int/inf.pr.

APPENDIX I

EDUCATION

Most aromatherapy courses on the market are intended for the lay public and have a recreational or esthetic approach, such as making perfumes, soaps, or cosmetics, or the aromatic content of the science of food additives. While these courses are interesting, they are not relevant to clinical practice.

CERTIFICATION

Certification can mean one of two things: the student has attended a course (although he or she may not have learned anything) or the student has attended a course and passed the required examination.

The term *certified* usually implies a student has passed the required examination and is therefore, in the mind of the certifying body (which may or may not be the school that set the examination), competent in that subject. A certified person is often described as licensed to use that training, as in the case of a certified lawyer or accountant. However, in the field of aromatherapy, there is no licensing body either in the United States or United Kingdom that can license an aromatherapist. The closest thing in the United Kingdom is a self-regulating body called the Aromatherapy Organization Council (AOC), which sets a core curriculum for aromatherapy training for lay people.

CHOICES OF TRAINING

There are three types of aromatherapy training: professional, academic, or within a specific discipline such as nursing. Any of these courses could have an esthetic or clinical focus.

Professional

National Association for Holistic Aromatherapy

The National Association for Holistic Aromatherapy (NAHA) is the largest aromatherapy organization in the United States with just under 1000 members. As NAHA is a membership organization, it cannot offer certification itself. However, NAHA does set guidelines for a national curriculum and approves schools and educational programs that heed these guidelines. A list of NAHA-approved schools and programs can be obtained from their Web site: www.naha.org.

NAHA-approved training is divided into Level One and Level Two. Level One requires 30 hours of training and covers a minimum of 10 essential oils. Level Two requires 200 hours of training, but the number of essential oils to be covered is not stated. Level Two also includes "the clinical science of at least five common ailments for each system covered." The systems listed are reproductive, circulatory, nervous, endocrine, lymphatic, musculoskeletal, and digestive. Students must write a 5-10 page research paper, complete 10 case histories, and pass an examination offered by the school. NAHA does not inspect schools or approve the exam.

Aromatherapy Registration Council

The Aromatherapy Registration Council (ARC), a not-for-profit organization in the United States, was set up in 2000 to mirror the work of the AOC in England. The ARC has a curriculum and national examination. The exam is held four times a year in different locations and is run by the Professional Testing Corporation (PTC). The curriculum content is available from the PTC. Areas covered on the examination are given as follows: 20% basic concepts of aromatherapy, 30% scientific principles, 35% administration, and 15% professional issues. There are no prerequisites to the examination but "a completion in a program of aromatherapy or one year of full-time experience in aromatherapy is recommended." For more information, see www.aromatherapycouncil.org.

PTC runs certification tests for different modalities. For information on the PTC, please see their Web site: www.ptcny.com. At the time of writing, the aromatherapy exam does not involve any specific clinical questions because the exam is open to lay people. I am an active and supportive member of ARC and helped set the ARC exam. It is hoped that in time the exam will include an optional clinical section specifically for licensed health professionals.

Academic Training

University Programs

Academic credit is given for some aromatherapy courses. One credit is equivalent to 11-15 hours of class at a particular level. The level at which the learning occurs will also be taken into account (undergraduate versus postgraduate) and will be reflected in the cost of each credit. Some aromatherapy courses are in the process of being accredited by a university. My own course, Aromatherapy for Health Professionals, is at the time of writing this book (2002) in the accreditation process. Several universities are beginning to look at creating aromatherapy programs. Academic training may concentrate on theory or research review and have wonderful library access, but unless the instructors are clinicians with years of experience and the students are given sufficient hands-on training, academic courses may not produce clinically qualified practitioners. The curriculum may or may not conform to ARC guidelines. Look for a well-rounded course with lots of hands-on practice directed by experienced instructors. An added bonus in a university program is the chance to carry out research.

The University of Minnesota began a four-credit program in 2001 aimed at "providing foundational knowledge in therapeutic uses of essential oils for health science students and professionals, including skills in critiquing the aromatherapy research literature. The focus is on 33 specific essential oils as well as general principles and chemistry." This is a Web-based course sequence with 2 days each semester on campus. Grading criteria include participation (including online discussion assignments), a written exam, case studies, and a report on an essential oil. Other universities that offer aromatherapy courses include Washington State University, University of Indiana, The College of New Rochelle, Bastyr University, and New York University.

State-Approved Schools

While it is encouraging that some schools teaching aromatherapy are state approved, this does not mean the content of the aromatherapy courses taught at that school is approved. State approval usually only means the school complies with regulations regarding safety and insurance.

Distance Learning

Discussing theory and analyzing research is excellent, but practical experience is irreplaceable—particularly with a therapy that involves smell and touch. However, distance-learning courses are an excellent way to begin and acquire base knowledge, and I have created a short home-study and on-line course myself (www.rjbuckle.com).

Education within a Specific Discipline (relevant to licensed health-care professionals)

Courses are being set up in complementary medicine for many health-care disciplines. These may or may not include separate training in aromatherapy.

Clinical Competency

To show clinical competency, licensed health professionals need to have completed an educational program recognized by their licensing body. Ideally, this should involve a course endorsed by a professional body or that at least gives continuing-education units (CEUs) for their professional modality.

Testing should be via a method that demonstrates clinical competency. Because clinical competency is involved, the instructor should be someone recognized as a health professional. To ensure fair and objective marking, the examination or testing should involve someone other than the person who taught the course.

Endorsed Programs

This means that the course *content* has been approved by an external accrediting body such as the American Holistic Nurses Association. One example is my course, which is a 250-hour CEU program endorsed by the American Holistic Nurses Association. For details on training in United States, Australia, Korea, and Japan, please visit www.rjbuckle.com, which is listed in *resources*. Training in South America, Korea, and Australia is expected to start in 2004.

Approved Providers

An approved provider means that the educational organization creating the aromatherapy course is approved by an accrediting body to give CEUs to physicians, nurses, massage therapists, pharmacists, and so on. One CEU is equivalent to 50 minutes of classroom teaching. There are several training programs that provide nursing or massage therapy CEUs, such as The Institute of Integrative Aromatherapy, The Institute of Dynamic Aromatherapy, The Atlantic Institute of Aromatherapy, The Pacific Institute of Aromatherapy, The Australasian College of Aromatherapy, and my company, R J Buckle Associates, among others. Some hospital groups approve specific educational providers to teach aromatherapy to their employees. R J Buckle Associates is an approved educational provider to the Planetree Hospital Group.

Specific Training for Nurses

The Royal College of Nursing (RCN) in England issued guidelines for nurses wanting to use aromatherapy. These state that a nurse "should know his/her subject and have received training." There is no requirement that the aromatherapy course should be nursing based. However, if aromatherapy is to be used to enhance nursing, the instruction probably should be clinically based and nurse centered. Nurses in the United Kingdom who use aromatherapy are part of nursing care are covered under RCN insurance for up to £3 million. To date, no claims have been made.

The guidelines for using aromatherapy issued by the RCN include the following:
- Supervised practice;
- Anatomy, physiology, pathology, and pharmacology;
- Practical and theoretical examination;
- Holistic approach;
- Supervised clinical practice;
- Counseling/communication and self-development skills training;
- Appropriately qualified teachers;
- Support for the trainee therapist;
- A sensible tutor/pupil ratio (Royal College of Nursing 1993).

REFERENCES

Royal College of Nursing. 1993. Choosing a complementary therapy. London: Complementary Therapies in Nursing Special Interest Group, Royal College of Nursing Department of Nursing Policy and Practice.

Appendix II

Policies, Protocols, and the Occupational Safety and Health Administration (OSHA)

Sample Hospital Patient Care Policy and Procedure

Most health facilities require a health-safety policy in place. If aromatherapy is to be integrated into a facility, this is the first thing that needs to happen. I am appreciative of the hospitals that worked with me to create policies and protocols and to those facilities that shared their documentation with me.

Purpose

To outline the management of patients receiving aromatherapy treatment.

Definitions

Clinical aromatherapy is the controlled use of essential oils to enhance health and well being, which targets a specific symptoms.

Topical application refers to the "m" technique, light massage, a compress with water, carrier oil, or gel (spore or bacteria free) on cotton squares directly over the affected area, or a bath (hand, foot, sitz, or full).

Inhalation can be indirect or direct, differentiated as follows:
- **Direct inhalation** means applying two to five drops of essential oil to a tissue and breathing normally for up to 15 minutes, applying two to five drops of essential oil on a cotton ball placed under the pillowcase, or floating two to five drops of essential oil on a bowl of hot water and inhaling the aroma for up to 10 minutes. Patients should remove spectacles and keep eyes closed.
- **Indirect inhalation** means using an electric nebulizer or battery-operated diffuser to diffuse fine particles of essential oil within a room.

Carrier oil is a cold-pressed vegetable oil. The most frequently used is sweet almond oil. Carrier oils have specific properties. Culinary oils are not suitable.

Patch testing is the process used to determine if a person is sensitive to potential allergens in an essential oil. Two drops of the mixture at double the concentration to be used are put on an adhesive bandage, attached to the patient's upper arm, and left for 12 hours.

Goals
- To promote a sense of well being
- To promote relaxation and reduction of stress
- To reduce or alleviate physical, emotional or spiritual symptoms

Indications
- Stress and related disorders
- Anxiety, depression, sadness, grief, anger
- Insomnia
- Digestive disorders, cramping, nausea
- Pain
- Muscular problems
- Inflammation
- Infection
- Mental agitation
- Premenstrual syndrome, menopausal problems
- Slow wound healing

Contraindications
- Use with caution in pregnancy, epilepsy, hypertension, estrogen-dependent tumors, and patients with sensitivities and allergies.

Policy
- Essential oils should be used in a clinical setting by a licensed health professional trained in the use of essential oils. Such training should be clinical and should be acceptable to the establishment where the health professional works. Such training should cover safety precautions, potential side effects, and contraindications related to the use of each essential oil (see Table A2-2 and Box A2-2).
- Treatments should be offered after consultation with the patient and after receiving their verbal consent or that of their family when applicable.
- Aromatherapy does not require medical order except for perceived prescriptive use. Nurses need to check with their Board of Nursing (see Chapter 6).
- Treatment will vary according to each patient and his or her needs (see Table A2-1).
- Essential oils used should be limited to the attached list (see Table A2-3).
- Full botanical name will be used.
- Aromatherapy will be offered in addition to conventional treatments.
- The dignity of the patient will be respected at all times.

- A Material Safety Data Sheet (MSDS) and Gas Chromatography/Mass Spectrometry (GCMS) is available for each essential oil used (see Box A2-1).

A health professional using aromatherapy as part of patient care will do the following.

- Check with patients about skin reactions to nuts, essential oils, perfumes, cosmetics, or pharmaceuticals
- Know how to take a proper case history to decide if the patient has a condition or is taking a drug that might contraindicate specific essential oils
- Know how to perform a patch test and use this in appropriate cases
- Ensure all undiluted essential oils (singles or mixtures) used by patients are adequately labeled and in bottles with integrated drop dispensers
- Advise patients not to ingest essential oils (except as part of specified treatment given by a person with prescription authority)
- Have sufficient knowledge of clinical practice to know when to avoid a particular procedure and when to obtain further medical assistance

Table A2-1 ❧ *Sample Protocol and Policy*

Procedure	Important Points
Assess patient Obtain history, including allergies, medications, skin integrity, and liked and disliked aromas.	Be aware of patient sensitivities: see safety guidelines.
Explain the procedure.	Provide information about aromatherapy.
Select essential oil and identify method to be used. Advise about photosensitivity when relevant.	Effects of inhalation are rapid; topical action is slower. Choice to be determined by patient's condition and targeted outcome.
Ensure patient privacy. Provide treatment.	Be sensitive about others in the room.
If a skin reaction occurs, remove essential oil with milk or carrier oil, wash the area with unscented soap and water, pat dry, and leave in open air for 10 minutes.	Complete an occurrence report and notify the appropriate staff. Provide follow-up care.
Evaluate the patient's response and document the treatment in the medical records.	Documentation includes assessment, choice of essential oil, method, and outcome.

Practitioner Safety

Practitioner safety measures should include the following.
• Maintain good ventilation in treatment areas.
• Air the treatment room between treatment sessions.
• Wash hands before and after patient contact.
• Take a minimum of 5 minutes to breathe fresh air after each treatment.
   An algorithm can be a simple and clear way to explain a thought process. Please see Fig. A2-1 for an algorithm exploring the use of lavender as a sleep aid.

Box A2-1 Sample Material Safety Data Sheet (MSDS)

Individual Safety Data Form for Specific Essential Oil

HP's name	*Patient's name*	*Date*	*Time*
Florence Nightingale	John Doe	11/11/96	3 p.m.

Essential oil: Melaleuca alternifolia CT terpineol
Number of drops: 1-5

Known Hazards	*Risks*
Xn: Cat 3 carcinogen	R10/22/38
$LD_{50} = 190$ mg/kg	Flammable, harmful if swallowed, not irritating to the skin

Safety	*Other safety data*
S24/25	No sensitization (Ford 1988)
Avoid contact with skin and eyes	No phototoxicity (Ford 1988)
	Nonirritant

Emergency Treatment:
• If swallowed, drink full-cream milk and seek medical attention.
• If in eye, irrigate with vegetable oils or full-cream milk followed by water, then seek medical attention

Application Method	*Contraindications*	*Precautions*
Topical, inhalation	—	Avoid using teatree with high 1,8-cineole content

Other Information:
• Can be used neat on insect bites/stings/zits
• Can be used in gargle and mouthwash (1–2 drops)
• Can be used vaginally diluted in carrier oil
• Insoluble in water: dissolve in alcohol/milk
• Ensure correct chemotype = low cineole. Cineole can be a mucous-membrane irritant.

Sources: AMA Council on Medical Service Report "Growing Nursing Shortage in the USA." South Florida Business Journal; California Nurses Association

Table A2-2 ❧ Accident Procedures

Problem	Answer
Essential oil in the eye	Irrigate the eye with milk or carrier oil, then with water. Keep the bottle to show which essential oil was being used. Seek medical assistance.
Used an undiluted essential oil (high phenols), skin burned	Dilute with carrier oil, then wash with non-perfumed soap and water and dry. Seek medical assistance.
5 ml (or more) essential oil taken orally	Give milk to drink, and keep the bottle. Seek medical assistance. Essential oils, when taken in amounts greater than 5 ml by mouth, should be treated as poisons.
Bottle of essential oil dropped and broken, essential oil and glass on floor	Use a paper towel to soak up essential oil and collect the glass. Put mixture in more paper. Dispose in double-sealed plastic bag.

Box A2-2 General Safety

Storage
All essential oils should be stored as follows:
- Locked up
- Out of reach of children
- In a cool place
- In tightly closed containers
- Away from food, drink, or animal feed
- Away from heat
- Away from naked flames

Labeling
All bottles containing essential oils should be clearly marked with indelible labels that include the following:
- Full botanical name
- Relevant safety information
- Quantity of oil
- Company name and address

Packaging
- All essential oils should be packaged in colored glass bottles that include an integral dropper of standard (20 drops per ml) size.

Continued

BOX A2-2 GENERAL SAFETY—CONT'D

Procedures
- Essential oils should only be used in a clinical setting by a member of the staff or an outside contractor qualified in aromatherapy and who has permission to use them.
- Whenever possible, essential oils should be used in enclosed areas to prevent the aromas from spreading.
- All essential oils used should be documented in the patient-care plan.
- The positive and negative effects of essential oils should be evaluated and noted.
- Use topically in 1%-5% dilution, except in specific situations as recommended by safety guides.
- When used in a bath with the elderly or small children, essential oils should be dissolved in a small amount of milk to avoid possible corneal damage during splashing.
- Essential oils that carry a high risk should be avoided. They are listed in safety guides (Tisseland, Balass 1995). A suggested list of safe oils can be found in Table A2-3.

Clothing
- No special clothing is required, but some essential oils such as German chamomile may leave stains.

Disposal
Essential oils are highly flammable and carry intense aromas. They should be disposed of in a sealed, polythene bag.

Table A2-3 ❧ *Some Essential Oils Suitable for a Clinical Setting*

Common Name	Botanical Name
Yarrow	*Achillea millefolium*
Angelica	*Angelica archangelica* (root)
Frankincense	*Boswellia carteri*
Ylang ylang	*Cananga odorata*
Roman chamomile	*Chamomelum nobile*
Bergamot	*Citrus bergamia*
Mandarin	*Citrus reticulata*
Neroli	*Citrus aurantium* var. *amara flos*
Petitgrain	*Citrus aurantium* var. *amara fol*
Myrrh	*Commiphora myrrha*

Table A2-3 ✤ *Some Essential Oils Suitable for a Clinical Setting—cont'd*

Common Name	Botanical Name
Cypress	*Cupressus sempervirens*
Palma rosa	*Cymbopogon martini* var. *motia*
Lemongrass	*Cymbopogon citratus*
Blue gum	*Eucalyptus globulus*
Gully gum	*Eucalytpus smithi*
Lemon gum	*Eucalyptus citriodora*
Fennel	*Foeniculum vulgare*
Everlasting flower	*Helichrysum italicum*
Juniper	*Juniperus communis*
True lavender	*Lavandula officinalis*
Spike lavender	*Lavandula latifolia*
Lavandin	*Lavandula hybrida* CT grosso
German chamomile	*Matricaria recutita*
Tea tree	*Melaleuca alternifolia*
Melissa	*Melissa officinalis*
Peppermint	*Mentha piperita*
Basil	*Ocimum basilicum* (European)
Marjoram	*Origanum majorana*
Geranium	*Pelargonium graveolens*
Black pepper	*Piper nigrum*
Rose	*Rosa damascena*
Rosemary	*Rosmarinus officinalis*
Clary sage	*Salvia sclarea*
Sandalwood	*Santalum album*
Clove bud (only use diluted)	*Syzygium aromaticum*
Thyme	*Thymus vulgaris* CT linalol
Vetiver	*Vetiveria zizanioides*
Ginger	*Zingiber officinale*

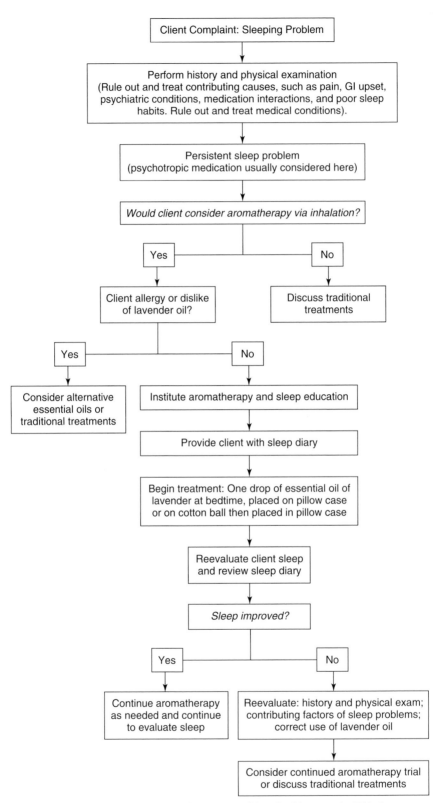

Figure A2-1 Nonpharmacological Approach to Sleep Problems in the Elderly. Kindly supplied by Sherry Simpson (2001).

Regulations and Health

In the United States, the two most important groups of regulations aromatherapy needs to address are those proposed by OSHA and JCAHO. For more information about JCAHO, see their Web site at www.jcaho.com. The most interesting part of the site for aromatherapy is the section on mind/body, spirituality, cultural, and psychosocial needs of patients.

OSHA is concerned with the transport, storage, and spillage of quantities of hazardous material. Essential oils fall into this category, particularly in large amounts. OSHA requirements go well beyond those normally required for aromatherapy use. However they are presented here in the unlikely event they might be needed. The people most likely to use this chapter are those preparing the MSDS for various essential oils.

The latest information on OSHA can be obtained from their Web site: www.osha.gov. A wide variety of materials including standards, interpretations, directives, and more can be purchased on a CD-ROM from the US Government Printing Office. To order, apply to

Superintendent of Documents
PO Box 371954
Pittsburgh, PA 15250-7954.

OSHA is divided into 10 regions. OSHA requires that MSDS be completed for any substance used on or with the public. Their toll-free compliance-assistance number is 1-800-321-OSHA(6742) or (202) 693-2100. Alternatively, a contact number may be sent to OSHA and their Compliance Assistance Phone Service will contact you, if you are located in the United States. To send a daytime contact number, forward your message to DCPContact@osha.gov.

A formal letter describing the particulars of the workplace and question also can be mailed to:

Department of Labor—OSHA
200 Constitution Avenue NW
Room N3603
Washington, DC 20210

OSHA

OSHA was created for the following purposes.

- Encourage employers and employees to reduce workplace hazards and to implement new, or improve existing, safety and health programs
- Provide for research in occupational safety and health to develop innovative ways of dealing with occupational safety and health problems
- Establish "separate but dependent responsibilities and rights" for employers and employees for the achievement of better safety and health conditions
- Maintain a reporting and recordkeeping system to monitor job-related injuries and illnesses

- Establish training programs to increase the number and competence of occupational safety and health personnel
- Develop mandatory job safety and health standards and enforce them effectively
- Provide for the development, analysis, evaluation, and approval of state occupational safety and health programs.

OSHA does not cover self-employed people, farms that only employ family members, or working conditions regulated by other federal agencies. OSHA is concerned with safety and risk management of potentially hazardous substances in the workplace. Hazardous substances include essential oils, as they are flammable and in some cases are skin irritants or sensitizing. The object of OSHA for aromatherapy is to assess and evaluate risk, thereby reducing the possibility of harm for those using essential oils either directly or indirectly. Risk and safety phrases to be used are listed in the material safety data sheet (MSDS). By standardizing them in this way, anyone looking at an OSHA document on an essential oil will immediately recognize its potential risk. MSDSs are required by OSHA. Some parts of the documentation may help health professionals and health administrators make an informed judgment about the safety of each essential oil in a clinical setting. However, much of the data involves estimates, not actual exact evidence.

OSHA assessment requires the person wanting to use essential oils to be aware of any potential hazards and risks involved. Essential oils that are defined as dangerous (corrosive, irritant, or toxic), need to be clearly identified as to the maximum exposure limit and the occupational exposure limit of any given essential oil. This will indicate the toxicity of an essential oil. Toxicity is measured by the oral dose needed to kill 50% of experimental animals (LD_{50}). It is expressed in milligrams per kilogram of body weight (mg/kg). The dose needed to kill 50% of experimental animals when taken other than orally is the lethal concentration(LC_{50}). Degrees of toxicity are listed in Table A2-4.

Essential oils are classified simply with a T (for toxic) hazard sign. An essential oil classified in this way will also have specific risk phrases on its labeling such

Table A2-4   *Degrees of Toxicity*

Extremely toxic	Up to 1 mg
Highly toxic	1-50 mg
Moderately toxic	50-500 mg
Slightly toxic	0.5-5 g
Virtually nontoxic	5-15 g
Relatively harmless	Up to 15 g

as "toxic if inhaled, toxic if swallowed, toxic if in contact with the skin," or "harmful if inhaled, harmful if swallowed, harmful if in contact with the skin," and specific safety phrases. Lists of essential oil classifications/guidelines are available that grade essential oils by giving them hazard symbols and acceptable risk (R) and safety (S) phrases. Some essential oils, such as cedarwood, clary sage, and geranium, have no hazard symbol or R and S number. Some, like grapefruit and lemongrass, have no hazard symbol and no safety phrase but carry a risk phrase such as R10, which means flammable, or R38, which means irritating to the skin. An MSDS identifies potential hazards of transporting and storing essential oils and is intended to warn people of any risk factors. It will include the features listed in Box A2-3. A list of organizations that give registration numbers is in Table A2-5.

Essential oil product identification includes the plant material, physical constants, registrations (usually in the form of numbers), and safety and toxicity considerations such as the flash point (the temperature at which an essential oil will ignite). This information should be available from the essential-oil dealer. Sample MSDS is shown in Box A2-4.

Flavor and Extracts Manufacturers Association

The Flavor and Extracts Manufacturers Association (FEMA), the oldest and largest national association of the flavor industry, produces many data sheets on essential oils (as well as flavor data sheets). They can be obtained in sets. The

---

Box A2-3 INFORMATION FOUND ON MATERIAL SAFETY DATA SHEETS (MSDSs)

1. Identification of the substance/preparation and company
2. Composition/information on ingredients
3. Hazards identification
4. First-aid measures
5. Fire-fighting measures
6. Accidental-releases measures
7. Handling and storage
8. Exposure controls/personal protection
9. Physical and chemical properties
10. Stability and reactivity
11. Toxicologic information
12. Ecologic information
13. Disposal considerations
14. Transport information
15. Regulatory information
16. Other information

Product Identification

Name	Tea tree
Botanical name	*Melaleuca alternifolia*
Chemotype	Terpineol
FEMA number	
CAS number	68647-73-4
Extraction	Steam distillation of the leaves

Specifications

Odor	Fresh, eucalyptus type, herbaceous, antiseptic
Origin	Australia
Appearance	Clear to faintly yellow

Analytical Data

(1) Physical constants	Specific gravity: 0.895–0.905 g
	Optical rotation: @ 20°C + 6.5 − +9.5
	Refractive index: @ 20°C 1.476 to 1.481
	Solubility: 1 vol of oil in 0.75 vol of 85% ethanol
(2) Chemical composition	See GLC

Toxicity

Low cineole content > 6% (as used for medicinal and dental purposes) reported to be nonirritant. LD_{50} = 400 mg (Ford 1988)

Flash Point

57–61°C

Table A2-5 ✿ *Organizations that Give Registration Numbers*

CAS	Chemical Abstracts Service
EINECS	European Inventory of Existing Chemical Substances
FEMA	Flavor and Extracts Manufacturers Association
IFRA	International Fragrance Association
RIFM	Research Institute for Fragrance Materials
CTFA	Cosmetic Toiletry and Fragrance Association
INCI	International Nomenclature of Cosmetic Ingredients
EFFA	European Flavor and Fragrance Association
IOFI	International Organization of the Flavor Industry
FDA	Food and Drug Administration
AIS	Association Internationale de la Savonnerie et de la Detergence
USES	Uniform System for the Evaluation of Substances

Table A2-6 ❦ *Other Important Organizations within the Fragrance Industry*

IFEAT	International Federation of Essential Oils & Aroma Trades
COLIPA	The European Cosmetic, Toiletry and Perfumery Association
NAFFS	National Association of Flavors and Food-Ingredient Systems
FF	Fragrance Foundation

Table A2-7 ❦ *Example:* **Citrus reticulata blanco** *Regulatory Numbers*

REFM	250
FEMA	2657 (GRAS)
FDA	182.20
CAS	8008-31-9

Research Institute for Fragrance Materials (RIFM) was established in 1966 and is a not-for-profit. The expert panel is independent of any manufacturing interests. RIFM collects and researches raw perfumery materials. The information is submitted to the International Fragrance Association (IFRA) (established in 1973). The IFRA produces guidelines for individual fragrance ingredients and is involved in risk management. IFRA publishes a "banned list" of 50 substances, and a further 58 have limitations for use. Some essential oils have many more regulatory numbers. Other important fragrance organizations are in Table A2-6. Opdyke's monographs on fragrance raw materials (1978) are also a good source of information.

Risk phrases give an indication as to how flammable an essential oil may be, if it is harmful when swallowed, if there is a risk of eye damage, if it may cause birth defects, etc. Safety phrases provide an indication of how to store the oil and dispose of it and what it will mix with. Both phrases are expressed as numbers. Mandarin has risk phrase number R10 (flammable) and safety phrase number S3 (keep in a cool place). R65 relates to the potential of a substance to cause lung damage after swallowing and is concerned with substances that contain more than 10% of aliphatic, alicyclic, or aromatic hydrocarbons. This is a relatively new risk hazard that only came into being in May 1988. An example of the different numbers given to one essential oil is in Table A2-7.

Some essential oils are not on the list of any of the fragrance organizations mentioned. Ravensara is one such example. When an essential oil is not listed, it should be possible to evaluate its risk and safety issues based on the chemical components within the essential oil. Therefore the simplest thing is to look them up in a phytochemical database or a reference book such as *Essential Oil Safety*. (Tisserand & Balacs 1995). While this section has gone into tremendous detail, the important thing to remember is essential oils are safe when used correctly.

REFERENCES

Burfield T. 2001. Toxicity myths. www.aroma-science.com. Sept. 2002.

Ford R. 1988. Tea tree oil. Food and Chemical Toxicology. 26: 407.

Opdyke D. 1978. Monographs on fragrance raw materials. Food and Cosmetics Toxicology. 16: 783-784.

Simpson S. 2001. Personal communication.

Tisserand R, Balacs T. 1995. Essential Oil Safety. London: Churchill Livingstone.

APPENDIX III

THE WHITE HOUSE COMMISSION ON COMPLEMENTARY ALTERNATIVE MEDICINE POLICY

The White House Commission on Complementary Alternative Medicine Policy (WHCCAMP) was created on March 8, 2000, by executive order. The 2-year commission will ultimately report to the president with legislative and administrative recommendations to ensure US public policy will maximize the benefits of complementary and alternative medicine (CAM) (Gordon 2002). The commission includes 20 members who represent a diverse range of experts in biomedical, medical, and CAM fields. The chair, James Gordon, MD, is helped by the following commissioners.

Bernier, George, MD	Kerr, Charlotte, RSM, RN, MAC
Bresler, David, PhD	Larson, Linnea, LCSW
Chappell, Thomas	Low Dog, Tieraona, MD
Chow, Effie, PhD	Ornish, Dean, MD
DeVries III, George	Paz, Conchita, MD
Fair, William, MD	Pizzorno, Joseph, MD
Fins, Joseph, MD	Rolin, Buford
Guttierrez Veronica, DC	Scott, Julia
Jonas, Wayne, MD	Tian, Xiaoming, MD
	Warren, Donald, DDS

The National Center for Complementary Alternative Medicine (NCCAM), which is part of the National Institutes of Health (NIH), divides CAM is divided into five categories. These categories are alternative medical systems, mind-body interventions, energy therapies, manipulative and body-based methods, and biologically based treatments (see Table A3-1).

Testimony indicated that coverage of CAM had been included by some employer-sponsored health plans as a direct response to employee requests. The commission held meetings in Washington DC, Seattle, San Francisco, New York, and Minneapolis, and spoke positively about encouraging rigorous research ($220 million was allocated for 2002).

Table A3-1 ❧ *Categories of Complementary Alternative Medicine*

Alternative Medical Systems: Acupressure, biologically based therapies, oriental massage, diet and nutrition (not herbs)

Mind-Body Interventions: Art, biofeedback, focused breathing, holistic nursing, humor, meditation, music, visual imagery, yoga

Manipulative and Body-Based Systems: Aromatherapy, cranial-sacral, deep-muscle massage, effleurage, Esalen, feldencras, friction, Heller work, infant massage, Lomilorri, lymphatic drainage, myofascial, neuromuscular, petrissage, reflexology, shiatsu, structural integration, Swedish massage

Energy Therapies: Healing touch, Reiki, therapeutic touch

Biologically Based Systems: Herbs

The commission reported on four key areas:
1. Education and training of health care practitioners
2. Research to increase training of health care practitioners
3. Provision of health care professionals and the public with reliable information
4. Guidance in appropriate access to and delivery of CAM

The report was filed after 14 meetings lasting over 18 months, in which submissions were heard from 1700 people and organizations from groups as diverse as the National Heart Lung and Blood Institute, the National Cancer Institute, the Food and Drug Administration, Blue Cross/Blue Shield, and the Journal of the American Medical Association, as well as many CAM practitioners and their organizations. It has 29 recommendations and 100 action items—too many to list here. But the response to the commission's recommendation by Dr Tieraona Low Dog MD and Joseph Fin MD is available at www.whccamp.hhs.gov/sfc.html.

NURSE PRACTICE ACTS

While the use of complementary therapies, including aromatherapy, has increased in the last few years, there is little reference in any published articles to the state practice laws and how they impact the professional use of CAM. However, licensure laws do affect the use of CAM. Sparber (2001) reports on a study of state Boards of Nursing (BON) policy conducted for WHCCAMP, the National Center for Complementary Alternative Medicine, and the Health and Human Services Bureau of Health Professions. The study found that liberalization of licensure laws to practice CAM has been associated with a significantly increased use by physician and non-physician CAM providers. CAM was viewed as representative of the "integrative nature of nursing practice rather than as an alternative method of care." The report suggests nurses are in a unique position to bridge the gap between orthodox, Western health care and CAM.

The Louisiana BON www.lsbn.state.la.us defines CAM as a "broad domain of healing resources that allow registered nurses to promote and/or enhance care supportive to or restorative of live and well being." Sparber (2001) has written an important document that clarifies the situation for many nurses. BONs are required to monitor the scope of practice issues and protect the public through licensure and practice acts. Employers also have a role in safe practice. Anecdotal reports indicate that although some nurses may consider certain complementary therapies to be questionable, professional nurses who use these therapies report their patients do experience an "increased level of comfort and well being"(Sparber 2001). The fifth WHCCAMP category was not included in the article as it is concerned with the prescriptive authority for herbal and other natural products. However, some boards did have recommendations for advanced nursing practice.

At the time of writing, 47% of BONs had taken a position that allows nurses to practice a range of complementary therapies. Thirteen percent were in the process of deciding on their policy, and 40%, although they did not have any formal policy, did not discourage nurses from using complementary therapies as part of their care (Table A3-2). Some states, noticeably Minnesota, have recently passed policies that cover the use of CAM by nonlicensed health professionals (www.minnesotanatucalhealth.org). Sturn and Unutzer (2001) write that the existence of a practice act that gives nonphysicians specific rights to deliver CAM is likely to increase the supply of persons practicing CAM.

The first state BON to issue a formal statement on CAM was Arizona (1991). This BON states that a nurse may hold dual professional licensure/certification, but the nurse will be held to the standard of the highest nursing credential he or she holds. "A professional, practical or advanced practitioner who has acquired or developed a specialized knowledge base in complementary therapies will be held to the standard of care for the nursing credential" (www.azboardofnursing.org). Kentucky followed in 1996, after several inquiries from nurses wanting to know if they could use their complementary-therapy skills to enhance nursing care (www.kbn.state.ky.us). In 1997, Massachusetts (www.state.ma.us/reg/boards/rn) and Pennsylvania (www.dos.state.pa.us) made general-position statements describing complementary therapies as being "within the scope of nursing practice" but noting that "the nurse had responsibility for safe practice."

Most BONs agree that the very nature of nursing lends itself to a framework that welcomes these noninvasive, complementary practices, and that much of the thinking behind nursing is similar to that underlying complementary therapies (Sparber 2001). What has come out of the WHCCAMP report is the need for documented training that clearly shows skills, knowledge, and competency in a CAM discipline. Credentialing is recommended to ensure safe practice and to indicate to other health professionals that nurses have learned another discipline. It is suggested that nurses do not use titles such as "nurse massage therapist" unless they are certified in massage. However, some states disagree with this. The New York BON says nurses "cannot hold themselves out to be nurse reflexologists— but they can say that reflexology is a service included as part of their overall care" (O'Brien 2001). New York requires nurses who wish to use CAM to have

Table A3-2 🦅 *CAM Policies of Individual US States and Territories*

Board of Nursing Has Issued Statement Permitting Practice of CAM

Arizona	Maryland	Ohio
Arkansas	Massachusetts	Oregon
California	Mississippi	Pennsylvania
Connecticut	Missouri	South Dakota
Illinois	New Hampshire	Texas
Iowa	New York	Vermont
Kansas	Nevada	West Virginia
Louisiana	North Carolina	
Maine	North Dakota	

Board of Nursing is Deliberating Practice of CAM

Delaware	Minnesota	Washington
District of Columbia	New Jersey	
Georgia	New Mexico	

Board of Nursing Has No Formal Position, but Does Not Necessarily Discourage CAM

Alabama	Kentucky	Tennessee
Alaska	Michigan	Utah
Colorado	Montana	Virginia
Florida	Oklahoma	Virgin Islands
Georgia	Puerto Rico	Washington
Hawaii	Rhode Island	Wisconsin
Idaho	South Carolina	Wyoming
Indiana		

"received special training or education in this area and have received a certificate of competency" (O'Brien 2001). The Oregon BON has stated that "complementary therapies fit within the definition of the practice of nursing" (Amdell-Thompson 2001). For up-to-date information on all State Boards of Nursing, see the web site of the National Council of State Boards of Nursing (www.ncsbn.org/public/regulation/boards_of_nursing_board.htm).

According to the WHCCAMP report, aromatherapy is accepted as part of nursing care in over half the states in the United States. What is also clear is that while there are many types of touch, there only appears to be one kind of aromatherapy, and that is the one associated with topical applications. This is a little strange as much of the psychological impact of essential oils will be from inhalation.

The American Holistic Nurses Association (AHNA) has for many years been the standard bearer for a more holistic approach to nursing care and more recently has embraced complementary therapies in nursing. In 1994, the AHNA approached me and asked me to create a course in clinical aromatherapy for nurses in the USA. The course, Aromatherapy for Health Professionals was endorsed by the AHNA in United States. In 2000, I worked with the AHNA to produce the following statement on complementary therapies in nursing:

> Nursing Complementary and Alternative Modalities (NCAM) offer therapies that supplement conventional nursing care. NCAM encompasses a broad range of healing resources that allow registered nurses to integrate such therapies into the nursing process, which can interface with traditional medical and/or surgical therapies in order to enhance and promote preventive, supportive, or restorative care.

AHNA is an organization of professional nurses dedicated to the promotion of health and healing of the whole person: body, mind, emotions, behavior, and spirit. Holistic nurses utilize nursing interventions that can impact body, mind, emotions, behavior, and spirit. Holistic nurses integrate nursing theory and practice models for health care that:

1. Promote and enhance health and well being, or support peaceful dying so that the person is as independent as possible
2. Manage prescribed care directed toward the prevention and complications of illness
3. Guide the healing of self and others.

For further information, see the *AHNA Standards of Holistic Nursing Practice* by Frisch et al (2000) and *Holistic Nursing: A Handbook for Practice* (Keegan et al 1999).

The AHNA believes in the integration of NCAM into conventional nursing care so the client can derive benefit from the best of all interventions available. The National Institute of Health Center on Complementary and Alternative Medicines groups CAM practices into five major domains (National Center for Complementary and Alternative Medicine 2000):

1. **Alternative medical systems** are complete systems of theory and practice developed outside the Western biomedical approach (examples include acupuncture and Oriental medicine).
2. **Mind-body–based modalities** include behavioral, psychological, social, and spiritual approaches to health.
3. **Biologically based modalities** include natural and biologically based practices and holistic nursing interventions, such as special diets/nutrition, biochemical monitoring, and aromatherapy.
4. **Manipulative and body-based methods**
5. **Energy therapies**

The AHNA recognizes the major domains of CAM as modalities that fall within the realm of holistic nursing practice, except for Alternative Medical Systems, which may require additional preparation to practice. The AHNA believes nurses must fulfill the educational and licensing/certification qualifications required by those disciplines.

The AHNA believes the integration of CAM into conventional practice offers opportunities for a higher quality of care. However, the AHNA does not equate the practice of a CAM modality with holistic care. Rather, holistic care is defined as the interventions built upon basic nursing practice. Nursing practice is defined and built upon by three standardized languages for classifying what and how nurses practice nursing. They are as follows.

1. **Nursing Interventions Classification (NIC):** is a comprehensive standardized nomenclature describing treatments nurses perform: more than 486 direct and indirect interventions (McCloskey & Bulechek 1999).
2. **Nursing Diagnoses Definitions & Classifications** (NANDA Association, 2000)
3. **Nursing Outcomes Classification** contains treatment outcomes representing all nursing-practice settings and clinical specialties (260 nursing-sensitive patient outcomes organized in seven domains and 29 classes)

Federal law governing the practice of nursing requires registered nurses to practice within the scope appropriate to their educational level, knowledge, skill, and abilities. It allows registered nurses to perform additional acts (such as NCAM) recognized within the standards of nursing practice and that are authorized by the nurse's state BON. Furthermore, registered nurses may employ and initiate such therapies as part of an overall plan of nursing care to meet nursing and patient goals (provided the patient has granted informed consent). Goals for the patient include pain reduction, improved comfort, relaxation, improved coping mechanisms, reduction or moderation of stress, modification of unhealthy behaviors, and enhancing a sense of well being. In all practice settings, the registered nurse must have written policies and procedures in place that guide the performance of such modalities. For more general questions on nursing, complementary therapies, and their legality, contact www.legalnurse.com.

References

Amdell-Thompson M. 2001. State boards of nursing (BONs)—Oregon. Retrieved April 2, 2003 from Mary.AMDELL-THOMPSON@state.or.us

Frisch N, Dossey B, Guzzetta C, et al. 2000. AHNA Standards of Holistic Nursing Practice. Gaithersburg, MD: Aspen.

Gordon J. 2002. Interim Progress Report. Alternative Therapies. 7(6) 32-40.

McCloskey J, Bulechek G. (eds). 1999. Nursing Interventions Classification (NIC). London: Harcourt.

National Center for Complementary and Alternative Medicine. 2000. Five-Year Strategic Plan. June 26. Retrieved October 2001 from http://www.niccam.nih.gov.

O'Brien L. 2001. State boards of nursing (BONs)—New York. Retrieved April 2, 2003 from Lobrien@mail.nysed.gov.

Sparber A. 2001. State Boards of Nursing and Scope of Practice of Registered Nurses Performing Complementary Therapies. Online Journal of Issues in Nursing. August 13. Retrieved October 2002 from http://www.nursingworld.org/ojin/topic15.

Sturn R, Unutzer J. 2001. State legislation and the use of complementary and alternative medicine. Inquiry 37:423-429.

Appendix IV

Recommended Essential-Oil Distributors

There are many essential oil distributors that sell good essential oils, and it would be impossible to list them all. Instead I have listed a few companies I have used for many years. There are the five companies I use in my certification program and others I use for my courses.

Companies Used in Certification Program
Florial France
42 Chemin Des Aubepine
06130 Grasse, France
www.florihana.com
US Distributors:
Lisa Roth
2653 Blackhoof Train
Milford, OH 45150
Tel: 513-576-9944
Email: danannscrossing@yahoo.com
   and
Kari Morford
9418 14th Avenue SW
Seattle, WA 98106
Tel: 206-768-2568
Email: karimorford@go.com

Fragrant Earth Ltd.
Orchard Court, Magdelene Street
Glastonbury, Somerset BA6 9EW UK
www.fragrant-earth.co.uk

Northwest Essence
Director: Cheryl Young
PO Box 428
Gig Harbor, WA 98335 USA
Tel: 253-858-0777
Email: northwestessence@earthlink.com

Nature's Gift
1040 Cheyenne Boulevard
Madison, TN 37115 USA
Tel: 615-612-4270
www.naturesgift.com

Companies Used for Other Courses
Essentially Oils Ltd.
8-10 Mount Farm, Junction Road
Churchill, Chipping Norton, OX7 6NP UK
www.essentiallyoils.com

Elizabeth Van Buren, Inc.
PO Box 7542
Santa Cruz, CA 95061 USA
Tel: 800-710-7759
www.evb.aromatherapy.com

Therapeutic Essentials
5 Michelle Court
Edgewood, NM 87015
Tel: 505-281-9547
Email: Ther1Ess1@aol.com

Springfield Aromatherapy
Unit 2, 2 Anella Avenue
Castle Hill, NSW 2154
Australia
(2)9894-9934
www.springfieldsaroma.com

Enfleurage
321 Bleeker Street
New York, NY 10014 USA
888-387-0300
www.enfleurage.com

APPENDIX V

USEFUL ADDRESSES, DATABASES, AND WEB SITES

A search on www.google.com or using one of the following databases is a great way to begin a search for studies on aromatherapy. For botanical sites, use an individual essential oil, either botanical or common name, as your search term is likely to bring up more studies than using *aromatherapy*. For more information on databases please see Wootton's Directory of databases for research into alternative & complementary medicine (1997) in the *Journal of Alternative & Complementary Medicine*. One of the best places to start for aromatherapy searches is Bob Harris's database, www.aromatherapy.database.com. This is a privately owned database you can subscribe to that has abstracts of over 800 studies and is excellent value.

DATABASES

Agricola (National Agricultural Library database) www.nal.usda.gov
American Indian Ethnobotany Database www.umd.umich.edu
Biosciences Information Service of Biological Abstracts www.csfs.ca
Current Awareness Topics/Alternative & Allied Medicine Database (CATS/AMED) www.bl.uk
Cumulative Index to Nursing and Allied Health (CINAHL) www.cinahl.com
EMBASE/Excerpta Medica Secondary Publishing Division http://library.dialog/bluesheets/html
EthnobotDB (Dr. Duke's Phytochemical Ethnobotanical database) www.ars.grin.gov
Focus on Alternative & Complementary Therapies (FACT); follow links through www.pubmed.com
Food Science & Technology Abstracts www.ifis.org
Herb Research Foundation www.herbs.org
IBIS: The Interactive BodyMind Information Service www.ibismedical.com

The Indian Medicinal Plant Distributed Database Network (INMED-PLAN); access through www.rosenthal.hs.columbia.edu/databases

International Pharmaceutical Abstracts (IPA) www.csa.com/csa

Journal of National Herbalists published by the National Institute of Medical Herbalists www.ejhm.co.uk

Medline National Library of Medicine www.ncbi.nim.nih.gov/PubMed

Medicinal Plants of Native America Database (MPNADBP) www.ars-grin.gov/duke

NAPRALERT (NAtural PRoducts ALERT) www.ag.uiuc.edu/~ffh/rapra.html

National Library of Medicine www.nim.nih.gov

Occupational Therapy Index/AMED www.bl.uk/services/information/amed.html

Phytodok (index of worldwide scientific journals) www.phytopharm.org/en/science.html

Pubmed www.ncbi.nim.nih.gov/PubMed

Review of Aromatic & Medicinal Plants Journal www.cabi-publishing.org

Science Citation Index; follow links from www.isinet.com

Social Science Citation Index; follow links from www.isinet.com

World Research Foundation www.wrf.org

PLANETREE MEDICAL CENTERS AND FACILITIES

Planetree facilities are patient-centered and use complementary therapies including aromatherapy in all their facilities. My company, R J Buckle Associates, is an approved educational provider in aromatherapy and the "m" technique for the Planetree Hospitals. For a list of their 45 facilities in the United States, go to www.planetree.org.

REFERENCES

Wootton J. 1997. Directory of Databases for Research into Alternative & Complementary Medicine. Journal of Alternative & Complementary Medicine. 3(2) 179-190.

Appendix VI

Hospitals and Other Institutions Employing Aromatherapy in Treatment

USA

Desert Samaritan Medical Center, Mesa, Arizona

Fountain Valley Hospital, Fountain Valley, California
Orange Coast Memorial Hospital, Fountain Valley, California
Saddleback Medical Center, Laguna Hills, California
Midway Hospital, Los Angeles, California
Children's Hospital and Health Center, San Diego, California
San Diego Hospice, San Diego, California
California Pacific Medical Center, San Francisco, California
O'Connor Hospital, San Jose, California

Aspen Valley Hospital, Aspen, Colorado
Memorial Hospital, Colorado Springs, Colorado
St. Anthony Hospitals, Centura Health, Englewood, Colorado
Gunnison Valley Hospital, Gunnison, Colorado

Griffin Hospital, Derby, Connecticut
St. Francis Medical Center, Hartford, Connecticut
Windham Community Memorial Hospital, Willimantic, Connecticut

Holy Cross Hospital, Sunrise, Florida

Northside Hospital, Atlanta, Georgia

North Hawaii Community Hospital, Kamuela, Hawaii

Advocate Good Shepherd Hospital, Barrington, Illinois
St. James Health and Wellness Institute, Chicago, Illinois
Advocate Heathcare, Oakbrook, Illinois

Deaconess Hospital Evansville Indiana
Riverview Hospital, Noblesville, Indiana
Memorial Health System, South Bend, Indiana

403

Charlton Health System, Fall River, Massachusetts

St. Luke's Health Care System, New Bedford, Massachusetts

Morton Hospital and Medical Center, Taunton, Massachusetts

Tobey Health Systems, Wareham, Massachusetts

Barbara Ann Karmanos Cancer Institute, Detroit, Michigan

Bronson Methodist Hospital, Kalamazoo, Michigan

Mercy Hospital Group, Port Huron, Michigan

St. John's Health, Warren, Michigan

Children's Hospital, St. Paul, Minnesota

Regions Hospital, St. Paul, Minnesota

St. Peter Community Hospital St Peter, Minnesota

Woodwinds Health Campus, Woodbury, Minnesota

Barnes-Jewish Hospital, St. Louis, Missouri

St Luke's Hospital. Chesterfield, Missouri

Bergen Mercy Medical Center, Omaha, Nebraska

St Rose Dominican Hospital, Henderson, Nevada

Wentworth-Douglas Hospital, Dover, New Hampshire

Cooper Hospital/University Medical Center, Camden, New Jersey

St. Barnabas Health Care System, Hackensack, New Jersey.

Mountainside Medical Center, Montclair, New Jersey

Bellevue Women's Hospital. Albany, New York

St Peter's Medical Center, Albany, New York

Northern Westchester Hospital Center, Mount Kisco, New York

Columbia Presbyterian Medical Center, New York, New York

Bellevue Women's Hospital, Niskayuna, New York

Morgan Stanley Children's Hospital, New York, New York

New York-Weill Cornell Children's Hospital, New York, New York

Hugh Chatham Memorial Hospital, Elkin, North Carolina

Iredell Memorial Hospital, Statesville, North Carolina

Children's Hospital Medical Center, Akron, Ohio

Alliance Community Hospital, Alliance, Ohio

Cleveland Clinic Health System, Chagrin Falls, Ohio

UHHS Bainbridge Health Center, Chagrin Falls, Ohio

University Hospitals' Health System, Cleveland Ohio

Mercy Health Center, Oklahoma City, Oklahoma

St. Charles Medical Center, Bend, Oregon

Mid-Columbia Medical Center, The Dalles, Oregon

Elk Regional Health Center, Elk, Pennsylvania

St. Peter's Hospital, Jeanette, Pennsylvania

Windber Medical Center, Windber, Pennsylvania

Highline Community Hospital Burien, Washington

Elmbrook Memorial Hospital, Brookfield, Wisconsin
St. Michael Hospital, Milwaukee, Wisconsin
Shawano Medical Center, Shawano, Wisconsin

Canada

Children's Hospital of Western Ontario. London, Ontario
Toronto Hospital, Toronto, Ontario
Trinity Health Center, Windsor, Ontario

UK

BUPA Hospital Group, nationwide

London

Edgware Hospital, Edgware, London,
Guy's and St Thomas' Hospital NHS Trust London
Hammersmith Hospital NHS Trust London
King's College Hospital Caldecot Centre, London
London Bridge Hospital, London
The Royal London Homoeopathic Hospital, London
St George's Hospital, London
St Thomas' Hospital, London
University College Hospital NHS Trust, London

Northern England

Bolton NHS Trust, Bolton, Lancashire
Bridlington Hospital, Bridlington, East Yorkshire
Hereford Hospitals NHS Trust, Hereford, Herefordshire

Leeds General Infirmary, Leeds, Yorkshire
Liverpool & Broadgreen University Hospitals NHS Trust, Liverpool
Newcastle General Hospital, Newcastle, Durham
Nottingham City Hospital NHS Trust, Nottinghamshire
Smallwood Day Hospital, Redditch, Worcestershire
The Queen Elizabeth Hospital, Birmingham

Southern England

Crowborough War Memorial Hospital, Crowborough, Sussex
Heatherwood Hospital, Ascot, Berkshire
Moorgreen Hospital, Southampton, Hampshire
Mount Vernon Hospital, Northwood, Middlesex
Musgrove Park Hospital, Taunton, Devon
Poole Hospital, Poole, Dorset
Royal Surrey Country Hospital NHS Trust, Guildford, Surrey
Royal South Hants Hospital, Southampton, Hampshire
Southend Hospital NHS Trust, Southend, Essex
Swanage Hospital, Swanage, Dorset
West Suffolk Hospital HNS Trust, Suffolk
Dorset Cancer Centre, based at Poole Hospital, Dorset
Queen Victoria Hospital NHS Chartham, Kent

Scotland

Borders Community Hospital Group thru-out Scotland
Western General Hospital, Edinburgh,

Western General Hospital in Edinburgh

Northern Ireland

Thompson House Hospital, Lisburn, Antrim, Northern Ireland
St Francis Private Hospital, Mullingar, Co Westmeath, Northern Ireland

IRELAND

Galway University College Hospital, Galway
Stewarts Hospital, Dublin

AUSTRALIA

Calvary Health Care, Kogarah, New South Wales
Prince of Wales, Randwick, New South Wales

St Vincent's Hospital, Sydney, New South Wales,

Mater Private Hospital, Brisbane, Queensland
Royal Brisbane Hospital, Brisbane, Queensland
St Andrew's Hospital, Toowoomba, Queensland

Cabrini Hospital, Malvern, Victoria
Myrtleford Hospital, Myrtleford, Victoria
St. Vincents & Mercy Private Hospital, Melbourne, Victoria
Swinburne Hospital, Swinburne, Victoria

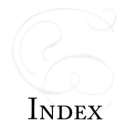

INDEX

Note: Page numbers followed by f indicate figures; those followed by t indicate tables.